Developments in Qualitative Psychotherapy Research

This book examines developments in qualitative psychotherapeutic research. It focuses on different methods and aspects of clinical practice. These range from the experiences of service users and clinicians, examining in detail different aspects of how therapy gets done in practice, to critiquing the politics and ideologies of psychotherapy practice. It aims to reflect the diversity that characterises this developing field and to represent practice-based research carried out in different clinical settings, from different perspectives and in different sociocultural contexts.

The wide range of research projects presented arise from a network of clinicians and psychotherapy researchers who have established an international transdisciplinary forum for dedicated qualitative research on a range of topics in the field of mental health, using a variety of methodologies and theoretical approaches. In the spirit of dialogue, this book further provides chapters written by key practitioners in the field of qualitative research in mental health discussing these contributions.

This book was originally published as a special issue of the *European Journal of Psychotherapy & Counselling*.

Del Loewenthal is Professor of Psychotherapy and Counselling and Director of the Research Centre for Therapeutic Education at the University of Roehampton, London, UK. He is an existential-analytic psychotherapist, photographer and chartered psychologist, with a particular interest in phenomenology. His books include *Existential Psychotherapy and Counselling after Postmodernism* (Routledge, 2017).

Evrinomy Avdi is Associate Professor in Clinical Psychology at the Aristotle University of Thessaloniki, Greece. She is a clinical psychologist, dramatherapist and psychodynamic psychotherapist. Her research interests lie in discursive approaches to psychotherapy research and the exploration of the links between deconstructive research and clinical practice.

Developments in Qualitative Psychotherapy Research

Edited by
Del Loewenthal and Evrinomy Avdi

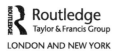

LONDON AND NEW YORK

First published 2019
by Routledge
2 Park Square, Milton Park, Abingdon, Oxon, OX14 4RN, UK

and by Routledge
52 Vanderbilt Avenue, New York, NY 10017

First issued in paperback 2020

Routledge is an imprint of the Taylor & Francis Group, an informa business

British Library Cataloguing-in-Publication Data
A catalogue record for this book is available from the British Library

ISBN 13: 978-0-36-758748-2 (pbk)
ISBN 13: 978-1-138-61403-1 (hbk)

Typeset in Times New Roman
by codeMantra

Publisher's Note
The publisher accepts responsibility for any inconsistencies that may have arisen during the conversion of this book from journal articles to book chapters, namely the possible inclusion of journal terminology.

Disclaimer
Every effort has been made to contact copyright holders for their permission to reprint material in this book. The publishers would be grateful to hear from any copyright holder who is not here acknowledged and will undertake to rectify any errors or omissions in future editions of this book.

Contents

Citation Information   viii

Notes on Contributors   xii

Introduction   1
Del Loewenthal and Evrinomy Avdi

PART I

1 Interventions in everyday lives: How clients use psychotherapy
  outside their sessions   12
  Ole Dreier

2 Eating disorders in the course of life: A qualitative approach
  to vital change   27
  Félix Díaz Martínez, Natalia Solano Pinto, Irene Solbes Canales
  and Sonsoles Calderón López

3 Exploring the meaning in meaningful coincidences: An
  interpretative phenomenological analysis of synchronicity in therapy   42
  Elizabeth C. Roxburgh, Sophie Ridgway and Chris A. Roe

4 Mirroring patients – or not. A study of general practitioners and
  psychiatrists and their interactions with patients with depression   60
  Annette Sofie Davidsen and Christina Fogtmann Fosgerau

5 The person-centred approach as an ideological discourse: a
  discourse analysis of person-centred counsellors' accounts on
  their way of being   77
  Sophia Sflakidou and Maria Kefalopoulou

6 Reading qualitative research   92
  John McLeod

CONTENTS

7 Whose voice are we hearing, really?   104
   Rachel Waddingham

PART II

8 Therapeutic community for children with diagnosis of psychosis:
   What place for parents? The relation between subject and the
   institutional 'Other'   114
   Katia Romelli and Giuseppe Oreste Pozzi

9 Hurting and healing in therapeutic environments: How can we
   understand the role of the relational context?   131
   Simon P. Clarke, Jenelle M. Clarke, Ruth Brown and Hugh Middleton

10 Mental health care and educational actions: From institutional
    exclusion to subjective development   148
    Daniel Magalhães Goulart and Fernando González Rey

11 Displaying agency problems at the outset of psychotherapy   165
    Jarl Wahlström and Minna-Leena Seilonen

12 How do people cope with post traumatic distress after an
    accident? The role of psychological, social and spiritual coping
    in Malaysian Muslim patients   181
    *Rafidah Bahari, Muhammad Najib Mohamad Alwi, Nasrin
    Jahan, Muhammad Radhi Ahmad and Ismail Mohd Saiboon*

13 Communities, psychotherapeutic innovation and the diversity of
    international qualitative research in mental health   199
    David Harper

14 Everyday life, manifesto-writing and the texture of human agency   213
    John McLeod

PART III

15 'Not dead ... abandoned' – a clinical case study of childhood and
    combat-related trauma   222
    Julianna Challenor

16 A shift in narratives: From 'attachment' to 'belonging' in
    therapeutic work with adoptive families. A single case study   238
    Ferdinando Salamino and Elisa Gusmini

CONTENTS

17 Critical incidents in mental health units may be better understood
   and managed with a Freudian/Lacanian psychoanalytic framework   259
   Gerard Patrick Moore

18 The impact of professional role on working with risk in a home
   treatment team   277
   Maxine Sacks and Maria Iliopoulou

19 From victimhood to sisterhood part II – Exploring the
   possibilities of transformation and solidarity in qualitative research 289
   Leah Salter

20 'Let me in! A comment on insider research'   303
   Helen Ellis-Caird

21 The researcher in the field – some notes on qualitative research
   in mental health   313
   Jarl Wahlström

   Index   327

Citation Information

The following chapters were originally published in the *European Journal of Psychotherapy & Counselling*, volume 17, issue 2 (June 2015). When citing this material, please use the original page numbering for each article, as follows:

Chapter 1
Interventions in everyday lives: How clients use psychotherapy outside their sessions
Ole Dreier
European Journal of Psychotherapy & Counselling, volume 17, issue 2 (June 2015) pp. 114–128

Chapter 2
Eating disorders in the course of life: A qualitative approach to vital change
Félix Díaz Martínez, Natalia Solano Pinto, Irene Solbes Canales and Sonsoles Calderón López
European Journal of Psychotherapy & Counselling, volume 17, issue 2 (June 2015) pp. 129–143

Chapter 3
Exploring the meaning in meaningful coincidences: An interpretative phenomenological analysis of synchronicity in therapy
Elizabeth C. Roxburgh, Sophie Ridgway and Chris A. Roe
European Journal of Psychotherapy & Counselling, volume 17, issue 2 (June 2015) pp. 144–161

Chapter 4
Mirroring patients – or not. A study of general practitioners and psychiatrists and their interactions with patients with depression
Annette Sofie Davidsen and Christina Fogtmann Fosgerau
European Journal of Psychotherapy & Counselling, volume 17, issue 2 (June 2015) pp. 162–178

Chapter 5

The person-centred approach as an ideological discourse: a discourse analysis of person-centred counsellors' accounts on their way of being
Sophia Sflakidou and Maria Kefalopoulou
European Journal of Psychotherapy & Counselling, volume 17, issue 2 (June 2015) pp. 179–193

Chapter 6

Reading qualitative research
John McLeod
European Journal of Psychotherapy & Counselling, volume 17, issue 2 (June 2015) pp. 194–205

Chapter 7

Whose voice are we hearing, really?
Rachel Waddingham
European Journal of Psychotherapy & Counselling, volume 17, issue 2 (June 2015) pp. 206–215

The following chapters were originally published in the *European Journal of Psychotherapy & Counselling*, volume 18, issue 4 (December 2016). When citing this material, please use the original page numbering for each article, as follows:

Chapter 8

Therapeutic community for children with diagnosis of psychosis: What place for parents? The relation between subject and the institutional 'Other'
Katia Romelli and Giuseppe Oreste Pozzi
European Journal of Psychotherapy & Counselling, volume 18, issue 4 (December 2016) pp. 316–332

Chapter 9

Hurting and healing in therapeutic environments: How can we understand the role of the relational context?
Simon P. Clarke, Jenelle M. Clarke, Ruth Brown and Hugh Middleton
European Journal of Psychotherapy & Counselling, volume 18, issue 4 (December 2016) pp. 384–400

Chapter 10

Mental health care and educational actions: From institutional exclusion to subjective development
Daniel Magalhães Goulart and Fernando González Rey
European Journal of Psychotherapy & Counselling, volume 18, issue 4 (December 2016) pp. 367–383

Chapter 11

Displaying agency problems at the outset of psychotherapy
Jarl Wahlström and Minna-Leena Seilonen
European Journal of Psychotherapy & Counselling, volume 18, issue 4
(December 2016) pp. 333–348

Chapter 12

*How do people cope with post traumatic distress after an accident? The role
of psychological, social and spiritual coping in Malaysian Muslim patients*
Rafidah Bahari, Muhammad Najib Mohamad Alwi, Nasrin Jahan, Muhammad
Radhi Ahmad and Ismail Mohd Saiboon
European Journal of Psychotherapy & Counselling, volume 18, issue 4
(December 2016) pp. 349–366

Chapter 13

*Communities, psychotherapeutic innovation and the diversity of international
qualitative research in mental health*
David Harper
European Journal of Psychotherapy & Counselling, volume 18, issue 4
(December 2016) pp. 401–414

Chapter 14

Everyday life, manifesto-writing and the texture of human agency
John McLeod
European Journal of Psychotherapy & Counselling, volume 18, issue 4
(December 2016) pp. 415–423

The following chapters were originally published in the *European Journal of
Psychotherapy & Counselling*, volume 19, issue 1 (March 2017). When citing
this material, please use the original page numbering for each article, as follows:

Chapter 15

*'Not dead ... abandoned' – a clinical case study of childhood and combat-
related trauma*
Julianna Challenor
European Journal of Psychotherapy & Counselling, volume 19, issue 1 (March
2017) pp. 6–21

Chapter 16

*A shift in narratives: From 'attachment' to 'belonging' in therapeutic work
with adoptive families. A single case study*
Ferdinando Salamino and Elisa Gusmini
European Journal of Psychotherapy & Counselling, volume 19, issue 1 (March
2017) pp. 22–42

Chapter 17
Critical incidents in mental health units may be better understood and managed with a Freudian/Lacanian psychoanalytic framework
Gerard Patrick Moore
European Journal of Psychotherapy & Counselling, volume 19, issue 1 (March 2017) pp. 43–60

Chapter 18
The impact of professional role on working with risk in a home treatment team
Maxine Sacks and Maria Iliopoulou
European Journal of Psychotherapy & Counselling, volume 19, issue 1 (March 2017) pp. 61–72

Chapter 19
From victimhood to sisterhood part II – Exploring the possibilities of transformation and solidarity in qualitative research
Leah Salter
European Journal of Psychotherapy & Counselling, volume 19, issue 1 (March 2017) pp. 73–86

Chapter 20
'Let me in! A comment on insider research'
Helen Ellis-Caird
European Journal of Psychotherapy & Counselling, volume 19, issue 1 (March 2017) pp. 87–96

Chapter 21
The researcher in the field – some notes on qualitative research in mental health
Jarl Wahlström
European Journal of Psychotherapy & Counselling, volume 19, issue 1 (March 2017) pp. 97–109

For any permission-related enquiries please visit:
http://www.tandfonline.com/page/help/permissions

Notes on Contributors

Evrinomy Avdi is Associate Professor in Clinical Psychology and Director of the Laboratory for Applied Psychology at the Aristotle University of Thessaloniki, Greece. She is a clinical psychologist, dramatherapist and psychodynamic psychotherapist. Her research interests lie in discursive approaches to psychotherapy research and the exploration of the links between deconstructive research and clinical practice.

Rafidah Bahari graduated with MB BCh BAO from the Queens' University of Belfast and is a Member of the Royal College of Psychiatrists in the UK. She is Assistant Professor of Psychiatry at Cyberjaya University College of Medical Sciences (CUCMS), Malaysia. Dr Bahari has developed a special interest in research into posttraumatic stress disorder and psycho-spiritual interventions. She is currently actively involved in research utilising both quantitative and qualitative methods. She is also Head of the Psychiatry Discipline in CUCMS.

Fernando González Rey is Professor at the University Centre of Brasília and Senior Associate Professor at the University of Brasília (Brazil). He is also coordinator of the research group "Subjectivity in health and in education" at the University of Brasília. His research interests focus on education and psychology from a cultural-historical approach in three specific fields: 1) the development of the theory of subjectivity and the epistemological and methodological issues related to the study of subjectivity from a cultural-historical approach; 2) Learning as a subjective development process; and 3) Health and subjectivity: beyond the pathologization of life.

Daniel Magalhães Goulart is a Lecturer at the University Centre of Brasília, Brazil. He is a member of the research group "Subjectivity in health and in education", coordinated by Fernando González Rey at the University of Brasília. He is also a member of the Discourse Unit, Manchester, UK. His research interests focus on psychology and education from the cultural-historical approach of subjectivity in the fields of 1) mental health care; 2) subjective development and education; 3) institutional strategies beyond the pathologization of life.

Maria Iliopoulou is a clinical psychologist at the City and Hackney Crisis Service in London, UK. She trained at the Centre for Mindfulness, UMass

Medical School and has offered Mindfulness Based Crisis Interventions to people in crisis and their families over the past ten years. She is co-founder of Athens Mindfulness Centre in Greece. She works as the Clinical and Operational Lead for the SUN and SOS, a therapeutic community and an outreach service for people in crisis in London. She is visiting lecturer at the Division of Psychiatry and Behavioural Sciences, University of Crete.

Maria Kefalopoulou, PhD ECP, is trained in person-centered counselling and specialises in abuse. Her research interests include gender identity issues, study of violence and aggression as social phenomena, and the exploration of difference, diversity and multicultural issues. She is trainer, supervisor and Lecturer in the Counselling Department of ICPS and she is also Lecturer in the Psychology Department of ICPS, in Athens, Greece.

Nasrin Jahan MBBS (DU), MPH (AIIAS), MMSc(CUCMS) is a public health physician with wide experience in working with the UN, government, private and NGO sectors in Bangladesh and abroad. Dr Nasrin taught medical students in Malaysia and Bangladesh for many years. She is also a participatory development expert in planning, monitoring and evaluating different projects. Recently, she worked as protection coordinator for Myanmar Rohingya refugees in Cox's Bazaar, Bangladesh in a private organization/partnership with UNHCR.

Del Loewenthal is Professor of Psychotherapy and Counselling and Director of the Research Centre for Therapeutic Education at the University of Roehampton, London, UK. He is an existential-analytic psychotherapist, photographer and chartered psychologist, with a particular interest in phenomenology. His books include *Existential Psychotherapy and Counselling after Postmodernism* (Routledge, 2017).

Muhammad Najib bin Mohamad Alwi is an Associate Professor of Psychiatry and Director of the Research Resources Centre (RRC) at Cyberjaya University College of Medical Sciences (CUCMS), Malaysia. He has been involved in numerous training workshops and has been invited to speak on a variety of topics at local and international conferences, workshops and meetings. He has also been involved in several humanitarian missions locally and internationally and is actively involved in the teaching of Disaster Relief Medicine. His main research interests are in cognitive rehabilitation for mental illness, psychological aspects of disaster and evidence-based practice in complementary treatments.

Muhammad Radhi Ahmad is an Associate Professor at the Faculty of Medicine, Cyberjaya University College of Medical Sciences (CUCMS), Malaysia. Dr Ahmad worked at various hospitals as an orthopaedic surgeon before later becoming a lecturer at UKM, where he was awarded the prestigious Award for Service Excellence for the year 2008. He is Deputy Dean (Students Affairs) at the Faculty of Medicine of the CUCMS, where he also teaches and is active in research. He has been invited to speak at numerous workshops and conferences mainly in topics related to Emergency Medicine and Pre Hospital Care.

Sophie Ridgway graduated from Nottingham Trent University with a Masters in Psychological Wellbeing and Mental Health. She dedicated her early career to assisting with psychological research in anomalous experiences, supporting adults in mental health services and facilitating parent roles for children with complex needs. She has now found her calling as a musician/songwriter and hopes to inspire others to follow their dreams.

Elizabeth C. Roxburgh is Senior Lecturer at the University of Northampton, UK. She was awarded her PhD by the University of Northampton for research exploring the phenomenology and psychology of Spiritualist mediumship. She has worked for the National Health Service as an assistant psychologist in a variety of clinical settings, including mental health, forensic, and learning disability services. She is now a BACP Registered counsellor, course leader for a BSc Psychology and Counselling degree.

Maxine Sacks is Psychology Lead for the City and Hackney Directorate of the East London NHS Foundation Trust, in London, UK. Most of her work has been in secondary mental health including managing services in addiction and setting up an early intervention in psychosis service. She is interested in integrative approaches including CAT, which she teaches on clinical and counselling psychology training courses. She is co-ordinator of the London Bi-Logic Group which studies the work of Ignacio Matte Blanco and has contributed to several research projects using IPA.

Ismail Saiboon's research interests include Emergency Medicine, Pre-hospital care and Healthcare Simulation. He has written and published extensively in these fields both at local and international levels. He is Deputy Dean of Post Graduate Studies Faculty of Medicine, University Kebangsaan Malaysia (UKM), American Heart Association (AHA)'s Training Center Coordinator (TCC) and Training Center Faculty in ACLS-P & ACLS EP; Chairman of the Malaysian Society for Simulation in Healthcare (MaSSH), board member of the Pan Asian Society for Simulation in Healthcare (PASSH), and member to SSiH.

Minna-Leena Seilonen is a licensed psychologist and psychotherapist working in her private practice at Tampere, Finland. She is a trainer and clinical supervisor in training programmes for integrative psychotherapy at the University of Jyväskylä and the University of Helsinki. She is pursuing her doctoral studies at the University of Jyväskylä on the topic of constructions of agency in accounts of drunk driving at the outset of semi-mandatory counselling.

Jarl Wahlström, PhD, is Professor Emeritus in Clinical Psychology and Psychotherapy at the Department of Psychology, University of Jyväskylä, Finland. He has served as head of the national integrative postgraduate specialization programme in psychotherapy for psychologists. He has advanced training in family and systems therapy, and longstanding experience as a clinical psychologist, family therapist, trainer and consultant, in addition to his vocation as a university teacher. His main research interest is in discursive and narrative processes in psychotherapeutic encounters and their relation to the (re)constitution of agency positions and sense of agency as outcome of psychotherapy.

Introduction

Del Loewenthal and Evrinomy Avdi

In 'What have current notions of psychotherapeutic research to do with truth, justice and thoughtful practice?' (Loewenthal, 2015), one of the editors of this book wrote how he was becoming disillusioned with qualitative research, suggesting that the psychological therapies, through clinical supervision and the presentation of clinical case studies, have a tradition of exploring our work's *physis* for something that comes out of itself and therefore should not be determined by externally imposed research methods.

So on this basis, can any development in qualitative research ever really be of help to us or our clients/patients? We thought a good place to find out would be from papers presented at the fifth and sixth Qualitative Research on Mental Health Conferences (held in Chania, Greece in 2014 and 2016, respectively), which the other editor of this book, Evrinomy Avdi, co-organised. These conferences have been established in the hope of providing an international transdisciplinary forum for dedicated qualitative research on a range of topics in the field of mental health, using a variety of methodologies and approaches. As co-editors, we invited conference participants to contribute to three special issues of the *European Journal of Psychotherapy & Counselling* (2015, 2016, 2017) with studies that are pertinent to psychotherapy and counselling. As a result, this book is in three parts with each part consisting of five chapters followed by two chapters of invited responses.

To develop the initial argument further, the following is a conversation between the editors, Del Loewenthal and Evrinomy Avdi.

Del Loewenthal

Some time ago I was asked by a publication to name what research has been most helpful to me as a psychotherapist. It was then that I had to face my growing realisation that there was nothing currently regarded as research that influenced how I work as a practitioner. Not only positivistic quantitative research but, since then, qualitative research continues to go down in my estimation. I can see that my students gain what might be a useful personal discipline, but this is of little use to anyone else as well as providing little opportunity for comparative research, etc.

Can I square all this up with being the founding chair of two national psychotherapeutic research bodies, responsible for two other books on research, one of the first journal editors-in-chief to establish a research section and continuing to co-edit this and other special issues of the *European Journal of Psychotherapy & Counselling* on research?

I have for a long time been interested in phenomenology, but I've always been concerned that 'phenomenological research' is a misnomer – surely 'phenomenology' is research? When I became the first chair of the United Kingdom Council for Psychotherapy (UKCP) research committee I was aware of many psychotherapists writing about theoretical considerations, but then, as in other areas of enquiry, the culture changed and the name 'research' changed to only mean 'empirical research'. Furthermore, UK universities, for one, endorsed this with an ever-increasing bias in National Research Assessment Exercises for empirical research, as with an increasing number of disciplines, anything else being labelled 'scholarship'! This has developed to the extent that several years later when, as a member of that UKCP committee, I asked how something was defined I got a response 'but that is philosophy!' Also, on another occasion when asking a similar question at an Economic and Social Research Council meeting I got the reply 'We don't know how to define it Del, but we think we know how to measure it!'.

I have consequently come to see research, as with counselling and psychotherapy, as cultural practices (Loewenthal, 2016). I still suggest to my master's and doctoral students that they carry out whatever is currently regarded as (usually qualitative) research so they can come alongside current research cultural practices and critique them. However, though I am still very much interested in questions of methodology as well as recent developments in research methods (as in this book), I am increasingly concerned that most research, along with the training for it, is for the most part a waste of time and can better be seen as attempts at professional legitimising rituals.

Evrinomy Avdi

I found myself struggling to respond to Del's position of critique, and, reflecting upon why this might be the case, I realised that one important reason for this is that very different versions of research came to mind when I was trying to respond to his arguments. It is almost impossible to discuss 'research', or even 'qualitative research' in counselling and psychotherapy as a unitary entity, given that the context of where research is carried out, by whom, for what reason(s), from what position, with what aims and in what manner are some of the, many, factors that affect its quality – and usefulness.

I agree with Del's position that research as well as psychotherapy and counselling are cultural practices – that occupy different positions of validity and legitimisation in different European countries and local contexts. Moreover, as a social and cultural practice psychotherapy research is entangled with power, and as such not all research is seen to have the same validity. For example, although there is more than ample evidence from outcome studies that so called 'common factors' are key to the outcome of therapy, the majority of outcome research is still engaged in defining the 'best' therapy approach for specific 'conditions' – with significant implications for the public funding, training and legitimisation of psychotherapy.

Given this diversity, 'research' in counselling and psychotherapy can include a vast range of activities and cultural productions, which are borne from different needs, rely on different theories, follow different ideologies and serve different functions. Given this, I will outline some of the conditions which I have found in my own experience help make research, at its best, useful.

I agree with Del that engaging in research can be extremely useful and enriching for clinicians, and I would argue that this is potentially the case at all stages in our professional development, despite the fact that we often only engage in research during training. I believe that at its best, engaging in research can enhance our reflexivity, promote rigour, foster an open and questioning attitude towards our assumptions and can work towards creating a culture of enquiry in our services and local contexts. In my own attempts to carry out research on psychotherapy, I have found that working closely with clinicians at all stages of the research endeavour – from formulating the questions to discussing issues of design and ethics to the collection, analysis and interpretation of the research material – enriching, stimulating and productive, if not always a smooth process. For example, in a recent project I have been involved in, we spent several hours watching and discussing videos of couple therapy sessions with the therapists in the service; in addition to better understanding the processes of engagement we were interested in, these dialogues produced changes in both the service itself and in the ways in which we are conducting our research. Moreover, engaging in research might improve practice in unexpected ways – for example in the project mentioned, there were noticeably less drop outs in couples participating in the project than in the service, in general – arguably an indication of improved practice.

Similarly, research carried out with clients or by users of services is, in my mind, another very fruitful avenue towards useful research. There is a wide range of studies adopting such a framework, including studies focusing on and highlighting clients' views and experiences of helpful and unhelpful aspects of therapy, to research exploring how clients make use of therapy in the context of their everyday life, to studies that interview clients and therapists together about their work, to name but a few.

In brief, I think that one condition that can help make research useful is when it is designed and conducted collaboratively – including co-researchers from different positions.

Del

In my recent book (Loewenthal 2017), I label a section as 'Thoughtful Practice and Research'; perhaps it should have been titled 'Thoughtful Practice or

Research' as they seem to be increasingly mutually exclusive! Though, as mentioned, this depends on what is meant by 'research'.

Evrinomy: I hesitate writing this, but wasn't it the Greeks who enabled us to see that the *phusis/physis*, which is the root of our psychology and psychotherapy, is the natural what comes out of itself? Furthermore, as in our Greek notions of democracy, shouldn't evaluation criteria emerge from the particular situation? Thus any attempt to actually impose external evaluation criteria will always induce some form of violence. Indeed, as a case in point, recently a student who said she thought it was wrong to carry out an evaluation after each counselling session was told by her agency, who had introduced the policy in an attempt to secure funding, that she had to stop working there and then with all her clients!

However, with regard to your point of working collaboratively with clients and service users, this is a cultural practice that I would wish to consider, whether it be within a consulting room or more generally within our communities. However, can we measure the effect of clients being involved in working with their therapists empirically – perhaps we can measure their satisfaction at a moment in time but surely not their experiences of for example intimacy or love?

Evrinomy

For me, research is one way of knowing; as such it can, at best, answer only some questions and from a specific perspective, and I firmly believe that it should not be treated as representing truth with regards to psychotherapy – or any other aspect of human life. From this perspective, the primacy given in more and more European countries to research as the most legitimate and valid source of knowledge about psychotherapy is very problematic – and I agree with Del that it is an act of violence.

In my view research, of any type, can at its best illuminate only part of the complex picture of human suffering and psychotherapy. At the same time, I do think that it has a useful – yet perhaps overestimated – contribution to make to our understanding and practice.

Del and Evrinomy

We now both wish to consider what then is happening regarding developments in qualitative psychotherapeutic research that might contribute to our knowledge and such debates? As mentioned, we asked an international array of eminent researchers to provide examples of their most recent qualitative psychotherapeutic research. We then divided the resulting 15 chapters into three parts (as in the original journal issues), and we asked further prominent experts in our field to comment on each of the five chapters.

However, before outlining the chapters in Part I, we first wish to provide the initial conference briefs and make some observations. The focus of the 2014 conference was on the exploration, through divergent qualitative research approaches, of mental health as a set of practices. These included the professional practices implicated in defining and treating mental distress; the practices through which individuals in distress live with, make sense of and manage their experiences; as well as the wider sociocultural and institutional practices of understanding and dealing with human suffering. Researchers, from a variety of disciplines, clinicians and service users were invited to present studies that describe the various practices of mental health, investigate their functions and their effects, examine the discourses associated with them and explore how these practices are viewed and experienced by the parties involved. Broadly, the conference aimed to promote critical engagement with mental health practices through highlighting the personal and sociocultural processes that underpin them, as well as their intersections with gender, culture and social position. The sixth Qualitative Research on Mental Health Conference focused on relational perspectives in mental health research. More specifically, the conference aimed to explore the role of interpersonal, family and social relationships in fostering mental health; helping cope with life's stresses, and manage trauma and distress; as well as to investigate the role of the relationship between professionals and service users in providing appropriate and helpful services and avoiding harm. These issues were examined in the context of personal and sociocultural factors that support or hinder relationships, including gender, culture and social position. In addition, delegates were invited to explore different novel relational research methodologies, which focus on communication, dialogue, affective interaction, embodiment and the intersubjective processes involved in the mutual co-construction of meaning. Both conferences attracted strong international interest with over 300 participants in total, from a diversity of backgrounds, including service users, health and social care professionals, social scientists and health policy makers, and created a space for lively and enriching discussions.

The focus on practice was of particular interest as it potentially would concur with those who consider the psychological therapies as cultural practices (Heaton, 2010; Loewenthal, 2011; Wittgenstein, 1958). Here we might see Freud, Klein and others as having discovered practices that they later theorised about and where too much research might then be seen as attempting to legitimise these theories. Moreover, arguably, one of the contributions of qualitative research to psychotherapy is that it provides methods and tools to study aspects of actual clinical practice, the rationale being that it takes place in everyday clinical work (by examining, for example, audio- or video-taped therapy sessions). The knowledge that arises from such in-session research can be seen to foster clinician reflexivity as well as to provide more valid and clinically useful knowledge regarding what takes place in therapy, as compared to a research tradition that relies solely on questionnaire-based post-session reports.

The other particular attraction of this conference was that it focused on client/patient's experiences as well as that of psychological therapists and aimed to provide space for client/service users' perspectives and to foster the development of novel research approaches that may be better suited to this aim. However, very few of such studies were submitted to the special issue, and there appeared to be issues regarding the extent to which users can carry out research themselves that would be acceptable for academic journal review processes. This leads to important questions regarding the politics and ideologies of knowledge dissemination and research publication, as, for example, the question regarding the extent to which such barriers might be more to do with professionalisation processes rather than scientific merit. Some of these issues are discussed in the published response by John McLeod in Chapter 6.

It was interesting to note that the studies that are included in Part I represent different research methods and processes, such as Case Study, Narrative Analysis and Discourse Analysis, which might be seen as being amongst the more fluid and hermeneutic of research methods, as well as Interpretative Phenomenological Analysis and Conversation Analysis, which can be seen to be more method-driven. Yet the questions still remain as to the extent to which the research methods affect what research questions are chosen and the extent to which they actually pervert the experiences of individual users and psychological therapists?

In Part I of the book, we have attempted to replicate one of the intentions of the 2014 conference by asking a service user (Rai Waddingham) and an academic (John McLeod) to provide published response chapters. It will perhaps be interesting to explore further how users might find a way of providing feedback on their experiences which does not necessarily have to fit either our audit culture or current fashions in systematising research processes.

Ole Dreier's Chapter 1, entitled 'Interventions in everyday lives: How clients use psychotherapy outside their sessions', presents the key findings from a wider project which explored how clients make use of psychotherapy in their everyday lives and investigates the complex ways in which professional treatment practices and everyday life practices interact. This study cogently puts forwards the argument that we need detailed and systematic research on how clients make use of psychotherapy in their everyday lives. Importantly, Dreier argues that this research should adopt a decentred approach, in the sense of using methods that privilege clients' ordinary lived practices, rather than professional theories and practices.

The theme of privileging client perspectives in developing professional knowledge is further elaborated in Chapter 2 by Felix Diaz, Natalia Solano Pinto, Irene Solbes and Sonsoles Calderón, entitled 'Eating disorders in the course of life: A qualitative approach to vital change'. In this study, the authors explore biographical narratives about eating troubles and about change, with an aim to better understand the ways in which people themselves make sense of and face the difficulties they experience with regard to eating. The common narrative structures that emerge from the analysis are described and discussed in the light of the Transtheoretical Model of Change, a dominant professional discourse regarding problem change. This chapter is an example of attempts to synthesise the knowledge produced through examining client perspectives to professional theories and accounts.

In Chapter 3, which is entitled 'Exploring the meaning in meaningful coincidences: An interpretative phenomenological analysis of synchronicity in therapy', Elizabeth Roxburgh, Sophie Ridgway and Chris Roe shift the perspective on therapists' experience by investigating synchronicity experiences, a relatively rare and under-researched issue psychotherapy practice. In line with a phenomenological perspective, the authors strive to explore and describe the process and nature of synchronicity experiences from the perspective of the practitioner, whilst their findings are then discussed in the context of the existing literature. Their chapter provides an example of rigorous phenomenological research on participants' experience as a starting point for conceptualising the process of therapy as well as rethinking issues of training and practice.

Chapter 4, by Annette Sofie Davidsen and Christina Fogtmann Fosgerau, is entitled 'Mirroring patients – or not. A study of general practitioners and psychiatrists and their interactions with patients with depression'. This study focuses on client–professional interaction as it unfolds within routine clinical work of general practitioners and psychiatrists. The authors employ a conceptually driven qualitative analysis that follows the principles of conversation analysis and aim to examine and describe the clinical interaction, with a focus on the practice of mirroring, itself conceptualised within the framework of mentalisation theory. This study provides an example of research which starts from practice in order to then conceptualise clinical interaction.

The final chapter in Part I, Chapter 5, by Sophia Sflakidou and Maria Kefalopoulou is entitled 'The person-centred approach as an ideological discourse: a discourse analysis of person-centred counsellors' accounts on their way of being'. The authors critically examine how person-centred counsellors position themselves within the discourses that comprise the person-centred approach and examine the effects of theory – itself approached as ideology – on counsellors' experience and behaviour. This study is an example of how qualitative research attempts to provide links between practice, experience, ideology and power, with the hope of furthering critical reflection on the discourses within which we operate and reproduce through our practices.

In his commentary on Part I, John McLeod in Chapter 6 critically engages with questions that concern the perspective of the practitioners who read qualitative research studies on psychotherapy, thus addressing the very important issue of the contribution and usefulness of qualitative studies for actual clinical practice. He explores some of the limitations to the readability of these studies and proposes alternative avenues for the dissemination of research findings, such as the arts and fostering open access to research with the aim of fostering dialogue between researchers and readers.

In her response, Rachel (Rai) Waddingham, in Chapter 7, explores the degree to which qualitative research as described in our five papers conveys the voice and perspective of research participants. Rai draws out some of the tensions inherent in making interpretations and connections within research papers from a client/patient perspective and the impact this may have on the quality of any conclusions drawn. Rai also suggests ways of involving clients in a dialogue to minimise assumptions and theoretical frameworks further obscuring participants' involvement in future research.

The above chapters also raise fundamental ontological questions regarding the nature of being, which current qualitative research in the psychological therapies is misaligned with; and, as a consequence, may increasingly mis-align and mangle the fundamental nature of our project (Loewenthal, 2015)? There is a further related question, and this is the extent to which develop-ments in qualitative research approaches in the psychological therapies, as we have attempted to illustrate in this book, are in relation to developments in qualitative research in general. Indeed, we would like to end this introduction to the first part of this book with a question from a review of qualitative re-search in education:

> ... rethinking humanist ontology is key in what comes after humanist qualitative methodology. If we cease to privilege knowing over being; if we refuse positivist and phenomenological assumptions about the nature of lived experience and the world; if we give up representational and binary logics; if we see language, the human, and the material not as separate entities mixed together but as completely imbricated 'on the surface' – if we do all that and the 'more' it will open up – will qualitative inquiry as we know it be possible? (Lather & St. Pierre, 2013, p. 630)

Part II commences with Chapter 8, entitled 'Therapeutic community for chil-dren with diagnosis of psychosis: What place for parents? The relation between subject and the institutional 'Other'', by Katia Romelli and Giuseppe Pozzi. This chapter concerns parents' perspectives on, and relationships to, the insti-tutions involved in moving their child to a therapeutic community. Here the authors describe an interesting way of working with parents in order to make their relationship with such residential services less problematic and providing an original theoretical conceptualisation of the dynamics characterising this re-lationship from a Lacanian perspective. It makes an important contribution both in terms of clinical work with parents in the context of therapeutic communities and methodologically, in terms of the authors' creative use of Lacanian theory in analysing discourse.

Our second chapter in Part II is Chapter 9, 'Hurting and healing in therapeu-tic environments: How can we understand the role of the relational context?', which provides summaries of the findings of three studies using different meth-odologies that indicate key factors in the relational context of therapeutic envi-ronments. Here, with methods including narrative ethnography, grounded theory and a novel auto-ethnographic methodology, Simon Clarke, Jenelle Clark, Ruth Brown and Hugh Middleton identify the expression and containment of affect in a congruent environment, belonging and hope and fluid hierarchies of relational structures as key aspects of the relational context informing change.

'Mental health care and educational actions: From institutional exclusion to subjective development' by Daniel Goulart and Fernando González Rey is our Chapter 10. They propose the idea that subjective development from a cultural-historical standpoint can help address dichotomised notions such as social/ individual. This, they argue, can then inform institutions for mental health care and how they may move away from manualised care and an adherence to diagnostic categories and instead see mental health as a living process. This chapter provides a cogent articulation of a theoretical model for conceptualising subjectivity and mental distress that relies on the dialectical interplay of social context and subjective experience. It draws upon the authors' experience of mental health care in Brazil and discusses some of the implications of the model in relation to a case study. The paper is interesting as it pulls together in a coherent way Rubinstein and Vygotsky's views on mental life and proposes a theoretical approach to subjectivity, with reference to literature from post-structuralism and the anti-psychiatry movement.

Chapter 11, 'Displaying agency problems at the outset of psychotherapy' by Jarl Wahlström and Minna-Lena Seilonen, deconstructs how psychotherapy clients construct themselves discursively in terms of agency. They uniquely seek to describe a noted difference in subject construction between clients in voluntary vs. semi-voluntary therapy, with an illustration of the presence of aspects such as relationality, causal attribution, intentionality, historicity and reflexivity in psychotherapy.

Rafidah Bahari, Alwi Mohamad, Najib Muhammad, Nasrin Jahan, Muhammad Radhi Ahmad and Ismail Mohd Saiboon provide our Chapter 12, 'How do people cope with post traumatic distress after an accident? The role of psychological, social and spiritual coping in Malaysian Muslim patients'. This paper reports on their interesting qualitative study of coping with distress following road traffic accidents in a Malay Muslim population. It is particularly topical in view of recent findings by Brewin et al. that people in less affluent countries are less likely to suffer from post-traumatic stress disorder.

Our two published respondents for the above chapters of Part II are by David Harper and, again, by John McCleod. In 'Communities, psychotherapeutic innovation and the diversity of international qualitative research in mental health' (Chapter 13) David Harper helpfully discusses common themes in, and differences between, the chapters in Part II, speaking directly to the authors whilst exploring how all our work could easily be criticised. John McCleod, in 'Everyday life, manifesto-writing and the texture of human agency' (Chapter 14), provides some thought-provoking reflections on these chapters in Part II from the perspectives of a focus on everyday life, the tension between theorising and description in qualitative research and the nature of human agency.

For both published respondents, it would appear that they consider that research in psychotherapy and counselling presented in this issue is far from a waste of time. For David Harper, 'Reading the articles, it is clear that there is theoretically and rich research being conducted internationally, on a range of important social topics in mental health and psychotherapy'. For John McLeod, 'The articles... confirm the rigour and relevance of qualitative research in counselling, psychotherapy and related disciplines'.

The first chapter in Part III, Chapter 15, is entitled, '"Not dead ... abandoned' – A clinical case study of childhood and combat-related trauma'. Here, Julianna Challenor provides a thorough and reflective account of the therapist's work with a client, a soldier in his adult life, who had experienced intense and continuous physical and emotional abuse as a child. It is this attention to detail and the ability to deeply interrogate one's processes and motivations that makes the case study a potential research tool for psychodynamic (and other psycho-therapeutic) work.

'A shift in narratives: from 'attachment' to 'belonging' in therapeutic work with adoptive families. A single case study' forms our next chapter, Chapter 16, in which Ferdinando Salamino and Elisa Gusmini present a study grounded in clinical practice of a family therapy approach with adoptive parents and their adopted child that focuses not on repairing attachments but on new relational opportunities. They provide an interesting alternative to attachment-based therapies for adoptive families, specifically within a systemic epistemological framework, underpinned by core principles of the Milan Approach and its further developments.

Gerard Moore, in 'Critical incidents in mental health units may be better understood and managed with a Freudian/Lacanian psychoanalytic framework', provides Chapter 17. Here, he addresses the important topic of the need for institutional analysis of the phenomena of transference and countertransference in an acute mental health service. The overall aim of the paper is to help staff and policy-makers work better together for patients.

Chapter 18, 'The impact of professional role on working with risk in a home treatment team' usefully explicates the difficulties of working in Home Treatment Teams and the struggle of being a professional in this circumstance. The authors, Maxine Sacks and Maria Iliopoulou, illustrate the vulnerability of the professionals working in the team and raise important questions for the profession.

Our last research chapter, Chapter 19, 'From victimhood to sisterhood part II – Exploring the possibilities of transformation and solidarity in qualitative research' by Leah Salter, is a follow-up to an earlier paper by the same author on how women have 'gone on' following experiences of abuse and considers the process of being an insider researcher. It contains interesting and thoughtful reflections, drawing appropriately on the relevant literature. The author subtly asks questions of the reader in using very complicated systemic ideas, such as those from Shotter and Wittgenstein in a fluid and understandable way.

Our two published respondents for the above five chapters of Part III are by Helen Ellis-Caird and Jarl Wahlström. In Chapter 20, 'Let me in! A comment on insider research', Hellen Ellis-Caird provides an articulate and thoughtful critique of the methodological rigour and wider impact of the last five qualitative research chapters included in this book. The author adopts an outsider perspective (compared to the authors who she perceives as being on the 'inside') and employs Tracy's (2010) eight markers for good qualitative research so as to carefully illustrate whether the five chapters meet these criteria and can thus have a clear impact not only on researchers inside the authors' field of inquiry but also to a wider (outsider) audience too. Finally, in Chapter 21 Jarl Wahlström, in 'The researcher in the field – some notes on qualitative research in mental health', approaches the studies from an interesting perspective – i.e. as social practices – and highlights the issues implicated in generating knowledge and the tensions inherent in the various positions different researchers assume with regard to 'knowing' in research on mental health practices.

Our particular thanks go to these last two published respondents for being able to draw our attention to such aspects as a critique of the methodological rigour and approaching qualitative research as social practice. On our part, we have noticed a tendency with many recent qualitative research papers for focusing more on the findings from qualitative studies rather than on issues in qualitative research – relating, for example, to theory, epistemology, method, ethics, etc. Whilst we are impressed by the number of chapters we have received and their quality, we hope that in editing the *European Journal of Psychotherapy & Counselling* in the future we will also be able to consider papers that explore such methodological issues as to whether a new science of consciousness (and unconsciousness) is required, or whether it is ever possible to develop first-person methods that can adequately be used by third-person science (Blackmore, 2010).

It may be that you are more of Gadamer's (2013) view that if you want truth you cannot have method. However, whatever your thoughts on what is currently regarded as research we both can strongly recommend not only the following specific chapters according to your interests but our three sets of published respondents analyses of all chapters for anyone carrying out psychotherapeutic and counselling research.

References

Blackmore, S. (2010). *Consciousness.* London: Routledge.

Gadamer, H. (2013). *Truth and method.* London: Bloomsbury Academic.

Heaton, J. M. (2010). *The talking cure: Wittgenstein's therapeutic method for psychotherapy.* London: Palgrave Macmillan.

Lather, P., & St. Pierre, E. A. (2013). Post-qualitative research. *International Journal of Qualitative Studies in Education, 26*, 629–633. doi:10.1080/09518398.2013.788752

Loewenthal, D. (2011). *Post-existentialism and the psychological therapies: Towards a therapy without foundations.* London: Karnac Books.

Loewenthal, D. (2015). *Critical psychotherapy, psychoanalysis and counselling: Implications for practice.* London: Palgrave Macmillan.

Loewenthal, D. (2016). Therapy as cultural, politically influenced practice. In J. Lees (Ed.), *The future of psychological therapy: Managed care, practitioner research and clinical innovation* (pp. 11–25). London: Routledge.

Loewenthal, D. (2017). *Existential psychotherapy and counselling after postmodernism: The selected works of Del Loewenthal.* London: World Library of Mental Health.

Tracy, S. J. (2010). Qualitative quality: Eight "abig-tent" criteria for excellent qualitative research. *Qualitative Inquiry, 16*, 837–851. doi:10.1177/1077800410383121

Wittgenstein, L. (1958). *Philosophical investigations* (2nd ed.). tr. G.E.M. Anscombe. Oxford: Blackwell.

Interventions in everyday lives: How clients use psychotherapy outside their sessions

Ole Dreier

The purpose of psychotherapy is to help clients address and overcome problems troubling them in their everyday lives. Therapy can therefore only work if clients include it in their ongoing lives to deal with their problems. Detailed, systematic research is needed on how clients do so in their everyday lives outside their sessions. A design of exploratory case studies on this topic is presented in this article. The main outcomes of such a case study on family therapy are then laid out in general terms. They highlight how treatment practices and clients' ordinary everyday practices interact when clients change their everyday lives to overcome their troubles. They also highlight what it involves for clients to accomplish this. It is concluded that we need more research on how to understand intervention; on the interaction between interventions and clients' conduct of their everyday life; on sessions as a particular, secluded part of clients' ongoing everyday lives, and on how to consider therapists' procedures and conduct of sessions accordingly.

Psychotherapie hat zum Ziel, Probleme, die Klienten in ihrem Alltag begleiten und stören, aufzuzeigen und zu überwinden. Therapie kann deshalb nur gelingen, wenn Klienten die Erkenntnisse aus den Sitzungen in ihren Alltag integrieren, um mit ihren Problemen zurecht zu kommen. Eine differenzierte und systematische Forschung soll über die diversen Praktiken der Klienten außerhalb der Sitzungen Aufschluss geben. Ein allgemeines Forschungsdesign entlang explorativer Fallstudien wird hierzu in diesem Artikel vorgestellt. Die wesentlichen Ergebnisse einer solchen Studie im Rahmen der Familientherapie werden in allgemeinen Begriffen dargelegt. Sie zeigen, wie Praktiken innerhalb der Sitzungen und die Alltagspraktiken der Klienten aufeinander einwirken, wenn Klienten ihre Praktiken im Alltag ändern, um ihre Probleme zu überwinden. Sie streichen ebenfalls heraus, was es für die Klienten mit sich bringt, dies zu erreichen. Abschließend lässt sich sagen, dass mehr Forschung zum besseren Verständnis von Interventionen benötigt wird; zu den

Wechselbeziehungen zwischen Intervention und dem Klientenverhalten im Alltag; zu Sitzungen als einem speziellen, „abgeschlossenen Teil" im täglichen Leben der Klienten, und, entsprechend, die Betrachtung der Sitzungen des Therapeuten in Bezug auf dessen Methodik und Verhalten.

El objetivo de la psicoterapia es ayudar a los clientes a enfrentar y resolver los problemas que les aquejan en sus vidas cotidianas, por lo tanto la psicoterapia puede funcionar solamente si los clientes la incluyen en el curso de su vida diaria. Se necesitan investigaciones sistemáticas y detalladas acerca de qué hacen los clientes en su vida fuera de las sesiones. En este artículo se presenta un diseño exploratorio de estudio de casos. Se dan los resultados más importantes de tal estudio en terapia de familia; ellos destacan cómo el tratamiento y la vida diaria de los clientes interactúan cuando ellos efectúan cambios en su vida cotidiana para resolver sus problemas. Alzo destacan lo que esto implica por parte de los clientes. Se concluye que se necesitan más investigaciones acerca de: cómo entender las intervenciones, la interacción entre las intervenciones y cómo los clientes conducen su vida diaria, las sesiones como una parte aislada y particular en la vida de los clientes y acerca de cómo considerar los procedimientos y maneras de conducir las sesiones.

Lo scopo della psicoterapia è quello di aiutare i clienti ad affrontare e superare i problemi che li angustiano nel loro quotidiano. La terapia può quindi funzionare solo se i clienti la utilizzano nel concreto svolgersi della loro vita per affrontare le questioni problematiche. Al fine di comprendere come i clienti utilizzano la terapia nella loro vita quotidiana al di fuori delle sedute sono necessarie ricerche dettagliate e sistematiche. Questo articolo presenta uno studio di caso che esplora il tema. I principali risultati emersi dall'analisi di questo caso relativo ad una terapia familiare sono presentati in termini generali. Essi evidenziano come il trattamento interagisca con le pratiche ordinarie e quotidiane dei clienti quando essi cercano di cambiare la loro vita di tutti i giorni al fine di superare i loro problemi. I risultati evidenziano inoltre che cosa implica per i clienti attuare questa integrazione. In conclusione è sottolineato come debbano essere realizzate ulteriori ricerche per meglio comprendere le interferenze, l'interazione tra interventi e comportamenti della vita quotidiana dei clienti, le sedute come una particolare area separata dalla vita di tutti i giorni del cliente e, di conseguenza e coerentemente, come considerare le procedure dei terapeuti e lo svolgimento delle sessioni.

Le but de la psychothérapie est d'aider les clients à adresser et surmonter les problèmes qui les gênent dans leur vie de tous les jours. La thérapie ne peut alors être efficace que si les clients l'incluent dans leurs vies pour traiter leurs difficultés. Une recherche systématique détaillée est nécessaire afin de trouver comment les clients opèrent dans leur vie de tous les jours en dehors de leurs séances. Nous présentons dans cet article la structure générale des études de cas à visée de recherche concernant ce sujet. Les résultats principaux d'une étude de cas de thérapie familiale sont ensuite exposés en termes généraux. Ils montrent les interactions entre les pratiques propres au traitement et les pratiques ordinaires des clients dans leur vie quotidienne lorsqu'ils la modifient pour surmonter leurs problèmes. Les résultats montrent également ce que cela implique pour y parvenir. En conclusion, il est proposé que des recherches supplémentaires soient menées afin de comprendre l'intervention ; d'étudier les interactions entre les interventions et la façon dont les clients mènent leurs vies quotidiennes ; sur les séances comme partie particulière et isolée de la vie de tous les jours des clients et par conséquent sur la manière dont on doit considérer les procédures des thérapeutes et la conduite des séances.

Ο σκοπός της ψυχοθεραπείας είναι να βοηθήσει τους πελάτες να αντιμετωπίσουν και να ξεπεράσουν προβλήματα που τους ταλαιπωρούν στην καθημερινή ζωή τους. Ως εκ τούτου η θεραπεία μπορεί να λειτουργήσει μόνο εφόσον οι πελάτες τη συμπεριλάβουν στη ζωή τους, για να αντιμετωπίσουν τα προβλήματά τους. Κρίνεται αναγκαία η ενδελεχής και συστηματική έρευνα για το πώς οι πελάτες εφαρμόζουν την ψυχοθεραπεία στην καθημερινή ζωή τους, έξω από τις συνεδρίες τους. Στο παρόν άρθρο παρουσιάζεται ο σχεδιασμός των διερευνητικών μελετών περίπτωσης σχετικά με το θέμα αυτό. Στη συνέχεια παρουσιάζονται τα κύρια αποτελέσματα μια τέτοιας μελέτης περίπτωσης οικογενειακής θεραπείας. Τα ευρήματα της έρευνας αναδεικνύουν πως αλληλοεπιδρούν οι θεραπευτικές πρακτικές και οι συνήθεις καθημερινές πρακτικές των πελατών όταν οι πελάτες αλλάζουν την καθημερινή ζωή τους για να ξεπεράσουν τα προβλήματά τους. Επίσης, διαφαίνεται τι χρειάζεται να κάνουν οι πελάτες προκειμένου να επιτευχθεί αυτή η αλλαγή. Συμπεραίνεται ότι χρειαζόμαστε περισσότερη έρευνα για να κατανοήσουμε βαθύτερα την παρέμβαση, την αλληλεπίδραση μεταξύ των παρεμβάσεων και της δράσης των πελατών στην καθημερινή ζωής τους, τις συνεδρίες ως ιδιαίτερο, αποκομμένο τμήμα από την τρέχουσα καθημερινή ζωή των πελατών, καθώς και σχετικά με το πώς να προσεγγίσουμε τις θεραπευτικές διεργασίες και τη διεξαγωγή συνεδριών.

Research on mental health usually focuses on the professional practices of defining and treating mental distress. There is also a substantial body of research about clients' experiences of living with mental distress. But an important link between these two research areas needs to be investigated in depth. We need research on how clients use their treatments in their everyday lives.

This claim becomes most obvious when viewing treatment and mental distress in practical terms – as practices. Then, distress is not merely a mental state. It is something clients must do something about in practice in their everyday lives. Treatment is something clients use to overcome their distress in relation to other aspects of their everyday life. And clients are not just acted upon and bearers of experiences. They are also agents in relation to their everyday life and treatment.

This expands our view on treatment practices from encounters in sessions to interventions in everyday lives. Still, research on treatment generally focuses on sessions. It rests on the implicit, general belief that the effect of treatment is brought about in sessions and merely transferred by clients afterward into their everyday lives and applied so that what the clients got in sessions is what continues elsewhere afterward. This reflects a poor theory of human learning (Dreier, 2008b, in press; Lave, 1988). It also reflects a general feature of the arrangement of expert practices. Experts generally conduct their practice in a particular setting – be it a therapy room, health-care consultation, or hospital – which is set off and secluded from the ordinary everyday life of the persons they serve. So it seems that we must look in sessions if we want to consider the treatment effect as caused by the experts. But the belief in the session as the place where therapy works has unfortunate consequences. One is that it has not been researched in detail how these expert practices come to make a difference in the everyday lives of the persons they serve. Another is that, in order to work as intended in the ongoing lives of their clients, these practices must rely on client agency elsewhere. But what clients do elsewhere to make them work is not researched systematically and in detail.

For some years, I studied how clients make their therapy work in interplay between their therapy sessions and their ordinary everyday lives (Dreier, 1998, 2000, 2008a, 2011). To do so, I developed a type of exploratory qualitative case studies of *Psychotherapy in Everyday Life* (Dreier, 2008a). The theory and methodology behind this work, a review of the pertinent literature, and the outcomes of such a case study are laid out in detail in that book. This article focuses on what I found about the client processes of bringing about outcomes outside sessions. These findings are summarized and, to some extent, clarified and elaborated below.

Design and method

The project reported in the above-mentioned book was carried out at an outpatient unit of child psychiatry in Copenhagen. The design of the study was quite straightforward. It involved four long family therapies with me as a co-therapist. All sessions were audio taped, and a research assistant interviewed the families in their homes at regular intervals throughout the period of their therapy and until half a year after it terminated. The examined therapies ran up to one and a half years. In the interviews, the clients were primarily asked about their everyday lives with key questions like: 'What happened in your everyday life since your previous interview?' 'Did anything change?' 'If any changes occurred, how did they come about?' 'Which role did you play in these changes?' 'Did you do things differently compared to before?' 'Did your sessions matter in these changes?' 'If they did, how did they matter?' Only then were they asked about their experiences of their sessions and of their therapists and about their participation in the sessions. Finally, they were asked what they now believe they need sessions for. By repeating these questions in each interview, we could track changes in their practices and in their points of view on their lives, distress, and therapy. We also gained access to what triggered particular changes and to the course of bringing them about by means of their sessions and various situations and events in their ordinary everyday lives. The guide for these semi-structured interviews can be downloaded from my homepage http://psychology.ku.dk/emeriti/ole_dreier/downloads/inter viewguide_to_psychotherapy_in_everyday_life.pdf.

This design reflects a decentered understanding of therapy as seen from the perspective and locations of clients' everyday lives instead of from their sessions. After all, the clients' troubles arise in their everyday lives and must, in the end, be overcome there, among other things, by means of a therapy that takes place elsewhere. Participation in a therapy is, in fact, a temporary addition to the clients' ordinary everyday life. The design also lets us illuminate the clients' change processes and the role of their sessions in these changes by following their practice as they move from their home to the sessions and from there to their home, school, work, and other regular and occasional parts of their everyday lives. In the book, I analyze one project case in depth and detail. This case was chosen because it contains the richest materials. The case analysis is based on the clients' statements in their interviews and sessions.

Semi-structured interviews were chosen because we wanted to learn from the clients about their experiences and activities. But such projects about ongoing therapies are rare. We, therefore, took care to design and conduct the interviews so that they were in accordance with the general aim of their therapy and did not disturb it or become too much for them; should such complications occur, interviews let us discover and respond to them. So we instructed the interviewer how to avoid them and respond to them. Interviews also let us ask the clients about the meaning for them of being interviewed. All the clients in the project responded that they were interested in talking about their everyday life and treatment in the interviews because they were in the process of reconsidering and changing their everyday life and using their treatment to do so. We registered no instances of the disturbances we wanted to avoid. The interviews could, therefore, be conducted as intended in a collaborative and supportive manner as enquiries with and not on the clients (Holzkamp, 2013).

Using interviews in such a project has some limitations. Clients can only tell us what they experience so clearly that they can articulate it in conversation with the interviewer. On the other hand, repeated interviews let us register when an idea or issue becomes clear to them and in connection with what this happens. Having somebody else than their therapists interview, the clients at home rather than at the clinic also proved vital to gaining other perspectives and pieces of information than in their sessions. But, to some extent, it entailed a family-centered perspective on their everyday lives as a whole. Furthermore, the fact that all family members were present in the interviews made them support or object to each other's statements in ways that further illuminated many issues. And, finally, the special focus of therapy on problems affected which features of their everyday lives we came to know most about.

The analysis of the materials is theory guided and grounded in a theory of persons in social practice (Dreier, 2008a). They are grasped in the first person perspective of subjects situated in and moving across the various settings of their ongoing everyday lives. Core concepts refer to their activities in taking part in these settings, to their positions, concerns, and stakes in them, and to the meaning and realization of their situated possibilities. Further concepts refer to how they pursue concerns and possibilities across settings, including how they pursue changes and resolutions to problems in such trajectories.

The materials were read through carefully to capture and categorize the clients' statements about various aspects of the topic of this study across various situations in various settings and across the time period of the study. Similarities and differences between these situated phenomena across times and places were used to generalize about them. Patterns were searched in which features hang together with which other features, and which features replace a certain feature in connection with which other features. In doing so, close attention was paid to the clients' own categories, reasons, and patterns and to what did not fit into the emerging pattern of understanding and had to be incorporated into a more comprehensive grasp of the topic in order to do justice to the complexity of the case. Surprises in what the clients said and struggles in coming to grips with it were taken as chances to reconsider and develop the analysis. The study was, therefore, not only theory guided but also theory building. Concepts were added, revised, and elaborated to come to grips with incommensurate features. This, finally, resulted in a coherent, comprehensive analysis which identified and characterized, among other things, the themes to be reported in this article. In systematizing the analysis – and in writing it up – I, first, elaborated how the clients move across diverse settings in pursuit of their concerns. Second, I added the time dimension of their change processes as pursued across times and places. Third, I zoomed in on how the clients pursue resolutions to their problems across times and places. And, fourth, I linked how they changed their therapy-related problems to how they conduct their everyday lives.

Similar projects were later carried out in other related areas of practice such as youth counseling, genetic counseling, rehabilitation following brain injuries, cancer screening and with spouses to brain tumor patients. The main outcomes of these projects complement and corroborate those from the family therapy project. But we are only beginning to illuminate issues of treatments in clients' practices and much more work is needed. Some projects used other, less labor-intensive methods. For instance, Mackrill (2008a) used solicited diaries to track the relations between counseling sessions and everyday lives of young adults who grew up in alcoholic families.

Interactions between interventions and ordinary everyday practices

I shall now present some main outcomes from the family therapy case analysis about how treatment practices and clients' ordinary practices interact in the everyday practices of clients and, especially, when clients are changing their practice. The outcomes are presented in general terms and insights which only became clear to me in later work after the publication of the book are included.

Selective uses

Having access to transcripts from all sessions and from interviews about the clients' everyday lives and changes and comparing the two sets of data, makes one thing evident from the start. Much more is said, experienced, understood, and suggested in therapy sessions than it is possible for the clients to pursue elsewhere and later. The clients' uses of sessions elsewhere and later are necessarily selective (Dreier, 2008a, p. 94). A therapeutic intervention is a complex nexus from which the clients must pick some features and leave the rest behind. As seen from our position as therapists in sessions, we were often surprised by what the clients picked out and what they let be. Again, analyzing both sets of data, it becomes clear that the clients' selective uses of sessions are primarily grounded in what they believe may make a desired difference in their everyday lives with distress rather than by adhering to the therapeutic procedure and rationale. What they use, therefore, depends on the settings, relations, events, and range of opportunities of their ongoing everyday lives. In other words, the therapists cannot control what the clients use from their therapy and clients taking part in the same sessions can and will use different aspects thereof.

Emerging events

During the period in which the clients attend therapy, many events occur in their everyday lives. They do not foresee most of these events and/or they occur for other reasons which have nothing to do with their ongoing therapy. Nonetheless, some of these events become a filter and condition for the clients' uses of their therapy. An event may trigger them to use a particular feature from their sessions and affect the way in which they use it. It may even launch crucial steps of change. Had that event not occurred, their therapy would have taken another turn where they do not use this feature from sessions or use it in other ways in connection with other events which might have occurred. In other words, certain events occurring independently of their therapy may be important facilitators – or obstacles – of therapeutically assisted changes. And because the clients' everyday lives may be changing for other reasons, which then affect the dynamics and course of their ongoing therapy, we need to know how the clients combine therapeutic and other influences in changing aspects of their everyday lives.

Making up their minds

Before the clients begin therapy, they have tried in vain to temper or overcome their increasing troubles in various ways. Mackrill (2008b, 2008c) found that, during their therapy, clients continue to use more or less modified versions of the strategies for change they used prior to their therapy which then affects how they use their sessions. I found that the clients' prior attempts rest on various understandings of the reasons for their troubles and of what might be suitable possibilities for overcoming them. When these attempts fail, they increasingly come to believe that there is something about their troubles which they do not quite understand. They become more uncertain and confused about them. This affects how they relate to ideas and suggestions from sessions. Asked whether they apply things from sessions afterward when they get home, the clients respond, 'No, we have to think more about it first.' This, on the surface quite innocent, statement sums up that attending therapy makes them think much more about how to understand their troubles as well as what they can and want to do, and do not want to do, about them. After all, what they do may not only reduce their distress. It becomes part of their lives, affects it, and it becomes part of who they are. In many respects, the clients, therefore, have to make up their minds about where they stand on understanding their troubles and on what to do about them. They may go through long-winding processes of reconsidering and of finding out and changing their minds on where they stand in relation to their troubles and ongoing lives. Their sessions are an important source of these reconsiderations and their clarifications and reconsiderations of stances affect which features from sessions they select for later uses. Asked what they do if they do not agree with what their therapists say or suggest or with what they take to be a piece of advice from them, the clients respond, 'Then we just don't do it.'

Other sources

The clients also draw on other sources than their therapy in making up and changing their minds about their troubles and what they want to do in relation to them (see also Mackrill, 2008c). They talk to friends about it, and they get ideas or reservations about it from being in particular situations, reading books, seeing movies, and so forth. Getting out of their ordinary everyday life for some time also offers opportunities to change their minds, for instance, while being on holidays or in hospital. Likewise, issues of trust play a part in finding out what they are ready to believe from particular sources.

Negotiated changes

Furthermore, because the clients generally live with various other persons in various settings of their everyday lives, they must negotiate many changes with others. This can be demanding and tough, for instance, when they are not quite certain where they stand on them; when it is difficult for them to hold on to their stances in disagreements; when they do not want particular others to know (much or anything) about their troubles; or when they are afraid what they will think of them if they do. Relevant other persons must also be willing to negotiate and to do their part. How and when negotiations may take place and may become an issue too. Relevant others may prefer different ways of addressing and negotiating troubles. For instance, some prefer negotiating when they are in the middle, or at the end, of an instance of trouble while others need to think about it first and come back to it later after things have calmed down.

Conflicts over troubles and changes

The clients are also in conflicts with others over their troubles and over their therapy. Thus, members of this family in therapy quarrel at home about what they want to do here with their therapy; what they believe their therapists really think about them and their troubles; whom they believe their therapists really agree with; which pieces of advice they believe their therapists really gave; and how they believe these pieces of advice could be reinterpreted. The clients even turn their therapists, and what they do and say in sessions, into objects of conflict between them at home, using the authority of their therapists as a weapon in these conflicts without telling their therapists about it.

Changing joint arrangements

The clients must come to agree with each other on other ways of dealing with their troubles. This often implies that they must come to agree on other joint arrangements of how they live this shared part of their everyday lives together. Still, joint arrangements cannot last unless they leave room for differences among them in how they take part in their shared life. And only a small part of reaching such agreements and establishing such arrangements takes place in sessions. What is more, the clients' troubles have often led to increased distance and distrust between the members of the client family. That makes it necessary for them to 'find each other again,' as they put it. The difficult, multifaceted, often troublesome processes of succeeding in doing so are carried out in other ways at home than in sessions.

Seizing opportunities on the spot

In everyday life, it is often not possible to predict the occurrence of suitable occasions to pick up and pursue particular changes and rearrangements. At least, many occasions are unforeseen. The clients must, therefore, be able to recognize various occasions quickly as they occur and seize them on the spot before the ongoing practice moves on to something else. Becoming able to do so well, involves clarifications and learning. The clients' statement that they must think more about suggestions from sessions before using them also refers to becoming able to do this.

Discontinuous pursuits

Though the clients must pursue problem-related changes in their everyday life, they do not do so continuously. Their troubles and these pursuits are not always on their mind, though they come to mind easily for a period of time. This reflects a crucial difference between sessions and the practices of ordinary everyday life. Session practices concentrate on a topic at a time, while in ordinary everyday life, several things mostly go on at the same time and compete for their time and attention. So, the clients' pursuits of changes in everyday life are purposeful, but they are also discontinuous. They take place in-between much else and they are interrupted by other important, and not so important, matters. The clients must remember them and learn how and when to pick them up again and continue them, as well as how to avoid that they slide into the background, become neglected and perhaps forgotten. They must also trust each other's willingness to come back to them and continue them. Besides, in the intervals between these pursuits, they may have re-appreciated their troubles and pursuits so that they continue in a somewhat changed manner. This increases the issue of internal coherence in their changes. The duration of the interval between consecutive sessions easily triggers a corresponding rhythm of pursuits in everyday life so that the clients are more concerned with these pursuits shortly before and for some time after each session while they slide more into the background in the meantime. Some intervals are surprisingly long. For instance, this family set aside pursuits of changes to their troubles while being on summer vacation and only picked them up again when their sessions resumed afterward.

In-between much else

Like many other concerns, therapy-related concerns are pursued in-between much else. They are, in fact, pursued in varying ways together with or against varying other circumstances, opportunities, activities, and concerns. The clients, hence, face the challenge of finding out and learning how to pursue them in various situated ways. I shall now go further into the situated character of the clients' pursuits of changes.

Transforming concerted problem talk

The clients stress that there are major differences for them between participating in their therapy sessions and in the settings of their ordinary everyday life. In other places, they have never talked to each other like they do in their sessions. To them, their sessions offer a strange practice which they must learn to participate in to their advantage and to make use of in other places. Their sessions draw them into a 'strange intimacy' with 'intimate strangers' which is different from their intimacy at home or with close friends and which they must become familiar with. Still, they insist that in the course of their therapy they do not begin to talk with each other at home like they do in the concerted problem talk of their sessions. So they do not transfer the practice of session talk directly into their everyday life elsewhere and apply it there. Indeed, they stress that important differences between their session talks and their practices in other settings enable their therapy to work in their everyday life. In other words, their therapy would not have worked if their session talks had offered the same possibilities, relationships, and experiences as elsewhere in their everyday life. That differences between what the clients do in their therapy sessions and elsewhere are important, is already obvious from the fact that they must be able to transform the concerted problem talk of therapy sessions into various forms of situated activity aimed at changing their troubles in various settings.

Moving across different settings

After all, when the members of the family move from one setting into another, they take part in other ways. This is so when they move from at home into their therapy session and when they go home, to school, to work, and so forth afterward. A change of setting means that they then take part in another practice with other contents and purposes which are connected to other personal concerns of theirs, other scopes of possibilities and positions for them and other relationships to other persons. A successful participation then calls for other abilities, affords other experiences, and has other meanings to them. Their participation, abilities, and experiences are then more or less different.

Fitted into different settings

Accordingly, the clients must use ideas and suggestions from sessions in situated ways in the diverse settings of their everyday life where various things are at stake for them, also when they try to do something about their troubles. They must fit ideas and suggestions from sessions with their varying possibilities in relation to their varying co-participants in various settings. Only then do these particular aspects of the therapeutic intervention become usable for them. How an aspect of sessions may be used and what it takes to use it in different settings, therefore, varies.

In different ways across settings

In other words, the clients pursue changes in various, particular ways in their different settings. To make this clear, I very briefly mention two examples related to common difficulties. First, the father has difficulties in finding out and holding on to what he stands for in practices with others in their therapy sessions, at home, at work, and so forth. This difficulty does not mean the same to him in these different settings. In pursuing a resolution to this difficulty, his possibilities and what is at stake for him in doing so vary in these different parts of his life. Second, the twelve-year-old daughter suffers from sudden anxiety attacks. In the sessions, she talks about these attacks with her therapist. At home her parents help her out, do much to prevent them from occurring and to make them go away quickly, and they overwhelm and confuse her with all their talk and worry about it. In school and with her friends, she seeks to remain at the periphery of things because she is afraid to be harassed and excluded if they find out or if she tells them about it. She too has good reasons to pursue a resolution to her difficulty in different ways in these and other settings.

Learning about troubles across settings

When the clients do so, they discover the particular possibilities which the practices in these various settings offer them, and they learn to seize these different possibilities. Using session ideas and suggestions adequately then mostly involves learning, and they must often be modified or transformed in order to become usable in their particular settings. In fact, the clients modify and change their ideas and suggestions from sessions elsewhere and later, even in ways their therapists rarely come to know about and which we were surprised to see in the interviews. What is more, in their different settings, their troubles hang together with different other things. This lets the clients learn about other dimensions of their troubles and come to see, understand, and appreciate them differently. They develop a richer, more complex, and differentiated understanding of their troubles and of what they are related to. We might call the clients' understanding of their troubles a complex nexus. This nexus holds general features, say, of what anxiety is or of what adopting and holding on to stances is, together with various specific features of what it is related to and what it means and how it can be dealt with in their different settings. In these different settings, the clients then combine the general and specific features into varied, situated understandings of their troubles, what they mean to them, what they can do about them, and what is at stake in doing so for them.

Learning to combine different pursuits across settings

Besides learning to understand and pursue their troubles differently in different settings, the clients learn to pursue a resolution to them across their different settings, that is, into their sessions and out again into and across the everyday settings of their home, school, work, and so forth. They learn to take advantage of having possibilities for doing different things about them in different settings. And they learn to combine the particular contextual parts of such complex change processes into a coherent pursuit so that the various parts support and supplement each other rather than neutralize or counter each other. In this sense, they compose, direct, and conduct their pursuits of changes across settings. As they learn more about this, they become better at it and able to pursue changes across an increasing span of times and places.

Open-ended learning

As the clients' everyday life and their troubles change because of their uses of their sessions and/or for other reasons, they must change the ways in which they pursue changes and combine various steps in these pursuits. They must, then, learn to use their therapy in other ways. In fact, they must change their understandings and pursuits of changes many times because their ongoing lives continue to vary and change. This involves recurrent multi-faceted learning (Dreier, 2008b, in press), which also changes their understanding of which aspects of their practices the emergence and overcoming of their troubles are related to. Indeed, their changes of and learning about their therapy-related troubles are mostly open-ended, that is, they have no definite endpoint or solution from when on the clients need not concern themselves with them any longer.

Fitted into their conduct of everyday life

Finally, it is important to the clients, and to those they share their lives with, that addressing their troubles does not get in the way of, or disturb or overshadow all those things in their lives which they treasure most and which they must get done. Dealing with troubles should not take over their lives. They do not want their life to be centered on or occupied by troubles. In that sense, addressing their troubles must be kept within bounds and fitted into the way they conduct their everyday life.

Conclusion

I have argued that therapy only works if clients link it to features of their everyday lives and include it in their ongoing lives to deal with their problems. This is a basic, general feature of how therapy can work because of the general arrangement of therapy sessions as set off and secluded from the everyday lives in which they are to make a difference. We must, therefore, expect to find it working in varying ways in different forms of therapy and depending on the clients' particular problems, selective uses, events, and nexuses of everyday life. But we must also study in depth and detail what is involved when clients accomplish it in their everyday lives and we need much more research to illuminate this encompassing topic which qualitative methods are very well suited for. Practicing therapists will recognize much of what I wrote about interventions in everyday lives from their work with clients. That underlines the reality of these phenomena. But we were surprised by the extent and frequency with which they occurred and carried changes forward in the case I analyzed. They were normally involved and not just occasional occurrences.

As the title indicates, this article rests on a radically different view on intervention than the one adopted in, for instance, evidence-based research (Dreier, 2011). It argues that an intervention does not work as an effect of what an expert does when following a particular, specified therapeutic procedure in sessions. What happens comes closer to the literal meaning of the word to intervene as 'to come, be, or lie between' and 'to come between as an influence, as in order to modify, settle, or hinder some action, argument, etc.' (Webster's New World College Dictionary's, 1997, p. 707). To intervene means to get involved by getting in-between much else that is already ongoing. Psychotherapy research must recognize that therapy always works alongside and in interaction with other environmental influences and with responses and initiatives by clients and others in their ongoing everyday lives. We need to know how therapeutic and other influences interact and clients combine them in their everyday lives. To understand the practice of intervening, we need knowledge about how things hang together and work together and about ways of getting in between them.

The article also points to other research topics which it urges us to reconsider.

One topic concerns the relation between therapy and clients' conduct of everyday life (Dreier, 2008a; Holzkamp, 2013). In order to be sustained, changes must be built into the way in which clients conduct their everyday life. But an intervention may interfere with their conduct of everyday life and can then only work if they change it. An intervention may also be called for due to events, breaks, and troubles in clients' everyday lives so that they need to reestablish their earlier conduct of everyday life or change it. Besides, troubles make clients reconsider their lives and want to live differently in certain respects. They then reconsider and experiment with changing their conduct of everyday life and they may draw on their therapy in doing so.

Another topic concerns how to understand what goes on in sessions when we consider sessions as a particular, secluded part of clients' ongoing everyday lives.

And a third topic concerns how research on interventions in everyday lives may make us reconsider and change our understanding of the conduct and procedures of therapists in sessions.

Disclosure statement

No potential conflict of interest was reported by the author.

References

Dreier, O. (1998). Client perspectives and uses of psychotherapy. *The European Journal of Psychotherapy, Counselling & Health, 1*, 295–310. doi:10.1080/1364253980 8402315

Dreier, O. (2000). Psychotherapy in clients' trajectories across contexts. In C. Mattingly & L. Garro (Eds.), *Narratives and the cultural construction of illness and healing* (pp. 237–258). Berkeley: University of California Press.

Dreier, O. (2008a). *Psychotherapy in everyday life*. New York, NY: Cambridge University Press.

Dreier, O. (2008b). Learning in structures of social practice. In S. Brinkmann, C. Elmholdt, G. Kraft, P. Musaeus, K. Nielsen, & L. Tanggaard (Eds.), *A qualitative stance: Essays in honor of Steinar Kvale* (pp. 85–96). Aarhus: Aarhus University Press.

Dreier, O. (2009). Interview guide from the project "Psychotherapy in everyday life". Retrieved from http://psychology.ku.dk/emeriti/ole_dreier/downloads/interviewguide_ to_psychotherapy_in_everyday_life.pdf

Dreier, O. (2011). Intervention, evidence-based research and everyday life. In P. Stenner, J. Cromby, J. Motzkau, J. Yen, & Y. Haosheng (Eds.), *Theoretical psychology: Global transformations and challenges* (pp. 260–269). Concord, MA: Captus Press.

Dreier, O. (in press). Learning and conduct of everyday life. In A. Larraín, A. Haye, J. Cresswell, G. Sullivan, & M. Morgan (Eds.), *Dialogue and debate in the making of theoretical psychology*.

Holzkamp, K. (2013). Psychology: Social self-understanding on the reasons for action in the conduct of everyday life. In E. Schraube & U. Osterkamp (Eds.), *Psychology from the standpoint of the subject* (pp. 233–341). Basingstoke: Palgrave Macmillan.

Lave, J. (1988). *Cognition in practice*. New York, NY: Cambridge University Press.

Mackrill, T. (2008a). Solicited diary studies of psychotherapeutic practice – Pros and cons. *European Journal of Psychotherapy & Counselling, 10*, 5–18. doi:10.1080/ 13642530701869243

Mackrill, T. (2008b). Pre-treatment change in psychotherapy with adult children of problem drinkers: The significance of leaving home. *Counselling & Psychotherapy Research, 8*, 160–165. doi:10.1080/14733140802193341

Mackrill, T. (2008c). Exploring psychotherapy clients' independent strategies for change while in therapy. *British Journal of Guidance and Counselling, 36*, 441–453. doi:10.1080/03069880802343837

Webster's New World College Dictionary (3rd ed.). (1997). Boston, MA: Houghton Mifflin Harcourt.

Eating disorders in the course of life: A qualitative approach to vital change

Félix Díaz Martínez, Natalia Solano Pinto, Irene Solbes Canales and Sonsoles Calderón López

Eating disorders (EDs) have become one of the biggest mental-health problems in the last decades, especially among youth and women. The present study aims to analyse the suitability of Prochaska and DiClemente's Transtheoretical Model of Change when applied to the living experiences of people diagnosed with ED and their carers. For this purpose, we applied a narrative biographic approach to the ways in which people face their problems and vital development in the ED domain. Through the narrative analysis of these autobiographies, we aimed to study the patients' own notions of 'change', 'problem' and 'vital trajectory'. We focused on five autobiographic interviews of persons diagnosed as ED (four women and a man). The analysis yields three discourses which organize and give sense to our participants' vital transitions: a discourse of functional adaptation to events and experiences; one that pays attention to random events and people entering your life; and one that has the personal initiative and agency of an individual agent at its core. It also illuminates particular ways of understanding determination, contemplation and pre-contemplation. These ways of understanding change are shown to extend the possible ways of thinking about people's lives and ED patients' perspectives.

Essstörungen (ES) haben sich in den letzten Jahrzenten faktisch zu einem der größten psychischen Störungsbilder entwickelt, vor allem unter Jugendlichen und Frauen. Die vorliegende Studie untersucht, inwiefern sich das von Prochaska & DiClementes (1983) entwickelte „Transtheoretische Modell" (TMC) für die Analyse der bislang gemachten Erfahrungen von Menschen mit ES und ihren Betreuern eignet. Zu diesem Zweck haben wir einen narrativ-biografischen Ansatz ausgewählt, um mithilfe dessen den verschiedenen Wegen nachzuspüren, wie Menschen ihrer Essstörungs-Problematik begegnen und sich, in Anbetracht dessen, deren weitere Entwicklung gestaltet hat. Mithilfe der narrativen Analyse dieser Biografien zielten wir auf die den Klienten je eigenen Vorstellungen von „Veränderung", „Problemen" und „vitaler Verlaufskurve". Die autobiografischen Interviews umfassen fünf Personen mit Essstörungen (vier Frauen und ein Mann). Die Untersuchung konnte drei Diskurse ausmachen, die die (weitere) Entwicklung der Klienten strukturieren und für sie Sinn ergeben: Einen Diskurs der funktionalen Anpassung an Ereignisse und Erfahrungen; ein zweiter, der auf zufällige Ereignisse und Menschen, die in deren Leben eintreten, abstellt. Im Mittelpunkt des dritten Diskurses stehen die Handlungsfähigkeit und Eigeninitiative des Aktors. Die Untersuchung erläutert darüber hinaus bestimmte Verständnisweisen von Entschlossenheit, Reflexion und „Vorüberlegungen". Diese Formen des Verständnisses von Veränderungen werden aufgezeigt, um die vorhandenen Vorstellungen über das Leben anderer Menschen und die bislang verfügbaren Sichtweisen von Klienten mit Essstörungen zu erweitern.

Los trastornos de la alimentación se han convertido en uno de los mayores problemas en el campo de la salud mental durante las últimas décadas, especialmente entre los jóvenes y las mujeres. El objetivo del presente estudio es analizar si el Modelo de Cambio Transteórico de Prochaska y Di Clemente (1983), es adecuado para ser aplicado al estudio de las experiencias vividas por personas que han sido diagnosticadas con trastornos de la alimentación y a las personas que cuidan de ellos. Se aplicó un método biográfico narrativo para estudiar la manera en que las personas enfrentan sus problemas y su desarrollo vital en la esfera de los trastornos de la alimentación. A través del análisis narrativo de estas autobiografías nos propusimos estudiar las nociones de ''cambio'', ''problema'' y ''trayectoria vital'' en los propios pacientes. Nos focalizamos en cinco entrevistas autobiográficas con personas diagnosticadas con trastornos de la alimentación (cuatro mujeres y un hombre). El análisis produjo tres discursos que organizan y dan sentido a las transiciones vitales en nuestros participantes: 1, adaptación funcional a eventos y experiencias; 2, atención a eventos imprevistos y a personas que vienen a formar parte sus vidas y 3, iniciativa personal y modo de operar como centro en la vida del individuo. Pudimos apreciar formas particulares para entender determinación, contemplación y pre-contemplación. Estas formas de comprender el cambio parecen extender las posibles formas en que pensamos acerca de la vida de las personas y las perspectivas de los pacientes con trastornos de la alimentación.

Negli ultimi decenni i Disturbi del Comportamento Alimentare (ED) sono diventati uno dei più grandi problemi di salute mentale, in particolare tra i giovani e le donne. Il presente studio si propone di analizzare l'idoneità del Modello Transteorico sul cambiamento (TMC di Prochaska & Di Clemente (1983)) ad essere applicato alle esperienze di vita delle persone con diagnosi di ED e a chi di loro si prende cura. A questo scopo, abbiamo utilizzato un approccio biografico narrativo per analizzare il modo in cui le persone affrontano i loro problemi e i cambiamenti della vita in presenza di ED. Attraverso l'analisi narrativa di queste autobiografie, ci siamo proposti di studiare le nozioni che i pazienti hanno di 'cambiamento', 'problema' e 'traiettoria di vita'. Ci siamo focalizzati i sulle interviste autobiografiche di cinque soggetti (quattro donne e un uomo) con diagnosi di ED. L'analisi conduce a tre tipologie di discorso che organizzano e danno senso alle transizioni dei soggetti considerati: un discorso di adattamento funzionale a eventi ed esperienze; uno che pone attenzione a eventi casuali e persone che entrano nella vita del soggetto; uno che pone l'iniziativa personale e un singolo agente al suo centro. Si chiariscono anche particolari modalità di comprendere la determinazione, la contemplazione e la pre-contemplazione. Queste concezioni relative al cambiamento sono state presentate al fine di ampliare il modo di pensare alla vita delle persone con ED e alle loro prospettive.

Depuis quelques dizaines d'années, les troubles du comportement alimentaire (ED) sont devenus l'un des problèmes principaux de santé mentale, en particulier chez les jeunes et les femmes. Cette étude a pour objectif d'analyser la pertinence du modèle trans-théorique du changement (TMC) de Prochaska & DiClemente's (1983) lorsqu'il est appliqué à l'expérience vécue des personnes diagnostiquées avec des ED ainsi que celle de ceux qui prennent soin d'eux. A cet effet, nous avons adopté une approche narrative biographique de la façon dont les gens font face à leurs problèmes et aux développements cruciaux dans le domaine des ED. A travers l'analyse narrative de ces autobiographies, notre objectif était d'étudier les notions que les patients ont eux-mêmes du 'changement', du 'problème' et de la 'trajectoire vitale'. Nous nous sommes concentrés sur cinq interviews autobiographiques de personnes diagnostiquées avec un ED (quatre femmes et un homme). L'analyse a donné trois discours qui organisent et donnent sens aux transitions vitales de nos participants : un discours d'adaptation fonctionnelle aux évènements et aux expériences ; un autre qui est attentif aux évènements dus au hasard et aux gens qui entrent dans votre vie ; et un dernier centré sur l'initiative et la capacité d'action des agents individuels. L'analyse met également en lumière les façons particulières de comprendre la détermination, la réflexion et la pré-réflexion. Nous montrons que ces façons de considérer le changement prolongent les façons déjà existantes de comprendre la vie des gens et les perspectives des patients.

Οι Διαταραχές στην πρόσληψη τροφής (ΔΠΤ) έχουν γίνει ένα από τα μεγαλύτερα προβλήματα ψυχικής υγείας τις τελευταίες δεκαετίες, ιδιαίτερα μεταξύ των νέων και των γυναικών. Η παρούσα μελέτη στοχεύει να αναλύσει την καταλληλότητα του Διαθεωρητικού Μοντέλου της Αλλαγής (TMC) των Prochaska & DiClemente (1983), όταν εφαρμόζεται στις εμπειρίες της ζωής των ανθρώπων που διαγιγνώσκονται με ΔΠΤ και των φροντιστών τους. Για το σκοπό αυτό, εφαρμόσαμε μια αφηγηματική βιογραφική προσέγγιση για να μελετήσουμε τους τρόπους με τους οποίους οι άνθρωποι αντιμετωπίζουν τα προβλήματα και την ανάπτυξη της ζωής τους στον τομέα των ΔΠΤ. Μέσα από την αφηγηματική ανάλυση αυτών των αυτοβιογραφιών, στόχος μας ήταν να μελετήσουμε τις αντιλήψεις των ίδιων των ασθενών για την «αλλαγή», το «πρόβλημα» και «την πορεία της ζωής». Επικεντρωθήκαμε σε πέντε αυτοβιογραφικές συνεντεύξεις με ανθρώπους που είχαν διάγνωση ΔΠΤ (τέσσερις γυναίκες και ένας άνδρας). Η ανάλυση ανέδειξε τρία συστήματα λόγου, που οργανώνουν και νοηματοδοτούν τις μεταβάσεις της ζωής των συμμετεχόντων μας: το λόγο της λειτουργικής προσαρμογής σε γεγονότα και εμπειρίες, το λόγο που εστιάζει σε τυχαία γεγονότα και τους ανθρώπους που εισέρχονται ζωή και αυτόν που ενέχει στη βάση του την προσωπική πρωτοβουλία και κυριότητα του ατόμου. Επιπλέον, η ανάλυση αναδεικνύει ιδιαίτερους τρόπους κατανόησης των σταδίων του προσδιορισμού, του προ-συλλογισμού και του συλλογισμού. Αυτοί οι τρόποι κατανόησης της αλλαγής φαίνεται να επεκτείνουν τους πιθανούς τρόπους προσέγγισης της ζωής των ανθρώπων και των οπτικών των ασθενών με ΔΠΤ.

The Transtheoretical Model of Change

The Transtheoretical Model of Change (TMC) emerged through the 1980s (Prochaska, 1979; Prochaska & DiClemente, 1983) in the field of psychological assistance to persons engaged in 'problematic' behaviours. It classifies patients into those who do not perceive their behaviour as a problem (pre-contemplation stage according to the model); those who are conscious of having a problem, but would do nothing to solve it (contemplation phase); those who are fully conscious of having a problem and looking for some kind of solution (preparation phase); those taking specific action to change (action phase); and those who have abandoned the problematic behaviour and are keeping the changes attained (maintenance phase).

The TMC was first applied to smoking behaviour (Prochaska, Velicer, DiClemente, & Fava, 1988; Schorr et al., 2008), then to addictions (Prochaska, Diclemente, & Norcross, 1992) and later to other health domains including eating disorders (EDs) (Dunn, Neighbors, & Larimer, 2003; Hasler, Delsignore, Milos, Buddeberg, & Schnyder, 2004; Sullivan & Terris, 2001).

The model is not just explanatory, but also clinically oriented. Attempts have been made to assess so-called change processes. The ultimate aim is to identify the stage of change (SOC) a person or group of persons is in, and to provide clinical recommendations accordingly (Prochaska et al., 1988; Rosen, 2000; Whitelaw, Baldwin, Bunton, & Flynn, 2000).

One of the most cited attempts to find clinical applications for Prochaska and Diclemente's model has been the creation of what is called the motivational interview, which would integrate Prochaska and Diclemente's categories with notions inherited from humanism, namely, the relevance of centering intervention in the person and her process of change. The general aim of the interview is to reduce the latency in active participation in intervention, while the therapist assumes a passive role and becomes a companion who avoids confrontation with the suffering person (Martins & McNeil, 2009; Miller & Rollnick, 2002).

Some problems with the TMC

Interest in the TMC has produced an important amount of research with the aims, among others, of assessing, quantifying and predicting intervention success (Rodríguez-Cano, Beato-Fernández, & Segura Escobar, 2006). This research has been mainly quantitative. Some authors pose certain methodological and ethical problems (Littell & Girvin, 2002; Piper & Brown, 1998). Methodological problems include the difficulty to establish the ecological validity of the model; validity of claims relating the 'problem' behaviour to other negative behaviours (e.g. does smoking necessarily come with other damaging health behaviours?); and the validity of processes and SOCs. With respect to ethical problems, some authors consider that the model may be used coercively against persons in a pre-contemplation stage. In this sense, other authors argue for the use of qualitative methodology to give voice to those affected (Whitelaw et al., 2000).

Littell and Girvin (2002) reviewed 87 studies evaluating the validity of the model. They concluded that 'The assumption that there are common SOCs across a range of situations, problem behaviors, and populations is not borne out by empirical data'; 'Nor is there consistent or convincing evidence of discrete SOCs in relation to specific problem behaviors'; and 'To our knowledge, there are no published studies of progression through the entire stage sequence' (p. 252).

In most studies based on Prochaska and Diclemente's model, SOCs are assessed through an algorithm based on yes/no responses to questions about current behaviour, future intention and (sometimes) former attempts to change; or through scales composed of items referring to the assessment of various stages (Prochaska, Redding, & Evers, 1997). In Díaz, Solano Pinto, and Solbes (2013), we review some of these instruments, highlighting some features of the construct which lead to a methodological and conceptual critique.

In the first place, even though SOCs are theoretically independent of the existence of institutional treatment, some formulations in the instruments suggest an equivalence between 'changing to better' and formal psychological intervention, thus identifying 'change' with 'receiving psychological treatment'. This ambiguity affects content validity and relates to a crucial matter concerning 'pre-contemplation' as a construct that might be assessed through self-reports.

Of course, that is not the model's conception of pre-contemplation. In order to find somebody in a state of pre-contemplation, there must be a problem in their behaviour *according to another person*, while the person claimed to be in trouble does not appreciate the problem.

Another obvious limitation of the instruments is diffuse reference to 'problems'. The ambiguity persists in scales adapted to make reference to a domain of problems, such as ED (see Treasure & Schmidt, 2001). The problem is eating too much or too little? Eating what, or when? Being despised for being fat? We can suspect that problem-definitions by participants will not always equate with those conceived by the scale designers or its administrators. In fact, those who have applied the model to ED have been facing a problematic inherent to these disorders: what professionals consider 'symptoms', patients may consider sources of satisfaction or personal realization (Serpell, Treasure, Teasdale, & Sullivan, 1999; Vitousek, Watson, & Wilson, 1998).

But our purpose here is not to test or refute the construct validity of Prochaska and DiClemente's model. We understand that its relevance does not emerge from its technical or scientific validity, but from the extension and normalization it has reached in the domain of psychological intervention. We concur here with Davidson's (1992, p. 822) suggestion that just as people can take 'apparently illogical but comfortable decisions' about problematic behaviour, professionals can accept Prochaska and DiClemente's SOCs because they allow us to 'grasp at the heuristics and partial truths which make us feel most comfortable'.

The ambivalence concerning the question 'Who defines problems?' emerges from the double origin of the model. If SOCs emerge from the humanistic clinic, they are defined through a process of personal reflection guided by a therapist. If they emerge from the worries of health agencies to attend problems they know but their sufferers do not always admit, then they should be defined by health agencies. The contradiction is manifest in a double bond common in contemporary psychological care: 'I will support you with your problem; but I will tell you what the problem is'.

Analysing biographies of persons diagnosed with ED

Our discussion so far points to an irremediable tension between two incompatible ways of considering how people change in life: mapping this 'how' onto a classification designed from the institutional definitions of healthy behaviour; or describing it according to the perspective of the person involved, which may require abandoning the project of consolidating a construct to embrace the goal of providing suitable resources to support their specific processes of change.

On the other hand, it seems misguided to invest in the refinement of multiple-choice instruments addressed at assessing important vital questions full of subjective nuance in specific contexts, to aid a process of psychotherapeutic intervention which works precisely by talking about all that nuisance, near those contexts, with the person affected (Sullivan & Terris, 2001).

These reflections suggest the need to develop qualitative procedures to illuminate biographic change with relation to problems from the perspectives of sufferers. Rather than 'proposing a new model' or discussing the claims of the models at hand, the task would consist of attending to the experience of sufferers as they describe and narrate them, and taking it from there. Various authors have focused on EDs from narrative and biographic stances, using qualitative approaches to show how these methods contribute to a deeper understanding of problems and recovery processes. Chan and Ma (2003) analysed the experience of a Chinese anorexic patient through her life history. Three topics emerged in her justifications of control: saving, reserving food and losing weight. Dawson, Rhodes, and Touyz (2014) studied the recovery processes of eight women with chronic anorexia and emphasized the importance of aspects such as hope, motivation, self-efficacy and support from others in this complex process. Weaver, Martin-McDonald, and Spiers (2012) analysed personal documents written by an adolescent with anorexia, her mother and her therapist. They found that mother and daughter shared similar strategies to deal with anorexia and highlighted six emerging topics.

The thrust of this paper consists of an analysis of change processes in the autobiographies of five persons diagnosed with ED, four males and one female whose ages range from 16 to 47. This analysis is part of a wider study comprising 20 biographic interviews of 5 people diagnosed with ED and their corresponding main carers; and 5 people without diagnosis, with characteristics matched with participants in the clinical group, and their relevant relatives (analogous to the main carers for people in the clinical group). So the total sample is composed of a post-clinic sub-sample and a control sub-sample, and each sub-sample is comprised of five autobiographies and their corresponding biographies as told by another person closely related to them (whom we will call 'carers'). Clinical participants and their carers were recruited by the psychotherapist (second author). Non-clinical participants were selected intentionally. The post-clinic participants went through psychotherapy with the second author or another colleague, and were interviewed by their respective therapists. All participants provided written informed consent to participate in the study.

The interview was structured as a life history: The vital trajectory and biography of the interviewee (or the patient in the case of interviews with carers) were the basic organizing thread. We tried to structure the narration along markers such as places of residence, educational institutions, partnerships, family relations or workplaces. Apart from that only one question was common for all participants roughly formulated thus at the beginning of the interview: *Tell me the story of your life to date, the most important things that happened to you, the ones that made you the way you are, your process up to here.*

Once the narration started with this generic question, we guided the interview through open questions. The interviewer would rely on a flexible guide, written as a list of domains or topics linked to body image, inviting the participant to discuss them on occasion. The 20 interviews were audio recorded and transcribed.

Analysis: six biographical repertoires

The materials for this analysis are 10 biographical interviews: five autobiographical interviews with persons diagnosed with ED, and the corresponding five interviews where their carers told the diagnosed persons' lives in the third person. We first coded these interviews in Prochaska and DiClemente's SOC categories, or in a general 'biographic change' category. The coded text was then reviewed for ways of linking key events to key consequences, and rhetorical and narrative procedures articulated in the story plot. This analytical approach relies mainly on Potter and Wetherell's (1987) notion of interpretative repertoires, as discursive devices which are deployed by the speaker to make sense of events and account for them.

This coding procedure allows the contrasting of the applicability of the SOC categories with biography, letting other conceptions of change emerge through the process. Six categories emerged (*functional adaptation; chance and fate; personal agency and initiative; determination leads to action; prospective contemplation; pre-contemplation in retrospect/in the eye of another*) which recast Prochaska & Diclemente's conception of change and suggest different conceptions.

Three vernacular ways of understanding change

Functional adaptation

An emerging way of understanding change was what we call '*functional adaptation*', where the person changes as a reaction to former or ongoing events within a system. This includes short- or medium-term reactions to traumatic experience or to others' behaviour; changing through a learning process; coming to terms with experience; adjusting to social demands; using diet as a reaction to bodily shape; and problems emerging from the experience of suffering verbal abuse.

In the following extract, María makes reference to a couple of experiences in her childhood:

29 María: (…) So in that sad part of my life, on the one hand we have, body image is there because up to 10, I was a child, I got my first period, I developed, I developed before the rest, and what happens, well there comes the part where they abused me two or three times, where there's a part where it really hurt me, which is the one on the street, which I really think about it and I say 'they did touch me here and here', but in my mind, it was, 'maybe I got pregnant or whatever', I think that from then on I started to fatten and to cover everything uh, to cover all that.

30 Natalia: Were you 10, when-?

31 María: I think not, I think I was 11 or 12, but with a growing body, that you don't change coat, you stay with the same coat bursting it up, and that part improved, I told you, when I was with those friends in the Burger, I already told you, and each of them had suffered some abuse, they were four or three. Then I felt normal, and it was like … well, all that … or that weight disappeared, or it was like normal, I don't know how, that part, that part fell

In line 29, María is narrating a sequence whereby (1) she develops 'before the rest', (2) she gets abused two or three times and (3) she starts fattening and 'covering all that'. The sequence assumes that a girl who develops soon is more vulnerable to abuse; that abuse is especially harmful for a girl who does not understand its meaning; that fattening is linked to 'covering' the abuse experience. 'Covering', in particular, can be interpreted in two possible ways: fattening may be a way of avoiding the body image of a beautiful and desired woman, thus avoiding sexual attraction associated to abuse experiences and 'covering' her body; or 'covering' as avoiding the recalls of traumatic experience through loss of control over eating.

In line 31, she tells how in a meeting with friends, she disclosed former abuse experiences and other friends disclosed similar experiences. This helped her to feel 'normal', and meant releasing a 'weight'. Both short stories unfold as an adaptation process: Abuse leads to adaptive behaviour patterns to fatten and cover up; sharing the experience with friends helps to normalize it.

Chance and fate

A second way of understanding change in life draws attention to the random appearance of events or persons through life, highlighting the role of *chance and fate*. Especially, meeting persons who allow you to live special experiences, or professionals who turn out to be helpful; but also including persons you wish you had not met, and professionals who make things worse.

For example, María gives an account of how she moved out of her family house, to live with friends in Madrid. Once in Madrid, she presents her search for rooms to share as a game like playing lottery; she finds two very interesting roommates just by chance; she presents them as valuable people casually entering into her life.

Personal agency and initiative

A third biographical repertoire is based on the narrating self as a reflexive, conscious and stable agent who takes decisions through time with her own *personal agency and initiative*. This is possibly the subject preferred by the TMC, or even the subject the TMC takes as both pre-condition and objective of therapy: A rational, coherent and strategic subject searching for balance, with a personal programme based on constancy. Some of the narrative threads relying on this repertoire tell how the accumulation of suffering leads to taking personal decisions, or how the subject transforms her perspective on the world.

A good part of Ana's autobiography has to do with a problematic boyfriend whom she took a long time to get rid of. The following extract gives some indication of the relevance of a strong autonomous self through the management of this process:

157 Ana:	((laughing:)) but the more you try,	
158 Natalia:	That's very good	
159 Ana:	((laughing:)) The more you try, I think at the end you- you get it don't you? . And that time, (...) when I called my parents, 'Come over here I'm packing my things and leaving'. And when (.)	

> David finally came 'No don't leave me This can't be like this .
> Fuck no We have to find the solution Ana' . And so I let myself
> go for one more year. But it got to a point where (.) I was starting
> to see (.) at home that (.) that I was not going out not going out.
> And also that the quarrels we had were (.) more and more frequent
> . Before maybe (.) we had a big one every fortnight but then now
> it was every other day every other day . I had to make such efforts
> (.) to stay with his (family) on top of that it was a very- ((coughs))
> very closed family like- . We had to do everything together, every
> weekend I would come here to eat with them, . ((coughs)) (…)

The idea of trying over and over until you achieve an aim involves a constant reflexive subject. This fragment shows a vivid description of the moment when Ana's determination to leave her boyfriend turns into action (even if the decision and action taken are not the kind of problems the TMC draws our attention to). As a whole, the process of change is constructed as an alternation between experiencing a problematic relation and autonomously reflecting about it.

Typically, the paradigmatic movement *from determination to action* promoted in the TMC appears in our biographies invested with this kind of agentive discourse. So when patients speak about their initiative to search for psychological help, from family or professionals, and how it is triggered, it appears as the outcome of a personal emotional reflection process or internal dialogue. This often includes self-attributions of responsibility or at least agency in the development of the problem, and admitting having a problem as such.

In the following extract, Gema describes the crucial moment in which she decided to disclose her 'bulimia' to her parents, thereby starting her search for professional help:

114 Gema: My grandfather had to be disconnected from a machine which I didn't understand why it had to be disconnected. I mean like I don't know. I think it was many things together and I had a bad time and then I generated even more. I was already very bad well again I generated a lot of anxiety, vomiting, lots of laxatives, it was all like (3)[1] very brutal

115 (2)

116 Gema: and then I got scared. I got so scared, I got scared because I could see that I felt like kicking the bucket. I mean saying. I can't stand it anymore, this bitch is killing me so then I sat with my parents and nothing I told them 'dad, mum (2) I have bulimia and I need your help'. I think at that point my parents must have thought, 'what a funny girl, ha, ha, ha' ((ironic tone)) but I knew it, I knew it because among other things, I was studying at college and also I investigated if I was (2) a possible, well if I had that problem. You know? So nothing, they called my uncle and I started to go to hospital

The sequence starts with a description that suggests functional adaptation to a difficult emotional situation: the emotional tension associated with her grandfather's terminal illness leads to increasing purging behaviours and suicidal thoughts which alarm Gema herself. Fear of suicide leads to a resolution to share the problem with her parents, who call her uncle (to take advantage of his contacts in hospital).

The description also illustrates how Gema uses her knowledge from her psychology studies and investigates her condition, which involves a concerned and thoughtful agent. She attributes scepticism or puzzlement to her parents in the moment of hearing her disclosure. This suggests she feels alone or not understood in front of the people who will be helping her. Such feelings are common in the moment of disclosing mental suffering in general and EDs in particular, and are definitely an element that adds difficulty to the decision to disclose.

A closer view on contemplation and pre-contemplation

Contemplation, as understood in the TMC, i.e. a reflection about a problem being there without determination or disposition to do something about it, did not appear in our participants' stories. What we did find were comments about the prospective possibility of problems appearing at any time in the future. These reflections have to be understood taking into account that the interviews are held after completion of a therapeutic process in persons who acknowledge their diagnosis. They also show a recurrent conviction that the ED is chronic, persistent and never leaves you once it catches you. *'Prospective contemplation'* includes the consideration of possible future risky situations; current problems with social relations, body image or vital change as symptoms of illness; and doubts and contradictions concerning body image at present.

In our review of Prochaska and DiClemente's model above, we have proposed that *'pre-contemplation'* is a problematic concept, since, as opposed to the other SOC categories, it does not describe a state of mind or activity in the person but emphasizes the inexistence of cognitive activity which 'should be there', simply reflecting a contradiction between the perspective of the patient and that of the clinical institution. In our data, we did find two forms of existence for pre-contemplation as the localization of a failure in a person to notice a problem which, from a different perspective, could be there.

One possibility is *in retrospect*. In the following extract, Vero, the mother of Luis, gives an account of not reacting appropriately to her son's problems in the past:

9 Vero:		So, for us, it was hard, for example, to see his eating problem. For that I mean it was seen, (.) but it was hard for us to see it
10 Isabel:		mhmh,
11 Vero:		because he was in his own world, (.) and now, . I mean one day he can talk to you about thousands of things, and another day he can say 'Hello good morning good (afternoon), goodbye'. (…)

Vero is presenting Luis as an introverted character. In line 11, she provides some evidence for this, describing him as somebody 'in his own world', who does not always talk about his issues. This description serves to support the conclusion that it was difficult for Luis' parents to spot the 'eating problem'.

Another possibility is for *somebody else* to see the problem in the affected person, while the affected person ignores it. In the following extract, Natalia and María (speaking here as mother of Tania and about Tania's life) remember jointly the moment in which Natalia had to show that there was a serious problem that needed María's attention:

165 Natalia: But how do you conjugate that in your head, . Right? Uh those emotions like-

166 (1)

167 María: Well suffering from- It's my fault it's my fault it's my fault, . And then a lot of it, and that you know as well because you used to say it, that we couldn't see it

168 Natalia: mhmh

169 María: And you even had to say to us 'But she is ill and this and that' and I remember one of the times you said to me 'We won't get out of here without you' and I stayed, . 'Well what do I have to do then' So- I would often forget it . I really lived it in a different way. Now I can see it clearer every time . Cause when she was in the middle of the mess then playing with-

170 Natalia: But surely the mess was- was going out of hand. Wasn't it? Because she was ill

171 María: Yes you would say 'How is she getting on' . 'Very good' . (...)

Natalia and María recall the contrast between María not seeing her daughter's problem and Natalia (Tania's therapist) seeing it and calling her attention to it. They describe an epic moment in which Natalia appealed to María's collaboration, and María reacted adequately. In line 169, we can read a strong contrast between the past confusing moment in the midst of the trouble, and present clarity.

Discussion

Our aim in this paper has been to show the utility of oral biography to examine personal stages of change in the terms and narrative structures used by the subjects of change themselves. We described three implicit discourses which organize and give sense to their vital transitions: a discourse of functional adaptation to events and experiences; one that pays attention to random events and people entering your life; and one that has the personal initiative and agency of an individual agent at its core. These ways of understanding change are not incompatible with those promoted in Prochaska and DiClemente's model, but they extend the possible ways of thinking about people's lives.

With respect to the TMC, we showed how an 'individual agency' repertoire can be the template on which the transition from determination to action is constructed. Contemplation appears blended with a notion of the ED as a chronic, irremediable dependency. And we brought out aspects of how pre-contemplation is experienced as a recollection (while reviewing your own past after a process of intervention) or as a mutual warning (when a third person points out a problem).

At the same time, we have stressed the necessity to respect vernacular definitions of change objectives. Prochaska and DiClemente's model systematically takes for granted that the only issue requiring change in a person is defined by their clinical diagnosis. In the ED domain, the problem would be eating behaviour and the purpose of change would consist of restoring it to a healthy pattern.

But when we listen to the lives of the persons diagnosed, we learn about other issues which demand legitimate attention, such as gaining autonomy from the family, overcoming problematic relationships or changing body shape through diet. To understand processes of change, we need to attend to these issues without judging them, being the issues that structure the lives and concerns of the patients.

Through the last decade, autobiographies of women with EDs have been a common resource to elaborate personal experience, to help other sufferers confront the problem or to furnish and dignify its complexities before the general public (e.g. Bowman, 2007; Saukko, 2008). Autobiography gives us the chance to learn about a highly theorized issue from the terms and meaning structures provided by its main characters. Qualitative analysis takes distance from the technical sophistication of open-ended questionnaires and from the diffuse aesthetics of literature, giving us the chance to understand this experience with rigour, in its human contexts and close to its vernacular categories.

A deeper knowledge of ED, grounded in patients' perspectives and worldviews, requires more accurate assessment methods, where understanding emerges from the discursive environments which engender the relevant discourse (typically, verbal interaction environments). This should facilitate the adaptation of prevention and intervention strategies to the worldview of patients, and the improvement of professional training, to keep it in line with patients' concerns.

Acknowledgements

We are grateful to the nine participants who contributed their time and intimacy to this study, and to Isabel Quiñones, who interviewed two of them. This study is part of the project *Discourses of body image in population with and without an Eating Disorder Diagnosis,* partially funded by a research grant from the University of Castilla-La Mancha through 2010.

Disclosure statement

No potential conflict of interest was reported by the authors.

Funding

This work was supported by the University of Castilla-La Mancha.

Note

1. In the excerpts, numbers between brackets indicate pauses in seconds.

References

Bowman, G. (2007). *Thin: A memoir of anorexia and recovery*. London: Penguin.

Chan, Z., & Ma, J. (2003). Anorexic body: A qualitative study. *Forum Qualitative Sozialforschung/Forum: Qualitative Social Research, 4*, Art. 1. Retrieved from http://www.qualitative-research.net/index.php/fqs/article/view/758/1644

Davidson, R. (1992). Prochaska and DiClemente's model of change: A case study? *Addiction, 87*, 821–822.

Dawson, L., Rhodes, P., & Touyz, S. (2014). "Doing the impossible": The process of recovery from chronic anorexia nervosa. *Qualitative Health Research, 24*, 494–505. doi:10.1177/1049732314524029

Díaz, F., Solano Pinto, N., & Solbes, I. (2013). Autobiografía y anorexia: Una alternativa cualitativa al modelo de estados del cambio de Prochaska y DiClemente [Autobiography and anorexia: A qualitative alternative to Prochaska and DiClemente's states of change model]. *FQS, 14*, Art. 13.

Dunn, E. C., Neighbors, C., & Larimer, M. (2003). Assessing readiness to change binge eating and compensatory behaviors. *Eating Behaviors, 4*, 305–314.

Hasler, G., Delsignore, A., Milos, G., Buddeberg, C., & Schnyder, U. (2004). Application of Prochaska's transtheoretical model of change to patients with eating disorders. *Journal of Psychosomatic Research, 57*, 67–72.

Littell, J. H., & Girvin, H. (2002). Stages of change: A critique. *Behavior Modification, 26*, 223–273.

Martins, R. K., & McNeil, D. W. (2009). Review of motivational interviewing in promoting health behaviors. *Clinical Psychology Review, 29*, 283–293.

Miller, W. R., & Rollnick, S. (2002). *Motivational interviewing: Preparing people for change* (2nd ed.). New York, NY: Guilford.

Piper, S., & Brown, P.A. (1998). Psychology as a theoretical foundation for health education in nursing: Empowerment or social control? *Nurse Education Today, 18*, 637–641.

Potter, J., & Wetherell, M. (1987). *Discourse and social psychology*. London: Sage.

Prochaska, J. O. (1979). *Systems of psychotherapy: A transtheoretical analysis*. Homewood, IL: Dorsey Press.

Prochaska, J. O., & DiClemente, C. C. (1983). Stages and processes of self-change of smoking: Toward an integrative model of change. *Journal of Consulting and Clinical Psychology, 51*, 390–395.

Prochaska, J. O., DiClemente, C. C., & Norcross, J. C. (1992). In search of how people change. *Applications to addictive behaviors. American Psychologist, 47*, 1102–1114.

Prochaska, J. O., Redding, C., & Evers, K. (1997). The transtheoretical model and stages of change. In K. Glanz, B. K. Rimer, & K. Viswanath (Eds.), *Health behavior and health education, theory, research and practice* (pp. 97–121). San Fransisco, CA: Jossey Bass.

Prochaska, J. O., Velicer, W. F., DiClemente, C. C., & Fava, J. (1988). Measuring processes of change: Applications to the cessation of smoking. *Journal of Consulting and Clinical Psychology, 56*, 520–528.

Rodríguez-Cano, T., Beato-Fernández, L., & Segura Escobar, E. (2006). Influencia de la motivación en la evolución clínica de los trastornos del comportamiento alimentario [Influence of motivation on the clinical evolution of eating disorders]. *Actas Españolas de Psiquiatría, 34*, 245–250.

Rosen, C. S. (2000). Is the sequencing of change processes by stage consistent across health problems? A meta-analysis. *Health Psychology, 19*, 539–604.

Saukko, P. (2008). *The anorexic self: A personal, political analysis of a diagnostic discourse*. Albany, NY: State University of New York (SUNY) Press.

Schorr, G., Ulbricht, S., Schmidt, C. O., Baumeister, S. E., Rüge, J., Schumann, A., … Meyer, C. (2008). Does precontemplation represent a homogeneous stage category? A latent class analysis on German smokers. *Journal of Consulting and Clinical Psychology, 76*, 840–851.

Serpell, L., Treasure, J., Teasdale, J., & Sullivan, V. (1999). Anorexia nervosa: Friend or foe? *International Journal of Eating Disorders, 25*, 177–186.

Sullivan, V., & Terris, C. (2001). Contemplating the stages of change measures for eating disorders. *European Eating Disorders Review, 9*, 287–291.

Treasure, J., & Schmidt, U. (2001). Ready, willing and able to change: Motivational aspects of the assessment and treatment of eating disorders. *European Eating Disorders Review, 9*, 4–18.

Vitousek, K., Watson, S., & Wilson, G. T. (1998). Enhancing motivation for change in treatment resistant eating disorders. *Clinical Psychology Review, 18*, 391–420.

Weaver, K., Martin-McDonald, K., & Spiers, J. (2012). Mirroring voices of mother, daughter and therapist in anorexia nervosa. *Forum Qualitative Sozialforschung/ Forum: Qualitative Social Research*, 13, Art. 6. Retrieved from http://nbn-resolving.de/urn:nbn:de:0114-fqs120363

Whitelaw, S., Baldwin, S., Bunton, R., & Flynn, D. (2000). The status of evidence and outcomes in stages of change research. *Health Education Research, 15*, 707–718.

Exploring the meaning in meaningful coincidences: An interpretative phenomenological analysis of synchronicity in therapy

Elizabeth C. Roxburgh, Sophie Ridgway and Chris A. Roe

Synchronicity experiences (SEs) are defined as psychologically meaningful connections between inner events (e.g. thought, dream or vision) and one or more external events occurring simultaneously or at a future point in time. There has been limited systematic research that has investigated the phenomenology of SEs in therapy. This study aimed to redress this by exploring the process and nature of such experiences from the perspective of the practitioner. Semi-structured face-to-face interviews were conducted with a purposive sample of nine practitioners who reported SEs in their therapeutic sessions (three counsellors, three psychologists and three psychotherapists), and focused on how participants make sense of their experiences of synchronicity in therapy. Interpretative phenomenological analysis was used to identify three superordinate themes: sense of connectedness, therapeutic process, and professional issues. Findings suggest that SEs can serve to strengthen the therapeutic relationship and are perceived as useful harbingers of information about the therapeutic process, as well as being a means of overcoming communication difficulties, as they are seen to provide insights into the client's experiencing of themselves and others, regardless of whether or not the SE is acknowledged by the client or disclosed by the therapist.

Synchronizitätserfahrungen (SEs) sind definiert als psychologisch-expressive Verbindungen zwischen körperlichen Ereignissen (z.B. Gedanken, Träume, Visionen) und einem oder mehreren externen Ereignissen, die entweder gleichzeitig oder zu einem bestimmten Zeitpunkt in der Zukunft stattfinden. Zu SEs im Rahmen der Psychotherapie wurde bislang nur bedingt systematisch geforscht. Die vorliegende Studie wollte dem Abhilfe

Data from this research was presented at the 18th Annual British Association for Counselling and Psychotherapy (BACP) Research Conference in 2012 and at the 5th Qualitative Research and Mental Health Conference in 2014.

schaffen, indem sie den Prozess und das Wesen solcher Erfahrungen aus der Sicht des Praktikers untersuchte. Hierfür wurden insgesamt neun teilstrukturierte Interviews mit verschiedenen Fachkräften erhoben (drei Berater, drei Psychologen und drei Psychotherapeuten), die SEs in ihren Sitzungen dokumentierten und darauf abstellten, wie sich Klienten diese Erfahrungen der Synchronizität erklären. Die interpretativ-phänomenologische Analyse (IPA; Smith, Flowers & Larkin, 2009) wurde hierfür herangezogen und es konnten drei übergeordnete Themenbereiche ausgemacht werden: Das Gefühl der Verbundenheit, der therapeutische Prozess und fachspezifische Themen. Die Ergebnisse weisen darauf hin, dass SEs eine stärkere therapeutische Beziehung fördern können und als nützliche Vorläufer von Informationen über den therapeutischen Prozess fungieren und darüber hinaus Kommunikationsprobleme überwinden helfen, da sie Einblicke in die Erfahrungswelt des Klienten über sich selbst und andere bietet - und das alles ungeachtet der Tatsache, ob die SE vom Klienten bekräftigt oder vom Therapeuten offen gelegt wird.

Las experiencias de sincronicidad (ES) se definen como conexiones significativas entre eventos internos (pensamientos, sueños, visiones) y uno o más eventos externos los cuales ocurren simultáneamente o en el futuro. Las investigaciones fenomenológicas sistemáticas de ESs en psicoterapia han sido pocas. Este estudio trata de corregir ésto explorando el proceso y la naturaleza de tales experiencias desde la perspectiva del terapeuta. Se condujeron entrevistas semi-estructuradas cara a cara con una muestra de nueve terapeutas quienes informaron acerca de ESs en sus sesiones (tres orientadores psicológicos, tres psicólogos y tres psicoterapeutas) enfocándose en cómo los participantes le dan sentido a estas experiencias. El análisis interpretativo fenomenológico (IPA; Smith, Flowers and Larkin, 2009) se utilizó para identificar tres temas, uno dentro de otro: sentido de estar en contacto, proceso terapéutico y aspectos profesionales. Los resultados sugieren que las ESs pueden servir para reforzar las relaciones terapéuticas y son percibidas como heraldos de útil información acerca del proceso terapéutico, así como también un medio para superar las dificultades en comunicación ya que son vistas como poseedoras de insight en cómo los clientes se perciben a ellos mismos y a otros, sin tomar en cuenta si la ES es reconocida por el cliente o puesta al descubierto por el terapeuta.

Esperienze di Sincronicità (SEs) sono definite come connessioni psicologicamente significative tra gli eventi interni (ad esempio pensieri, sogni o visioni) e uno o più eventi esterni che si verificano nello stesso tempo o in un momento futuro. Scarse sono le ricerche sistematiche che hanno indagato la fenomenologia delle SEs in terapia. Il presente studio si pone l'obiettivo di porre rimedio a questa lacuna, esplorando il processo e la natura di tali esperienze dal punto di vista del professionista. Sono state condotte Interviste semi-strutturate dirette (faccia a faccia) su un campione mirato di nove professionisti che hanno sperimentato SEs nelle loro sedute terapeutiche (tre counsellors, tre psicologi e tre psicoterapeuti), le interviste sono focalizzate sulle modalità con cui viene attribuito significato alle esperienze di sincronicità nella terapia. È stata utilizzata l'Analisi Interpretativa Fenomenologica (IPA, Smith, Flowers, & Larkin, 2009) per identificare tre temi sovraordinati: senso di connessione, processo terapeutico e questioni professionali. I risultati suggeriscono che le SEs possono servire a rafforzare la relazione terapeutica e sono percepite come mezzo di informazioni utili sul processo terapeutico, oltre ad essere uno strumento che consente di superare alcune difficoltà di comunicazione, in quanto possono suggerire intuizioni circa l'esperienza del cliente relativa a se stesso o agli altri, indipendentemente dal fatto che la SE sia riconosciuta dal cliente o spiegata dal terapeuta.

Les expériences de synchronisme (SE) se définissent comme étant des connexions significatives entre des évènements internes (pensées, rêves ou visions) et un ou plusieurs évènements externes qui surviennent de manière simultanée ou dans le futur. La recherche systématique de la phénoménologie des SEs en psychothérapie est limitée. Cette étude a pour objectif de remédier à cette lacune en explorant le processus et la nature de telles expériences du point de vue du praticien. Des entretiens semi-directifs de recherche ont été menés avec un échantillon ciblé de neuf praticiens qui font état de leur expérience de SEs au cours de leurs séances (trois counsellors, trois psychologues et trois psychothérapeutes). Ces entretiens étaient centrés sur le sens que les participants attribuent à leurs expériences de synchronisme en thérapie. La méthode IPA (analyse phénoménologique interprétative, Smith, Flowers, & Larkin, 2009) a été utilisée et a permis d'identifier trois thèmes principaux : sentiment de connectivité, processus thérapeutique et problèmes professionnels. Les résultats suggèrent que les SEs peuvent servir à renforcer la relation thérapeutique et sont perçues comme signes avant-coureurs d'informations utiles quant au processus thérapeutique. Elles sont également un moyen de surmonter les difficultés de communication en tant qu'elles sont conçues comme fournissant un aperçu de l'expérience que les clients ont d'eux-mêmes et des autres, et ceci que les SEs soient ou non reconnues par le client et/ou dévoilées par le thérapeute.

Οι εμπειρίες συγχρονικότητας (ΕΣ) ορίζονται ως συνδέσεις, που έχουν κάποιο ψυχολογικό νόημα, μεταξύ εσωτερικών γεγονότων (π.χ., σκέψη, όνειρο ή όραμα) και ενός ή περισσότερων εξωτερικών γεγονότων που συμβαίνουν ταυτόχρονα ή σε κάποια μελλοντική χρονική στιγμή. Η συστηματική έρευνα που έχει ερευνήσει τη φαινομενολογία των ΕΣ στη θεραπεία είναι περιορισμένη. Για το λόγο αυτό, η παρούσα μελέτη είχε ως στόχο τη διερεύνηση της διεργασίας και της φύσης αυτών των εμπειριών από τη σκοπιά του επαγγελματία. Πραγματοποιήθηκαν ημι-δομημένες συνεντεύξεις με ένα επιλεγμένο δείγμα εννέα επαγγελματιών που ανέφεραν ότι είχαν ΕΣ στις θεραπευτικές συνεδρίες τους (τρεις σύμβουλοι, τρεις ψυχολόγοι και τρεις ψυχοθεραπευτές), επικεντρώθηκαν στο πώς οι συμμετέχοντες κατανοούν την εμπειρία τους της συγχρονικότητας στη θεραπεία. Χρησιμοποιήθηκε ερμηνευτική φαινομενολογική ανάλυση (Smith, Flowers, & Larkin, 2009) και προσδιορίστηκαν τρία κυρίαρχα θέματα: το αίσθημα σύνδεσης, η θεραπευτική διεργασία και επαγγελματικά ζητήματα. Τα ευρήματα δείχνουν ότι οι εμπειρίες της συγχρονικότητας μπορεί να χρησιμεύσουν στην ενίσχυση της θεραπευτικής σχέσης και γίνονται αντιληπτές ως χρήσιμοι προάγγελοι πληροφοριών σχετικά με τη θεραπευτική διεργασία. Επιπλέον αποτελούν μέσο για να ξεπεραστούν τυχόν δυσκολίες στην επικοινωνία καθώς προσφέρουν στοιχεία σχετικά με τον τρόπο που ο πελάτης βιώνει τον εαυτό του και τους άλλους, ανεξάρτητα από το αν η εμπειρία συγχρονικότητας (SE) αναγνωρίζεται από τον πελάτη ή αποκαλύπτεται από το θεραπευτή.

In this study, we were interested to explore whether synchronicity experiences (SEs) that occur or are reported during therapy sessions might be perceived as having some beneficial function in the practitioner–client therapeutic interaction. The classic definition of synchronicity describes it as a psychologically meaningful connection between an inner event (e.g. thought or dream) and one or more external events occurring simultaneously (Jung, 1952/1973). Jung also proposed a broader definition in which SEs could involve a coincidence between an inner event and an outer event occurring at either a distant place or a future point in time, which is similar to parapsychological experiences, such as clairvoyance (gaining information by 'seeing' objects or events beyond what it is possible with normal vision) and precognition (predicting events that later come true). Main (2007a) has also noted that SEs can occur between two or more inner events (e.g. two people reporting the same dream on the same night which has some sort of shared meaning between them) or two or more external events (e.g. a person finding several copies of a rare book in the same day which has particular relevance to them).

In the therapeutic setting, Hopcke (2009) distinguishes between 'in-session' synchronicity, 'in which what is happening within the psychotherapeutic session itself is interrupted or punctuated by an event that ends up being synchronistic' (p. 292), and 'out-of-session' synchronicity where external events are brought into the therapeutic setting. The most notable example of the therapeutic setting becoming part of the synchronistic event is the Scarab beetle incident (cf. Jung, 1952/1973).[1] In terms of out-of-session events, much of the literature has focused on understanding precognition in clients' dreams, which has often been interpreted as synchronistic phenomena in the form of a coincidence between an internal event (dream) and an external event occurring at a future point in time (where the dream is described as 'coming true' and is represented in an actual event). For example, clients have accurately described their therapist before meeting them for the first time from details in a dream they have had (Targ, Schlitz, & Irwin, 2000), and different clients have reported similar dreams (Ehrenwald, 1948) or have had dreams about the life experiences of the therapist that are later verified as correct (Peerbolte, 2003; Ullman, Krippner, & Vaughan, 2002). There have also been instances where the therapist has apparently acquired previously unknown information about the client in dreams (Ehrenwald, 1948; Orloff, 1996).

There is a growing body of literature that has either used survey methods to investigate the range and incidence of SEs (Bressan, 2002; Coleman, Beitman, & Celebi, 2009; Costin, Dzara, & Resch, 2011; Henry, 1993), or has explored the personality factors associated with coincidence-proneness (Coleman & Beitman, 2009; Meyer, 1989; Pasciuti, 2011). However, very few empirical studies have included therapist samples. In a survey study conducted by the authors (Roxburgh & Ridgway, 2012) to explore the incidence of SEs, we found 44% ($N = 100$) of the total sample ($N = 226$) had experienced synchronicity in the therapeutic setting. More specifically, 55 psychotherapists, 24 psychologists, and 21 counsellors said they had experienced synchronicity, suggesting that acknowledgement and reporting of SEs is not necessarily attributable to therapeutic orientation or training. In addition, 67% of the total sample felt that SEs could be useful experiences in therapy, and 31% felt they might be useful. This supports research which has proposed that SEs can be associated with personal growth (Nachman, 2009) and which emphasises their clinical value (Main, 2007b).

Marlo and Kline (1998) propose that SEs can facilitate the therapeutic process and may be more likely in the therapeutic setting given the openness to unconscious communication, the salience of the therapeutic relationship, and the development of symbolic thought. The emotional intensity of the therapeutic setting has been proposed as accounting for SEs, in particular when there is high transference (Beitman & Shaw, 2009; Hopcke, 2009), high dependency needs (de Carvalho, 1996), when patients are withdrawn and need to maintain a sense of connectedness with the therapist (Ullman, 2003) or when a critical turning point has been reached in therapy (Hopcke, 2009).

Despite an awareness of the factors that might be conducive to SEs and the reporting of such instances indicating an openness to SEs in the therapeutic setting and to their utility in providing material to encourage personal growth, there has been little systematic work to explore the phenomenology of SEs. Therefore, in this study, we were interested to explore the process and nature of these experiences from the perspective of the practitioner. An essential means of achieving these aims is to adopt a qualitative approach, that of interpretative phenomenological analysis (IPA), since this approach 'is committed to understanding how particular experiential phenomena (an event, process or relationship) have been understood from the perspective of particular people, in a particular context' (Smith, Flowers, & Larkin, 2009, p. 29).

Method

Design

IPA is a dual-facet approach: the phenomenological facet refers to the study of phenomena as they are perceived (their nature and meaning) regardless of whether what is experienced is objectively real; the interpretative facet acknowledges that things have visible *and* hidden meaning so maintains that access to phenomenology is best achieved through interpretation. As such, the researcher plays a key role in creating an understanding of participants' experiences and existing knowledge and experience is drawn upon to help make sense out of data. IPA is an ideographic approach which attempts to capture the quality and texture of *individual* experience, but it is also interested in convergences and divergences (what is the experience like for this person in relation to another person?). This qualitative approach was deemed to be the most suitable for our aims since we were interested in how practitioners make sense of their lived experience of synchronicity and the meaning they assign to these experiences in the context of the therapeutic setting. We were not concerned with establishing the role of language in the construction of reality or the development of a theory about SEs as might be the case with other qualitative approaches we could have selected from. No significant ethical issues in the research were encountered and the study was approved by the authors' University Research Ethics Committee.

Participants

Participants were purposively recruited to present a homogeneous sample of 'therapists' who reported that they had experienced synchronicity in the therapeutic setting. Participants had all taken part in a previous survey about the range and incidence of SEs in the therapeutic setting (Roxburgh & Ridgway, 2012) and expressed an interest in taking part in the interview study. Smith (2004, p. 42) has argued that 'it is only possible to do a detailed nuanced analysis associated with IPA on a small sample. Many studies have samples of 5–10'. Therefore, the sample consisted of three counsellors registered with the British Association for Counselling and Psychotherapy (BACP), three psychologists registered with The British Psychological Society (BPS), and three psychotherapists registered with the UK Council for Psychotherapy (UKCP). Five of the participants were female and four were male, ages ranged between 39 and 64 years, and length of time practising ranged between 5 and 22 years (see Table 1).

Data collection

Semi-structured face-to-face interviews were conducted by the second author. Participants were given the opportunity to view a copy of the schedule in advance of the interview. The interview schedule followed a 'funnelling' format, as outlined in Smith and Eatough (2006), whereby the first broad question asked participants to discuss their experiences of synchronicity and to

Table 1. Participant details.

Pseudonym	Gender	Therapist	Organisation	Duration of interview (mins)
Holly	Female	Psychotherapist	UKCP	60
Peter	Male	Psychotherapist	UKCP	70
Diana	Female	Psychotherapist	UKCP	47
Ruth	Female	Counsellor	BACP	51
Mark	Male	Counsellor	BACP	63
Kay	Female	Counsellor	BACP	80
Rose	Female	Clinical Psychologist	BPS	137
Walter	Male	Counselling Psychologist	BPS	108
Jack	Male	Clinical Psychologist	BPS	67

describe their most memorable experience(s). Further questions explored how therapists make sense of SEs (i.e. what do they mean to them, how do they identify a SE, what is the process and nature of SEs, how they thought SEs impacted on clients, and how are SEs understood?). Interviews took place in either the participant's home or place of work. The main aim during the interviews was to engage in a collaborative dialogue with participants so that they felt comfortable talking freely about their experiences. Therefore, some time was spent before the interviews in general conversation in an attempt to build a good level of rapport. After the interview participants were also given the opportunity to ask any further questions about the study.

Data analysis

The flexible guidelines to IPA analysis (e.g. Smith et al., 2009) were followed. Each interview was transcribed verbatim and participants' identities were protected by changing any potential identifying information within the transcript. The first step of the analytical process involved the authors immersing themselves in the data, reading the first transcript several times, in order to identify any interesting ideas and emerging themes. Initial themes from the first participant were then listed on a separate piece of paper, examined for connections, and organized into clusters. The next step involved reading the remaining transcripts to look for new emerging themes and to identify 'both convergence and divergence, commonality and nuance' (p. 79). A master table of superordinate themes and corresponding subthemes was then constructed (see Table 2).

Findings

Three superordinate themes, which all have consecutive subthemes, emerged from analysis of the data and reflect how participants made sense of the SEs they experienced whilst in therapeutic sessions with clients (see Table 2).

Theme 1: sense of connectedness

This superordinate theme reflects how SEs were seen as an expression of, or realisation of, an underlying sense of deeper interconnection. Participants

Table 2. Master table of superordinate themes and subthemes.

Superordinate themes	Subthemes
Sense of connectedness	• 'Moment of meeting' • 'Living the symbolic life'
Therapeutic process	• 'Communication catalysts' • 'It just cut through an awful lot of valleys' • 'It unites us in some way'
Professional issues	• Impact on the therapist • Disclosure decisions

discussed feeling a greater sense of connection to their clients and felt that the SE is connected to the client's presenting issues.

Moment of meeting

All of the participants except one described their SEs as being very profound moments whose meanings were instantly understood and shared, and so required no deeper discussion. There was something in the sharing of the experience that connected the client and therapist and brought them closer together:

> I felt this inner deep resonance of some, something's happened which is really profound and meaningful, and I felt a sense of the connection with my client (...) and that was an 'I-Thou' moment (...) That moment where we looked at each other and we saw each other and we saw that something very deep had happened, I saw him and he saw me. (Peter)[2]

Peter's client had been discussing, and trying to process, a painful bereavement when a picture in the therapy room fell off the wall. The picture was of members of Peter's family who had died in a concentration camp. On an emotional level, Peter describes the SE as an embodied one that was really felt at the core of his being. He was also aware on a cognitive level that the experience was very profound, and that something very meaningful and significant had occurred. All this seemed to happen in the flicker of a moment without anything being expressed verbally. The experience was a very moving one for Peter and it helped him to trust the work they were doing. He was also aware that something had shifted for the client who was very pleased that they hadn't talked about it too much or tried to analyse the event, rather they accepted something very deep had happened and trusted that without 'trying to dry it out and make it into some kind of intellectual concept'.

Similarly, Diana confirms the deep sense of connection that participants felt with their clients after experiencing synchronicity. She also expresses the heightened emotional context that was present and how difficult it was to put the experience into words. In her extract below it is almost as if the experience would be explained away or lose some of its meaning if it were put down on paper, instead the permanent record lives on in the intensity of the experience:

> I mean the connection, the unspoken connection happens at the most meaningful times and both the client and I would be in ... would have tears in our eyes and it's lovely and very powerful. You can't write it in a discharge summary letter very easily but it's a real feeling that we have connected at a level beyond words that will be permanent and memorable for both of us. (Diana)

Likewise, Walter stresses that words can sometimes get in the way of the relational depth that is felt when participants share a SE with their clients: 'We were connecting there at quite a deep level, I think, where words are often unnecessary, and sometimes just a bloody nuisance!'

Living the symbolic life

This theme reflects the connection between the inner world of the therapist and the outer world of the client in relation to what the client communicates or experiences. Synchronicity comes about through precognitive dreams, metaphors, imagery, or intuitive illuminations that are of relevance to the clients' issues:

> What I often find with things that pop into my mind or feelings I have in my body or memories that come up for me, or things that catch my eye is that, fifteen, twenty, thirty minutes later, the client makes some explicit reference to the same thing; happens over and over and over again. (Walter)

Diana spoke about a magpie (which is both 'black' and 'white') tapping on the window when discussing difference and identity issues with a mixed race client, which is reminiscent of Jung's Scarab beetle case in that the symbol appears in the form of a living thing that has some metaphorical meaning for the client. All of the six participants that mentioned synchronicity in symbolic form said that the imagery would just spontaneously emerge in consciousness without knowing where the imagery came from. For example, one participant mentioned seeing the image of an old Victorian house with a green door and Christmas wreath. She mentioned this to her client as the imagery was so insistent and the description exactly matched a memory of the client visiting their Grandparents' house which was significant in terms of her childhood experiences and the focus of the therapeutic session. Interestingly, experiencing synchronicity in symbolic form was not restricted to therapists with psychoanalytical training suggesting it is not simply a function of that training. Sometimes the imagery would not make sense to participants and they were hesitant to share it with their clients for fear that it wasn't relevant or wouldn't make any sense. However, most of the time the clients could relate to the symbolism and found it matched their experience of an issue:

> Sometimes the images are really out there, sometimes they don't seem to have much to do with the content and the client will say 'that's exactly right' ... They just pop up ... they appear, and they're really strong and powerful and worthwhile. (Kay)

Most participants described SEs occurring in symbolic form when they were attuned to the client or when they liked the client, but others also mentioned symbols to be prominent features of synchronicity at times of stress or transitional periods:

> I think that in terms of my having noticed meaningful coincidence in the past it's tended to happen at times when I've been more stressed or there's been a lot of change going on, my dream life's been very active as well at these times ... there's a pressure to get over something or for me to recognise something consciously, and that comes through in experiences in which I can see metaphors or a symbolism. (Jack)

Theme 2: therapeutic process

This superordinate theme represents how SEs served to draw attention to aspects or features of the therapeutic process that were valuable foci for reflection as well as functioning as reinforcers that the therapy was worthwhile or on the right track.

Communication catalysts

Most participants felt that SEs revealed salient issues that were crucial to the therapeutic process without the client having to use words to share particular aspects of themselves or communicate their distress with the therapist. Diana interpreted this as the unconscious becoming conscious:

> Maybe it's when the unconscious becomes conscious for both people at the same time and that's brought about by this intrusion from the outside world that something that has ... Something gets put into consciousness without having to be spoken. (Diana)

Participants talked about SEs being more likely to take place when there is difficulty in communicating; where there is resistance, or the person can't put something into words, or the recipient isn't willing or able to hear what's being said. Jack felt that synchronicity was more likely to be encountered in the therapeutic setting given the focus on communication and feelings of being connected or disconnected from one's self, others, or the world:

> It's all about communication and connection. I think given that that's the core feature of therapeutic interaction that it makes sense that that (synchronicity) would happen at a time when communication is disrupted or impossible in other ways ... they can and often do serve as triggers or sort of catalysts or facilitators of communication and understanding. (Jack)

Participants felt that SEs had the potential to maintain or re-establish connection and were opportunities to gain information about clients that turned out to be useful for the therapeutic process, as Walter stated: 'Often something comes up that's, you know, not in the manual, not in the textbook, and it proves to be rich and significant, opens a door, clarifies something, spurs somebody on'.

It just cut through an awful lot of valleys

All participants felt that SEs facilitated growth, pushed through resistance, or provided a turning point in the therapeutic process:

> It encapsulates a lot of things without having to find the words for them. So it can condense something. It can do far more than a whole raft of therapy sessions. It speeds things up in a way. (Diana)

Diana provided an example of synchronicity involving humour that facilitated a shift in a client who had become stuck. She mentioned being in a group therapy setting with a client who seemed to be taking a backwards step when suddenly a refuse lorry drove by outside, went into reverse, and announced on loud speaker 'Attention, this vehicle is reversing'. Diana continued to say that the whole group found the experience amusing and realised that the moment matched the juncture the client had reached in therapy. She felt that the SE provided an opportunity for something to be expressed in a safe way:

> The bin lorry was safer than me saying it, but it said what I would've liked to say, but it might have been more hostile coming from me, but because it was out there it was the comic timing of it that that made it so wonderful and I suppose it reminded me that people in that stuck place do respond well to a humour and a little gentle teasing. That can free something up and it came in from outside and helped me and still goes on helping because I remember the bin lorry when I'm working with (clients who are) stuck. (Diana)

Similarly, Jack felt that SEs could serve to push through defence mechanisms and could be a real turning point in the therapeutic process: 'It made a huge difference in terms of rapport and breaking through this resistance that had been apparent prior to that stage, and she went on to work extremely constructively and very openly'. Rose used exaggerated figures of speech, such as '3 million times' and 'massive revelation' to emphasise quite how much one SE impacted on the therapeutic process:

> What she gave us was this really juicy coincidence that meant we could run with it. So I had a therapeutic plan, but she gave us the much better, I mean 20 million times better therapeutic plan. She got us to where I wanted us to go but 3 million times more quickly (...) For her it was a massive revelation if you like, it kind of shifted her worldview slightly. It certainly shifted her view of me a lot and it shifted her view of herself a lot so she could work completely differently and more productively.

It unites us in some way

All participants, except one, commented on how SEs increased the therapeutic relationship and had showed them the way *to be with* their clients. They reflected on how the shared experience served to break down some of the barriers to intimacy and deconstructed some of the power imbalances that can sometimes be felt in the therapeutic process:

> I think an open discussion of experiences like that (synchronicity), particularly when they're shared, can have the effect of deconstructing some of the power imbalance between a therapist and client (...) The main change was that there was a very rapid increase in levels of rapport and that it felt as though things were much more comfortable, she was much more open with me from that point onwards, much more trusting in the process than she had been before. (Jack)

This subtheme also relates to the previous subtheme, 'It just cut through an awful lot of valleys', whereby participants felt a turning point in the therapeutic process had been reached as a result of the SEs, in that they also felt a turning point in the therapeutic relationship. In addition, they consistently mentioned attaining a 'deeper level' of relational depth when there has been the shared experience of synchronicity, which relates to the subtheme, 'Moment of meeting':

> I think that if there are those synchronous moments, they strengthen the bond ... and there's plenty of clients I've had ... still have, where there is not that synchronous moment, and the relationship continues ... but it doesn't maybe deepen in the same way. So it doesn't reach a deeper level. I'd say it's about engaging on a deeper level maybe when those moments happen. (Ruth)

Moreover, the sense of connection that participants felt with their clients after SEs is reflected in the development of the therapeutic alliance and the 'joining together' or 'attachment' of two individuals to make a strong bond:

> It was almost like it joined us together in a way to make sense of this strange event, it was like she became attached to me through it. So, erm, as a process it was a really important moment because from that moment on we could begin to work. She had got what I would describe as a therapeutic attachment with me. (Holly)

Theme 3: professional issues

This super-ordinate theme represents the implications SEs have for the therapist, for training, and for the supervisory process.

Impact on the therapist

All participants, except one, mentioned that SEs had a profound impact on them both personally and professionally. In making sense of their experiences, participants went through stages of initial shock, leading to a search for a conceptual model to explain the experience as it had challenged their concept of reality, and then reformulation of the experience; often accepting that there wasn't an explanation they were happy to adopt but feeling comfortable with the uncertainty that came with that, and feeling curiosity and excitement about experiencing synchronicity again. Often, the experience was shared with an understanding supervisor who helped to process the experience. This is best exemplified by Kay who uses hyperbole to accentuate the intensity of the SE, and to emphasise her astonishment:

> It was a massive shock, it was really, really, it was a huge shock (...) and I thought I'd jumped, I mean I literally thought I'd jumped because it was just such a surprise, but so many of the circumstances, the circumstances of their lives, were very, very similar to mine as well. That wasn't the only thing, there were just lots and lots of little things, and of course, once I'd noticed that, I started looking, I suppose I noticed them more. But what happened as a result, I mean on that session I kind of readjusted myself and the session continued, but I felt sort of curious afterwards, and I was a bit worried about it and talked to my supervisor.

Kay also mentioned that she had heard of such things happening and had been scared of them happening to her but that when one did occur 'it wasn't a terrible experience at all, it was a wonderful experience (participant laughs) ... it's made me un-scared. It's un-scared me!' Participants also felt that the experience was confirmation of their work and helped them to develop in ways that standard knowledge could not provide:

> So each time they happen it confirms something quite different that I've experienced before so it's adding to my repertoire of understanding and you can't get that understanding from reading a book and going to church. (Diana)

Disclosure decisions

Another subtheme that emerged, for all participants, was the dilemma of whether or not to disclose the SE to clients. Decisions to disclose varied amongst participants and depended on factors such as the personality and openness of clients, the therapeutic relationship, whether it would risk focusing the client on the therapist rather than themselves, clinical judgement, intuition, and in cases where synchronicity involved symbolism, how persistent the imagery was. Diana relied on her own inner feelings when deciding whether to disclose:

> I think if you are looking for them and start contriving things then that would be unhelpful, but the actual times when it's really synchronicity and it just feels right to use it, you just know it's the right thing to do and it always feels very rewarding. The other person's found it helpful as well and I've not found a negative experience from them myself. (Diana)

Participants agreed that even if they didn't feel it was appropriate to disclose the experience it could still be used for the benefit of the client:

> I can still notice it and use it for information to me about what's happening in the process, but I may not talk about it with the client, I may not open it with the client over concerns of his or her fragility. (Peter)

Discussion

Findings are comparable to previous research which proposes that synchronicity can have a positive outcome on the therapeutic process (Hopcke, 2009; Keutzer, 1984; Main, 2007a; Marlo & Kline, 1998; Nachman, 2009). Participants reflected upon how SEs resulted in a greater sense of connection between clients and therapists and provided valuable opportunities for working at relational depth (Mearns & Cooper, 2005). Hogenson (2009) refers to synchronistic encounters as 'moments of meeting', after research conducted by the Boston Process of Change Study Group (Stern et al., 1998). Stern et al. focused on the delicate process of negotiation between caregiver and infant and refer to moments of meetings as special moments of authentic person-to-person connection:

The key concept, the 'moment of meeting', is the emergent property of the 'moving along' process that alters the intersubjective environment, and thus the implicit relational knowing. In brief, moving along is comprised of a string of 'present moments', which are the subjective units marking the slight shifts in direction while proceeding forward. At times, a present moment becomes 'hot' affectively, and full of portent for the therapeutic process. These moments are called 'now moments'. When a now moment is seized, i.e. responded to with an authentic, specific, personal response from each partner, it becomes a 'moment of meeting'. (p. 6)

This resonates with Clarkson's (1995) *person-to-person relationship*, which concerns the authentic humanness shared by client and therapist as characterised by the here-and-now encounter between two people and the recognition that each is changed by the other. Participants also drew attention to the ineffable and numinous quality of synchronicity, which is comparable to Clarkson's *transpersonal relationship* as reflected in the spiritual, mysterious or currently inexplicable dimension of the healing relationship. Findings suggest that therapists may tap into this relationship when experiencing a shared silence or an intuitive illumination that culminates from synchronistic moments.

SEs often involved symbolism, persistent imagery, sensations, and metaphors that emerged into participants' awareness and that resembled the feelings or experiences of the client. In terms of the therapist, this has similarities with what Rogers (1986) described as *presence* when he stated:

I am perhaps in a slightly altered state of consciousness, indwelling in the client's world, completely in tune with that world. My nonconscious intellect takes over. I [nonconsciously] know much more than my conscious mind is aware of. I do not form my responses consciously, they simply arise in me, from my nonconscious sensing of the world of the other. (p. 206)

Moreover, it also relates to the concept of *co-presence*. This has been described by Cooper (2005, p. 17) as 'moments in which the client's presence to the therapist's presence, or the therapist's flow in response to the client's flow, creates a synergistic encounter that may not be reducible to the sum of its individual parts'. When synchronicity occurred, perhaps as a consequence of co-presence when both client and therapist were fully present with each other, and was recognised as such by both client and therapist, implicitly or explicitly, it had the effect of deepening the therapeutic relationship as it gave both the therapist and the client an opportunity to be experienced as authentic.

Participants also pointed out that synchronicity was likely to occur when communication was difficult for clients and that the experience could tap into the unconscious or express what was in conscious awareness but was difficult to speak. They felt that SEs had the potential to break through resistance and unite the client and therapist so that healing could take place. This relates to theories that propose synchronicity helps clients to feel more connected to their therapist (Ullman, 1949, 2003) and occurs at transitional periods in therapy (Hopcke, 2009). In terms of implications for practice we are reminded of expressive arts therapy in that some clients are more comfortable working with imagery, objects or symbolism to express inner states in outer form. It also supports Jung's proposal to assimilate SEs into consciousness, through explication and amplification, so that transformation and individuation can take place (Marlo & Kline, 1998).

Stern et al. (1998, p. 8) also state that when a *now moment* is entered they are 'unfamiliar, unexpected in their exact form and timing, unsettling or weird'. This has parallels with the surprise that was sometimes felt by participants in the current study when they experienced synchronicity in the therapeutic setting. In making sense of SEs, participants seemed to search for a conceptual model of understanding and went through stages of shock, reformulation, acceptance, curiosity and excitement. There was also the issue of disclosure in terms of deciding whether or not to discuss the SE if the client hadn't seemed to be aware of it or hadn't initiated discussion, the general consensus being that information could still be gleaned from the experience of use to the therapeutic process without necessarily having to disclose one's thoughts and impressions. Although some participants accepted the SEs as being something they could not explain, for others it was important to find an explanation. However, they also spoke about finding resolution by living with the uncertainty that accompanied the experience and by tolerating the 'unknown of the unknown' (Cayne & Loewenthal, 2007, p. 373).

In this study we did not attempt to engage with the ontology of SEs. However, as part of a larger research project on SEs, we also conducted a survey study to investigate explanations for SEs in the therapeutic setting. That study found differences between types of practitioners in terms of how they account for SEs but no differences in perception of when synchronicity events were likely to occur in the therapeutic setting (Roxburgh & Ridgway, 2012). Interested readers might also like to review the multiple perspectives that have been put forward for SEs (see, e.g. Storm, 2008).

Conclusion

Findings suggest that SEs can serve to strengthen the therapeutic relationship as participants felt a greater sense of connection to clients. Participants also perceived SEs as useful harbingers of information about the therapeutic process, as well as being a means of overcoming communication difficulties, as they are seen to provide insights into the client's experiencing of themselves and others, regardless of whether or not the SE is acknowledged by the client or disclosed by the therapist. Given that some participants were shocked by the SEs we feel that findings have important implications for the training and supervision of therapists in terms of acknowledging that such experiences are perceived to occur as a natural part of the therapeutic process. Further research is currently being conducted by the first author to explore whether therapists believe there is a need for specialist training to address such experiences. A limitation of this study is that we focused on practitioners' perspectives of SEs in the therapeutic setting and it would be interesting in future research to investigate the phenomenology of SEs from the perspective of clients. Additional areas for exploration include: Are some therapists more intuitive, relaxed, and open to SEs? Are some clients more likely to elicit SEs in their therapists? Does the experience of having one's own personal therapy enable a therapist to tune into SEs more?

Acknowledgement

We acknowledge a reviewer of this paper who made these thoughtful suggestions for further research. We would like to thank the participants who took part in this study and the Bial Foundation for financially supporting the project (grant number 82/10).

Disclosure statement

No potential conflict of interest was reported by the authors.

Funding

This work was supported by the Bial Foundation [grant number 82/10].

Notes

1. Jung recounts a therapeutic session in which a client who was resistant to change describes a dream (internal event) about a golden scarab beetle at the exact moment he heard a tapping on the window (external event), only to find that it was a beetle closely resembling the scarab. Jung considered this event as one in which an archetype was activated, seeing the scarab as an Egyptian symbol of rebirth, and discussed the coincidence with the client, which helped to bring about transformation.
2. Transcription notes: ellipses in the participants' quotes means there was a pause and round brackets with ellipses (…) indicates that text has been removed due to space.

References

Beitman, B. D., & Shaw, A. (2009). Synchroners, high emotion, and coincidence inter-pretation. *Psychiatric Annals, 39*, 280–286.

Bressan, P. (2002). The connection between random sequences, everyday coincidences, and belief in the paranormal. *Applied Cognitive Psychology, 16*, 17–34.

Cayne, J., & Loewenthal, D. (2007). The unknown in learning to be a psychotherapist. *European Journal of Psychotherapy and Counselling, 9*, 373–387.

Clarkson, P. (1995). *The therapeutic relationship*. London: Whurr Publishers.

Coleman, S. L., & Beitman, B. D. (2009). Characterizing high-frequency coincidence detectors. *Psychiatric Annals, 39*, 271–279.

Coleman, S. L., Beitman, B. D., & Celebi, E. (2009). Weird coincidences commonly occur. *Psychiatric Annals, 39*, 265–270.

Cooper, M. (2005). Therapists' experiences of relational depth: A qualitative interview study. *Counselling and Psychotherapy Research, 5*, 87–95.

Costin, G., Dzara, K., & Resch, D. (2011). Synchronicity: Coincidence detection and meaningful life events. *Psychiatric Annals, 41*, 572–575.

de Carvalho, A. P. (1996). Transference and possible spontaneous psi phenomena in psychotherapy. *Journal of the Society for Psychical Research, 61*, 18–25.

Ehrenwald, J. (1948). *Telepathy and medical psychology*. New York, NY: W. W. Norton.

Henry, J. (1993). Coincidence experience survey. *Journal of the Society for Psychical Research, 59*, 97–108.

Hogenson, G. B. (2009). Synchronicity and moments of meeting. *Journal of Analytical Psychology, 54*, 183–197.

Hopcke, R. H. (2009). Synchronicity and psychotherapy: Jung's concept and its use in clinical work. *Psychiatric Annals, 39*, 287–293.

Jung, C. (1952/1973). *Synchronicity: An acausal connecting principle*. Princeton, NJ: Princeton University Press.

Keutzer, C. S. (1984). Synchronicity in psychotherapy. *Journal of Analytical Psychology, 29*, 373–381.

Main, R. (2007a). *Revelations of chance: Synchronicity as spiritual experience*. Albany, NY: The State University of New York Press.

Main, R. (2007b). Synchronicity and analysis: Jung and after. *European Journal of Psychotherapy and Counselling, 9*, 359–371

Marlo, H., & Kline, J. S. (1998). Synchronicity and psychotherapy: Unconscious communication in the psychotherapeutic relationship. *Psychotherapy: Theory, Research, Practice, Training, 35*, 13–22.

Mearns, D., & Cooper, M. (2005). *Working at relational depth in counselling and psychotherapy*. London: Sage.

Meyer, M. B. (1989). *Role of personality and cognitive variables in the reporting of experienced-meaningful coincidences or "synchronicity"* (Unpublished doctoral thesis). Saybrook Institute, San Francisco, CA.

Nachman, G. (2009). Clinical implications of synchronicity and related phenomena. *Psychiatric Annals, 39*, 297–308.

Orloff, J. (1996). *Second sight*. New York, NY: Warner Books.

Pasciuti, F. (2011). Measurement of synchronicity in a clinical context. *Psychiatric Annals, 41*, 590–597.

Peerbolte, M. L. (2003). Parapsychology and psychoanalysis. In N. Totton (Ed.), *Psychoanalysis and the paranormal* (pp. 47–72). London: Karnac.

Rogers, C. R. (1986). Client-centred therapy. In I. L. Kutash & A. Wold (Eds.), *Psychotherapists' casebook: Theory, and technique in the practice of modern therapies* (pp. 197–208). San Francisco, CA: Jossey-Bass.

Roxburgh, E. C., & Ridgway, S. (2012, March 28–31). *An investigation into the prevalence and phenomenology of synchronicity experiences in the clinical setting*. Poster presented at The Bial Foundation 9th Symposium 'Behind and Beyond the Brain', Porto, Portugal.

Smith, J. A. (2004). Reflecting on the development of interpretative phenomenological analysis and its contribution to qualitative research in psychology. *Qualitative Research in Psychology, 1*, 39–54.

Smith, J. A., & Eatough, V. (2006). Interpretative phenomenological analysis. In G. M. Breakwell, S. Hammond, C. Fife-Schaw, & J. A. Smith (Eds.), *Research methods in psychology* (3rd ed., pp. 322–341). London: Sage.

Smith, J. A., Flowers, P., & Larkin, M. (2009). *Interpretative phenomenological analysis*. London: Sage.

Stern, D. N., Sander, L. W., Nahum, J. P., Harrison, A. M., Lyons-Ruth, K., Morgan, A. C., ... Tronick, E. Z. (1998). Non-interpretive mechanisms in psychoanalytic therapy: The 'something more' than interpretation. *The International Journal of Psychoanalysis, 79*, 903–921.

Storm, L. (Ed.). (2008). *Multiple perspectives on meaningful coincidences*. Pari: Pari Publishing.

Targ, E., Schlitz, M., & Irwin, H. J. (2000). Psi-related experiences. In E. Cardeña, S. J. Lynn, & S. Krippner (Eds.), *Varieties of anomalous experience: Examining the scientific evidence* (pp. 219–252). Washington, DC: American Psychological Association.

Ullman, M. (1949). On the nature of psi processes. *Journal of Parapsychology, 13*, 59–62.

Ullman, M. (2003). Dream telepathy: Experimental and clinical findings. In N. Totton (Ed.), *Psychoanalysis and the paranormal* (pp. 15–46). London: Karnac.

Ullman, M., Krippner, S., & Vaughan, A. (2002). *Dream telepathy*. New York, NY: Macmillan.

Mirroring patients – or not. A study of general practitioners and psychiatrists and their interactions with patients with depression

Annette Sofie Davidsen and Christina Fogtmann Fosgerau

For mentalization theorists, implicit mentalization is a key component of all forms of therapy. However, it has been difficult to grasp and to describe precisely how implicit mentalization works. It is said to take place partly by mirroring others in posture, facial expression and vocal tone. Based on studies of imitative behaviour within linguistics and psychology, we argue that interactional mirroring is an important aspect of displaying implicit mentalization. We aimed to explore if, and in that case how, mirroring is displayed by general practitioners (GPs) and psychiatrists in consultations with patients with depression. We wanted to see how implicit mentalizing unfolds in physician–patient interactions. Consultations were video-recorded and analysed within the framework of conversation analysis. GPs and psychiatrists differed substantially in their propensity to mirror body movements and verbal and acoustic features of speech. GPs mirrored their patients more than psychiatrists in all modalities and were more flexible in their interactional behaviour. Psychiatrists seemed more static, regardless of the emotionality displayed by patients. Implicitly mirroring and attuning to patients could signify enactment of implicit mentalization, according to how it is described by mentalization theorists. We discuss reasons for the differences between GPs and psychiatrists, and their implications.

Für Mentalisierungstheoretiker ist implizite Mentalisierung das zentrale Element jeglicher Art der Therapie. Dennoch ist es bislang schwierig gewesen, die Funktionsweise impliziter Mentalisierung begreiflich zu machen und sie detailliert zu beschreiben. Es heißt, dass es zum Teil durch das Spiegeln der Haltung des Gegenübers, dessen Gesichtsausdruck sowie dessen Klang der Stimme geschehen soll. Auf Grundlage von linguistischen und psychologischen Studien zu imitativem Verhalten gehen wir davon aus, dass interaktionales Spiegeln ein wichtiger Aspekt für die Darstellung implizierter Mentalisierung ist. Wir wollten in Erfahrung bringen, ob und in diesem Fall wie sich innerhalb des Beratungssettings zwischen Allgemeinmedizinern (AM) oder Psychiatern und Depressionserkrankten das Spiegeln darstellt und so, über den Weg der Arzt-Patienten Beziehung, verstehen, wie sich implizite Mentalisierung äußert. Die Treffen wurden per Videoaufzeichnung festgehalten und über eine Konversationsanalyse ausgewertet. AMs und Psychiater unterschieden sich dabei erheblich in ihrer Neigung, Körperbewegungen sowie verbale und akustische Merkmale der Sprache zu spiegeln. AMs spiegelten ihre Patienten in jeglicher Hinsicht mehr als die Psychiater und sie waren wesentlich flexibler in ihrem Beziehungsverhalten. Psychiater erschienen, ungeachtet der vom Patienten jeweils geäußerten Emotionen, eher statisch. Implizites Spiegeln sowie das sich einstellen auf den Patienten induzieren womöglich implizites mentalisieren - ganz im Sinne der Mentalisierungstheoretiker. Darüber hinaus werden die Gründe für die Unterschiede zwischen AMs und Psychiatern sowie die sich daraus ergebenden Konsequenzen diskutiert.

Para los teóricos de la mentalización, mentalización implícita es un componente clave en toda forma de terapia. Sin embargo, ha sido difícil captar y describir en forma precisa cómo ésta trabaja. Se dice que ocurre en parte al reflejar a otros en posturas, expresiones faciales y tono vocal. Basándonos en estudios de conducta imitativa en lingüística y psicología, argumentamos que la reflexión interaccional es un aspecto importante en mostrar mentalización implícita. Nuestro objetivo es explorar si y cómo los médicos generalistas y los psiquiatras emplean esta técnica con pacientes deprimidos, para ver cómo la misma se despliega en estas interacciones. Se grabaron consultas y se analizaron dentro del marco de trabajo de análisis de la conversación. Hay una diferencia sustancial entre los médicos generalistas y los psiquiatras en su propensión a reflejar los movimientos del cuerpo y las características acústicas del habla. Es mayor en los m médicos generalistas en todas las modalidades y fueron más flexibles en su conducta interaccional. Los psiquiatras fueron más estáticos, sin tomar en cuenta la emocionalidad que sus pacientes mostraron. Adaptarse a los pacientes y reflejar sus emociones podría significar aprobación de la mentalización implícita, de acuerdo como los teóricos la han descrito. Exponemos sus 'pros' y las implicaciones de las diferencias entre médicos generalistas y psiquiatras.

Per i teorici della mentalizzazione, la mentalizzazione implicita è un componente chiave in tutte le forme di terapia. Tuttavia, è difficile individuare e descrivere con precisione come la mentalizzazione implicita funzioni. Si è detto che, in parte, essa ha luogo nel rispecchiare l'altro nella postura, nell'espressione del viso, nel tono vocale. Sulla base di studi relativi al comportamento imitativo entro la linguistica e la psicologia, si afferma che il rispecchiamento interazionale è un elemento importante nel dare evidenza alla mentalizzazione implicita. Il nostro obiettivo è comprendere se, e in tal caso come, il rispecchiamento è presentato da medici generici (GPs) e da psiquiatri nelle consultazioni con i pazienti depressi, così da osservare come la mentalizzazione implicita si dipana nelle interazioni medico-paziente. Le consultazioni sono state video registrate e analizzate entro il modello dell'analisi della conversazione. GPs e psichiatri differiscono sostanzialmente nella loro propensione a rispecchiare i movimenti del corpo e le caratteristiche verbali e acustiche del discorso. I GPs rispecchiano i loro pazienti più di quanto facciano gli psichiatri in tutte le modalità e risultano più flessibili nel loro comportamento interazionale. Gli psichiatri sembrano più statici, indipendentemente dalla emotività mostrata dai loro pazienti.

Selon les théoriciens de la mentalisation, la mentalisation implicite est une composante-clé de toutes les formes de thérapie. Il a cependant été difficile, jusqu'à présent, d'appréhender et de décrire précisément la façon dont la mentalisation implicite opère. On dit qu'elle se manifeste en partie dans la réponse en miroir donnée aux autres (posture, expression faciale et ton de la voix). Nous fondant sur des études des comportements imitatifs dans le champ de la linguistique et de la psychologie, nous avançons ici l'argument que le comportement interactionnel en miroir est un des aspects de la manifestation de la mentalisation implicite. Nous souhaitions savoir si (et si c'est le cas, comment) les médecins généralistes (GPs) et les psychiatres expriment des comportements en miroir lors de consultations avec des patients dépressifs afin de voir comment la mentalisation implicite se déroule dans ces interactions physicien-patient. Les consultations ont été filmées et analysées selon la méthode de l'analyse conversationnelle. Les GPs et les psychiatres se différencient de manière substantielle dans leur propension à adopter une attitude en miroir envers les mouvements du corps et les figures de style verbales. Les GPs répondent davantage en miroir que les psychiatres pour toutes les modalités et se montrent plus flexibles dans leurs comportements interactionnels. Les psychiatres apparaissent plus statiques quel que soit le type d'émotions exprimé par les patients. Le comportement en miroir implicite et l'adaptation aux patients pourraient signifier la mise en acte d'une mentalisation implicite, selon les théoriciens de la mentalisation. Nous débattons dans cet article des raisons des différences entre GPs et psychiatres et des implications de ces différences.

Για τους θεωρητικούς της ψυχικοποίησης (mentalization), η άδηλη ψυχικοποίηση αποτελεί βασικό συστατικό όλων των μορφών θεραπείας. Είναι, όμως, δύσκολο να κατανοηθεί και να περιγραφεί πώς ακριβώς λειτουργεί η άδηλη ψυχικοποίηση. Έχει υποστηριχθεί ότι λαμβάνει χώρα εν μέρει μέσω της κατοπτρικής αντανάκλασης των άλλων μέσα από τη στάση του σώματος, την έκφραση του προσώπου, και τον τόνο της φωνής. Με βάση τις μελέτες της μιμητικής συμπεριφοράς στη γλωσσολογία και στην ψυχολογία, υποστηρίζουμε ότι η διαδραστική αντανάκλαση είναι ένας βασικός τρόπος μέσα από τον οποίο παρουσιάζεται η άδηλη ψυχικοποίηση. Στόχος μας ήταν να διερευνήσουμε εάν και πώς εμφανίζεται η αντανάκλαση στην κλινική πρακτική των γενικών ιατρών και των ψυχιάτρων με ασθενείς με κατάθλιψη, για να δούμε πώς η άδηλη ψυχικοποίηση εκτυλίσσεται σε αυτές τις αλληλεπιδράσεις γιατρού-ασθενή. Βιντεοσκοπήθηκαν συνεδρίες και αναλύθηκαν με τη χρήση της ανάλυσης συνομιλίας. Οι γενικοί ιατροί και οι ψυχίατροι διέφεραν σημαντικά στην τάση τους να αντανακλούν τις κινήσεις του σώματος όπως και τα λεκτικά και ακουστικά χαρακτηριστικά του λόγου. Φαίνεται ότι οι γενικοί ιατροί αντανακλούν τους ασθενείς περισσότερο από τους ψυχιάτρους σε όλα τα επίπεδα αλληλεπίδρασης και ήταν πιο ευέλικτοι στην αλληλεπιδραστική συμπεριφορά τους. Οι ψυχίατροι φαίνονταν περισσότερο στατικοί, ανεξάρτητα από το συναίσθημα που εξέφραζαν οι ασθενείς τους. Η έμμεση αντανάκλαση και η εναρμόνιση με τους ασθενείς θα μπορούσε να αποτελεί εκδραμάτιση της άδηλης ψυχικοποίησης, σύμφωνα με τον τρόπο που περιγράφεται από τους θεωρητικούς της ψυχικοποίησης. Συζητάμε τους λόγους και τις επιπτώσεις που προκύπτουν από τις διαφορές μεταξύ του των γενικών ιατρών και των ψυχιάτρων.

Introduction

Understanding of another person is established through the perception of the person's body and mind as an intertwined unity. Merleau-Ponty emphasized the influence of the body in the process of understanding each other. Linguistic communication draws upon a primordial bodily understanding, and it is through language that 'our perspectives slip into each other, we coexist in a single world.' (Merleau-Ponty, 2012, p. 370).

Other phenomenologists have noted the importance of empathy in intersubjective understanding. Empathy is thought of as a special irreducible intentionality which makes it possible to experience another person's emotions, beliefs, and desires, more or less directly, and it also involves embodiment (Husserl, 1983; Rudebeck, 2001; Zahavi, 2010). In psychotherapy, empathy is considered an important factor for outcome irrespective of the therapist's theoretical persuasion. Empathic therapists do not simply reflect on the content of the patients' words, but they also attend to what is not said and what is at the periphery of awareness (Norcross, 2010). In the main, empathy has included the affective components of understanding (Bohart, Elliot, Greenberg, & Watson, 2002), and it has focused on understanding the other. More recent developments in the concept of empathy have widened the focus and added the understanding of one's own contribution to the interaction and the involvement of mental states other than affective ones (Finset, 2010).

When these additional dimensions are included, empathy has a great similarity to the concept of mentalization, which means being aware of and understanding the mental processes of oneself and others (Allen & Fonagy, 2006). Mentalization reflects different mental processes, such as thoughts and feelings, but also additional facets, such as need, desire, imagination, belief and fantasy (Allen, Fonagy, & Bateman, 2008). Recent developments include the body (Luyten, van Houdenhove, Lemma, Target, & Fonagy, 2013; Shai & Belsky, 2011). Mentalization is described through four different dimensions, and each dimension is suspended between two poles (Bateman & Fonagy, 2012). One dimension moves between the explicit and the implicit poles. Explicit mentalization is controlled, reflective, and requires conscious attention.

Implicit mentalization is described as automatic, non-verbal, intuitive, and unreflective, representing the immediate emotional understanding (Allen et al., 2008; Fonagy & Luyten, 2009).

Mentalization theorists have given examples of when implicit mentalization takes place, but they have not accounted for how implicit mentalization can be identified or how it can be captured in interaction. Only explicit processes of mentalization have been investigated. In a comprehensive review of tests to assess mentalizing capacity, the authors exclusively refer to tests of the explicit dimension. The few available tests of implicit mentalization are at an experimental level (Bateman & Fonagy, 2012). Existing tests fail to capture implicit, interactive mentalization because they rely solely on verbal processes and they are not grounded in a dialogical approach to understanding mentalization processes. Nevertheless, implicit mentalization is said to be the most important factor in all forms of therapy (Fonagy, 2003). It is described as taking place in conversational turn-taking, when there is no apparent tension and no need to think explicitly about when to take the next turn (Bateman & Fonagy, 2012). It is also said to take place when perceiving and spontaneously responding to another person's emotional state, as when 'nodding sympathetically with a concerned look on our face as we listen to a friend talking about her child's frightening accident' (Allen, Bleiberg, & Haslam-Hopwood, 2014). Furthermore, it is repeatedly said to be typified by mirroring (Allen et al., 2008; Fonagy & Luyten, 2009), as when responding to another person's mental states by mirroring them automatically in posture, facial expression and vocal tone (Allen & Fonagy, 2006).

In psychotherapy research, different forms of non-verbal synchrony have been linked to relationship formation and empathic understanding, although real psychotherapeutic interactions have seldom been assessed directly (Ramseyer & Tschacher, 2011). Ramseyer and Tschacher (2011) showed that coordinated body movements influenced therapy process and outcome. The descriptions of implicit mentalizing as mirroring also seem to correspond to designations of imitative behaviour within linguistics and psychology as, for example, convergence, mimicry, interactional synchrony and accommodation (Toma, 2014). Studies show that the smoothness of an interaction is more highly rated when mirroring behaviour is increased (Babel, 2009; Chartrand & Bargh, 1999; Lakin & Chartrand, 2003), that convergence promotes establishment of rapport (Pardo, 2006), and that unconscious mimicry functions as social glue (Dijksterhuis, Chartrand, & Aarts, 2007). Couper-Kuhlen (2012) found that vocal expressions of affiliation were accompanied by prosodic matching; and in a psychotherapy study, Weiste and Peräkylä found that exhibiting similarity in prosody with the client's talk conveyed emotional empathy (Weiste & Peräkylä, 2014). Such observations of mirroring and convergence could be seen as being consistent with descriptions of implicit mentalization. Therefore, it seems probable that linguistic and psychological studies of the interactional phenomena of mirroring could be used to grasp whether the process of implicit mentalization takes place.

We chose to look at the interactions between patients with depression in consultations with general practitioners (GPs) and psychiatrists. Most patients with depression are treated in general practice, but in many countries, quality improvement initiatives aim at introducing collaborative care with psychiatric professionals (Kennedy, Lam, Parikh, Patten, & Ravindran, 2009; National Institute for Health and Clinical Excellence, 2009). Patients with depression are described as lacking mentalizing capacity themselves and as being difficult to mentalize. Targeted psychotherapeutic interventions are proposed (Fischer-Kern et al., 2013; Luyten, Fonagy, Lemma, & Target, 2012), and in Denmark, such an initiative is currently being implemented (Eplov et al., 2014).

By focusing on mirroring, we wanted to study whether professionals from the two sectors had the same approach to implicit, empathic understanding of their depressed patients. We aimed to explore if, and in that case how, mirroring was displayed by GPs and psychiatrists in consultations with patients with depression to see how implicit mentalizing processes unfolded in physician–patient interactions.

Methods

Consultations with patients suffering from depression were video-recorded and analysed within the framework of the sequential perspective of conversation analysis (CA).

Participants

Participants were purposively sampled to cover the range of demographic differences between selected doctors. Twelve GPs and 12 psychiatrists from Denmark participated in the study, all of whom were covered by collective agreement with the health authorities or employed at a public hospital. Gender distribution was equal in the two groups and age range was comparable: for psychiatrists, 45–62 years and for GPs, 43–66 years. All consultations with psychiatrists were outpatient appointments, thus ensuring an environment comparable to that of the GPs.

Videos

All participants made videos of consultations with patients with moderate depression, according to ICD-10 criteria. Twelve GPs made 13 videos, and 12 psychiatrists made 20 videos. The videos made by psychiatrists were on average longer (30–60 min) than those made by GPs (15–45 min), reflecting the different working conditions of the two groups of physicians. The physicians were asked to position the video camera so that as much as possible of the patients' and physicians' faces and bodies were visible. In one video with a psychiatrist, only the patient was visible and one GP was seen partly from the back, but the rest of the videos fulfilled the researchers' request. Informed consent was obtained from patients and physicians to use the videos for linguistic analysis. Based on assessment of the videos, patients in both the GP and the psychiatrist consultations appeared comparable in terms of psychopathology.

Conversation analysis

We used CA which has an established tradition for studying talk-in-interaction in meetings between doctors and patients in both general practice and psychiatry (Byrne & Long, 1984; ten Have, 1989; Peräkylä, Antaki, Vehviläinen, & Leudar, 2008). CA makes it possible to describe the systematic and structural organizations of the interaction. The conversation from the videos was transcribed according to established conventions in CA (ten Have, 2007, p. 215f). Both verbal and non-verbal interactions were noted.

CA was developed by Sacks, Schegloff, and Jefferson (1974) in the late 1960s. One of the fundamental analytic perspectives in CA is that interactants routinely establish intersubjectivity with each other and that this establishment is inherent in the structures that underlie the organization of talk (Goodwin, 1995; Schegloff, 1992). Interlocutors display their understanding in their interaction, and displays of understanding can be studied in the interactants' responses to each other.

Within the sequential framework of CA, it is possible not only to focus on the verbal modality but also to see understanding as an embodied and non-verbalized phenomenon. According to Mondada, 'understanding is constantly displayed in a multimodal way: participants manifest their current understanding in their gesture, gaze, facial expression, body position etc.' (Mondada, 2011, p. 545). All modalities are seen as equally important and as resources that do interactional work (Mondada, 2011; Stivers & Sidnell, 2005).

Analysis

Our analysis ran through different steps. First, both authors watched all videos to familiarize themselves with the content and to explore the ways in which mirroring was taking place. As we were interested in revealing implicit mentalizing processes, we then focused on sequences across the material where patients disclosed emotions (Davidsen & Fosgerau, 2014a). We identified sequences where a response from the physician could be characterized as mirroring the patient's body movements or behaviour, or language patterns. There is no unified definition of mirroring processes in interaction (Toma, 2014); therefore, there is no clear way of identifying them either. Building on the sequential perspective of CA, we defined mirroring as actions where the physician in the subsequent turn repeated either a body movement or behaviour, or a language pattern displayed by the patient (prosody, rhythm or tone of voice). The actions should be similar but displayed sequentially, not simultaneously, and assessed as conditional and displayed without conscious effort (Burgoon, Stern, & Dillman, 1995). Identification of mirroring actions was based on this definition and applied in relation to both verbal and non-verbal actions. To ensure that coding of these mirroring phenomena followed our definition, selection of the sequences where patients disclosed emotions and where the physician's response could be characterized as mirroring was discussed with a third member of our research group (a language psychologist) who had also seen the videos.

Mirroring was almost absent in the videos from psychiatrists, whereas it appeared frequently in the GPs' videos. We then selected two videos from GPs and two from psychiatrists for close CA analysis. The selection was based on the following criteria: in these videos, patients disclosed obvious emotions; both patient and physician were clearly visible, and the presence or absence of mirroring could be described in written language. Some mirroring phenomena in GP videos were subtle body movements that would demand demonstration of visual material, for which we did not have informed consent. Our selected videos featured both a male and a female GP and psychiatrist, all in their fifties. The second author performed detailed analysis of the identified sequences in the four selected videos. This analysis was rigorously discussed among the authors and the third member of our research group until we reached consensus.

In the whole corpus, we identified just over 100 sequences where patients disclosed emotions. The disclosures were equally distributed between GP and psychiatrist consultations, although consultations with psychiatrists were on average twice as long as consultations with GPs. In the four videos which we subjected to close CA, we identified four or five sequences in each video. The length of the sequences and the time spent on emotional talk varied. All sequences were analysed. Only GPs showed mirroring responses in these videos, whereas psychiatrists reacted with a monotonous, static attitude. We present results from the four videos. Based on our overall analysis of all the videos, we believe that the tendencies observed in these videos are transferable to the whole corpus.

Results

GPs and psychiatrists differed substantially in their tendencies to mirror the body movements and the verbal and acoustic features of their patients. GPs mirrored their patients in different modalities and were flexible in their interactional behaviour, adapting to the behaviours of the patients. In contrast, psychiatrists were more static, regardless of whom they were interacting with, what they were talking about, and the degree of emotionality displayed by the patients.

The GPs' mirroring of body movements took place throughout the conversation, but was most obvious at moments when patients displayed emotions, whether bodily, verbally, or acoustically. However, GP mirroring also occurred even when patients did not display obvious emotional engagement. The absence of mirroring of acoustic features and body movements characterized almost all consultations with psychiatrists. This absence was also apparent when patients displayed emotions, both positive and negative.

The differences are illustrated in the following examples.

GPs mirroring of acoustic features

GPs often mirrored patients by attuning the intensity of their voices to the patients' expressions and by mirroring the length of vowels or the emphasis on syllables. Extract 1 is from a consultation between a GP and a female patient in her thirties. The patient has been treated for depression for some time. In this consultation, the patient has said that she now feels better and that 'it is really nice'. The conversation continues as follows:

```
Extract 1:
1 PA:   but I can just feel that I ((nods and moves her body
2          along)) (.) I'm more relaxed a:nd
3 GP:   ((nods))
4 PA:   °well I just feel absolutely different°=
5 GP:   =°mm:: that sounds really great°
```

In line 4, the patient lowers the intensity of her voice describing how different she feels. The GP mirrors this lowering in her response in line 5 and acoustically attunes her talk to the patient's talk. The patient's nodding in lines 1 and 2 is also mirrored by the GP in line 3.

In CA terms, the GP is affiliating with the patient's talk (Stivers, 2008). The patient started the sequence by assessing her new mental state and saying 'it is really nice'. She continues by uttering 'I am more relaxed' and 'well I just feel absolutely different'. The GP responds by producing another assessment, 'that sounds really great', which agrees with the patient's assessment. In CA, responding to assessments by producing assessments which agree with those produced by a first speaker is considered a preferred action (Pomerantz, 1984). Preference refers to sequential properties of turns and the ways sequences are constructed, it is about a structural tendency in conversations describing that some first pair parts prefer specific second pair parts and that second pair parts can be delivered in preferred or dispreferred turn shapes (Schegloff, 1988). Preference is included in our analysis to point out that when the GP mirrors and agrees with the assessment produced by the patient, and when she does so by latching her agreement to the patient's assessment (indicated by the =) and thereby without any gaps or delays, she acts in an unmarked way and as people tend to when interacting with each other in everyday talk. GPs had a greater tendency than psychiatrists to produce these agreeing assessments when responding to patients' assessments.

Acoustic features were also mirrored by GPs when patients described and displayed negative emotional states. These features were related not only to turn units at the sentence level, but also to smaller phrasal units, such as the length of vowels, pitch pattern and (non-)stress on syllables. This is exemplified in extract 2, which is from the same consultation as extract 1.

Prior to extract 2, the patient told the GP that she has decided not to return to her job. Apparently, her employer supports this decision. While relating this, the patient shakes her head from side to side, takes deep breaths and turns her lips downward displaying distress and sadness. The GP asks her if this is 'hard to swallow', and the patient states with a low vocal intensity that it is 'hard to acknowledge that you are ill'. The GP responds by uttering 'yes' with low vocal intensity, mirroring the vocal intensity of the patient. The patient nods, and the nodding is mirrored by the GP. The patient continues as follows:

Extract 2:

```
1 PA:     ((sniffs)) but on the other hand (0.5) ((swallows)) (0.5) I also believe that, well °I've
2         been depressed ever since I sta:rted (.) that job [( ) ° ((nods)) ]
3 GP:            °[yes you ha:ve] ° ((nods))
```

The GP's reply in line 3 mirrors the lowered vocal intensity of the patient's speech at the end of line 1 and throughout line 2. A further elaboration of the acoustic attunement is seen in line 3. In line 2, the patient prolongs the vocal 'a' in 'sta:rted' This prolonging of 'a' is mirrored by the GP in the word 'have' in 'yes you ha:ve' in line 3. In addition, the pitch pattern expressed by the patient in 'since I started' is the same as the pitch pattern in the GP's 'yes you have'. Furthermore, in the patient's phrase, the syllable 'star' from the word 'started' is stressed, whereas the previous two syllables in the words 'since I' are non-stressed. This is mirrored by the GP in that 'yes you' are unstressed syllables, whereas 'have' is stressed. The rhythm of the patient's phrase is in this way mirrored by the GP. The expression 'yes you have', as in extract 1, can be seen as a display of agreement with the patient's revelation. Mirroring both the patient's nodding and linguistic patterns shows that the GP is simultaneously mirroring the patient in more than one modality.

Psychiatrists' non-mirroring of emotional displays

Psychiatrists did not attune their displays to the patients' displays. When patients displayed their emotions by acoustic means, the psychiatrists reacted in an emotionally unmarked way. They did not change the intensity of their voice, and they did not move any parts of their bodies. Extract 3 illustrates the moment when a patient expresses and displays a positive emotional experience, and the psychiatrist responds in an acoustically and bodily non-attuned way.

The patient, a middle-aged man, has had some consultations with the psychiatrist prior to this conversation. He used to be very fond of music and had been able to reproduce melodies from memory. While being depressed, he had lost this ability. Now that he has regained it, he describes the loss of his capacity:

Extract 3:

```
1 PA:          it's (.) it's been (.) so special
2 PS:          °mm°
3 PA:          .hh ((clenches left fist)) Anna I have (.) I have (0.7)
4              I have been (0.8) trying to whistle (0.6) ((shakes
5              head)) some melodies (.) and I just could not get them right (.)
6 PS:          °mm°
```

In line 1, the patient displays emotionality when describing the loss of his musical memory: he assesses how special this was and emphasizes with a 'so' which is uttered with stress. The psychiatrist responds with a continuer 'mm' with decreased vocal intensity (Gardner, 2001). Her emotionally unmarked response is not attuned to, but rather contrasts with, the patient's display of his mental state.

The psychiatrists did not often produce a second assessment in response to the patient's initial assessment. This was in contrast to the GPs, who frequently produced such assessments (as in extract 1). The psychiatrist in extract 3 does not verbally display that she agrees with the patient's assessment regarding the loss of his musical memory. Nor do her utterances display that she understands what the patient is saying. Possibly, as a consequence, and to evoke the response that he has made relevant, the patient intensifies his emotional display in line 3: he clenches his left fist and explicitly directs his telling to the psychiatrist by uttering her name. The psychiatrist once again responds with an 'mm' uttered with a low vocal intensity remarkably in contrast to the patient's displayed emotional engagement. In addition, the psychiatrist keeps her body quite motionless, which contrasts with the patient's intense movements. In what follows (not in extract), the patient continues his telling, still displaying emotionality, and still not receiving any response that is attuned to his emotional display, only 'mm's uttered with a contrastingly marked low vocal intensity. He then says:

```
Extract 4:
1 PA:       so I (.) I've been writing in my diary at home (.) yip:pee⤴
2           ((clenches his fists in front of his chest)) Y::ES (.) now I can do it again
3           [hee ] hee
4 PS:       [°mm°]
5 PA:       ((laughter decreases)) .hh well
6 PS:       °when did you discover ↑that°
```

In line 1 to 2, the patient enhances his engagement by uttering 'yippee' with a raise on the last syllable; he lifts his arms and clenches both fists in front of his chest and loudly utters 'yes', and then starts laughing. The psychiatrist once again responds with an 'mm' uttered with low vocal intensity. She does not attune her response to the patient's lively actions and loud outbursts, she does not move, and she does not mirror his laughter in line 3 either. Instead, in line 6, she changes the focus from the patient's emotional experience, to a factual question: 'when did you discover that', uttered with a lowered vocal intensity markedly in contrast to the patient's outbursts.

When patients displayed negative emotional states, the psychiatrists similarly displayed monotonic, uninvolved and non-mirroring ways of interacting. An example is given in extract 5. This is a female patient in her twenties who has had suicidal thoughts and self-harming impulses. The psychiatrist has seen her a couple of times. Prior to this extract, the psychiatrist asked how things were at the moment with 'thoughts about hurting yourself, about life and death', and they continue as follows:

Extract 5:

1 PA:		yeah well I still don't want to live (.) °I think it would be
2		a lot easier if I could just disappear°
3 PS:		mmhmm ((nods))
4 PA:		and it was the weekend before last the:n it was really bad=
5 PS:		=yes
6		(1.1)
7 PA:		where (.) I called my mother and Lotte and she came over
8		and so on
9 PS:		yes ((takes notes))
10		(2.2)
11 PA:		because I was in a really (.) terrible state ((voice filled with air
12		shivers, pulls her crossed arms forward))
13 PS:		yes
14		(1.8)
15 PS:		wha- what ab- (.) did it relate to

The patient says that she has no will to live, and she adds with a lowered vocal intensity that she would rather just disappear. The psychiatrist responds with a continuer 'mmhmm' uttered with an unmarked voice. He does not attune his response to the patient's emotional display. The patient continues by relating that things were really bad the previous weekend. She called her mother and her sister came to her house. The psychiatrist responds with 'yes' while taking notes, neither looking at nor showing attention to the patient (Ruusuvuori, 2001). The patient then takes turn in line 11 and relates that she felt awful. At this point, her voice is thick and breathless, and she signals being uncomfortable and troubled when moving her body. The psychiatrist once again answers with an acoustically unmarked 'yes' in line 13, displaying no signs of attunement to the difficulties she is having. His body is motionless, only moving his head when he looks at the paper he is writing on. After a long pause (1.8 s), he takes turn. He initially self-repairs and then asks a formal question. He does not give any display of intuitive sensitivity to the patient's mental state.

Mirroring of body movements

Just as their tones of voice maintained the same intensity throughout the consultations, regardless of how their patients behaved, the psychiatrists' body positions also appeared rigid. They generally kept their bodies still and in the same position during the consultations, no matter how much their patients moved. The psychiatrists rarely used gesticulations and did not mirror their patients' body language.

GPs used more flexibility in their body positions. Their bodies were more active, and they used much gesticulation. They tended to mirror their patients' postures and changed their position or moved their hands in synchrony with the patient. This is in accordance with the findings of Ramseyer and Tschacher (2011) in a study that uses more objective measures.

Discussion

The GPs and psychiatrists differed markedly as to whether or not they mirrored patients during their interactions with them. GPs displayed an active and mirroring attitude. Psychiatrists acted in an unanimated way and did not mirror or attune to patients' actions. In line with results from other studies on mirroring, GPs' mirroring could be seen as a display of pre-reflective emotional attunement to the patients' mental states, conveying empathy, rapport and smoothness in the conversation (Dijksterhuis et al., 2007; Weiste & Peräkylä, 2014). This form of attunement corresponds to mentalization theorists' description of implicit mentalization, expressed through mirroring of patients' verbal and acoustic activities and body movements (Allen et al., 2008; Bateman & Fonagy, 2012).

Mentalization theorists have not accounted for how implicit mentalization can be identified in interaction (Bateman & Fonagy, 2012). Recently, Shai and Belsky (2011) focused on this inadequacy. They suggest studying mentalizing as an embodied phenomenon, involving non-verbal aspects of interaction to grasp the implicit part of the interactive mentalizing processes. We argue that CA could be used to study interactional mirroring as an expression of implicit mentalizing processes.

We found that GPs showed a greater propensity to mirror their patients interactionally than psychiatrists, and we interpreted this as a greater inclination towards implicit mentalizing. They seemed to engage more with the patient as a person rather than as a patient with depression. GPs have been shown to have a different understanding of depression compared to psychiatrists (Chew-Graham, May, & Headley, 2000; Gask, Klinkman, Fortes, & Dowrick, 2008; Pilgrim & Bentall, 1999) (Davidsen & Fosgerau, 2014b). They consider context and social conditions as important for understanding and treating depression (Armstrong & Earnshaw, 2004; Chew-Graham et al., 2000). In addition, since GPs are responsible for dealing with all the problems that patients bring, including both somatic and mental illness, they must rely on an intuitive and open approach to patients in order to understand the patients' concerns in a broader and less focused way than psychiatrists. In contrast, psychiatrists need only relate to the psychiatric aspects of the patients' problems, and they could therefore be more oriented towards finding the right psychiatric diagnosis and treatment. The implication of this is that the intuitive approach to the patient is turned off and replaced with a search for specific symptoms which could confirm or disprove the diagnosis of depression. This more controlled, reflective, conscious and intellectual understanding of patients carries the risk of appearing more stiff and distanced, and of not mentalizing (Allen & Fonagy, 2006).

The contrasting ways in which GPs and psychiatrists relate to patients with depression in the primary and secondary care sectors could have implications for implementation of planned collaborative efforts. Initiatives are already in place where professionals from the two sectors are expected to cooperate on the treatment of patients with depression in general practice (May, 2013; Richards et al., 2013). The differences in approach might also affect patient outcome. Our findings provide fertile ground for future studies that focus on patient outcome in different implicitly mentalizing interactions. There is also scope for studies employing linguistic methods to explore different mirroring phenomena in order to identify when implicit mentalization takes place in interaction. However, we recognize that there is also a need for clarification on how a response is identified as a mirroring action in interaction analytical approaches, and for an examination of the ways in which the mirroring phenomenon brings the interaction forward.

Disclosure statement

No potential conflict of interest was reported by the authors.

References

Allen, J., Bleiberg, E., & Haslam-Hopwood, T. (2014). *Understanding mentalizing. Mentalizing as a compass for treatment.* Retrieved from http://www.menninger clinic.com/education/clinical-resources/mentalizing

Allen, J. G., & Fonagy, P. (2006). *Handbook of mentalization-based treatment.* Chichester: Wiley.

Allen, J. G., Fonagy, P., & Bateman, A. (2008). *Mentalizing in clinical practice.* Washington, DC: American Psychiatric Publishing.

Armstrong, D., & Earnshaw, G. (2004). What constructs do GPs use when diagnosing psychological problems? *British Journal of General Practice, 54,* 580–583.

Babel, M. E. (2009). *Phonetic and social selectivity in speech accomodation* (PhD thesis). University of California, Berkeley.

Bateman, A., & Fonagy, P. (2012). *Handbook of mentalizing in mental health practice.* Arlington, TX: American Psychiatric Publishing.

Bohart, A. C., Elliot, R., Greenberg, L. S., & Watson, J. C. (2002). Empathy. In J. C. Norcross (Ed.), *Psychotherapy relationships that work* (pp. 89–108). Oxford: Oxford University Press.

Burgoon, J. K., Stern, L. A., & Dillman, L. (1995). *Interpersonal adaptation. Dyadic interaction patterns*. Cambridge: Cambridge University Press.

Byrne, P. S., & Long, B. E. L. (1984). *Doctors talking to patients*. Exeter: The Royal College of General Practitioners.

Chartrand, T. L., & Bargh, J. A. (1999). The chameleon effect: The perception–behavior link and social interaction. *Journal of Personality and Social Psychology, 76*, 893–910.

Chew-Graham, C. A., May, C. R., & Headley, S. (2000). The burden of depression in primary care: A qualitative investigation of general practitioners' constructs of depressed people in the inner city. *International Journal of Psychiatry in Clinical Practice, 6*, 137–141.

Couper-Kuhlen, E. (2012). Exploring affiliation in the reception of conversational complaint stories. In A. Peräkylä & M. L. Sorjonen (Eds.), *Emotions in interaction* (pp. 113–144). New York, NY: Oxford University Press.

Davidsen, A. S., & Fosgerau, C. F. (2014a). General practitioners' and psychiatrists' responses to emotional disclosures in patients with depression. *Patient Education and Counseling, 95*, 61–68.

Davidsen, A. S., & Fosgerau, C. F. (2014b). What is depression? Psychiatrists' and GPs' experiences of diagnosis and the diagnostic process. *International Journal of Qualitative Studies on Health and Well-being, 9*, 24866. doi:10.3402/qhw.v9.24866

Dijksterhuis, A. P., Chartrand, T. L., & Aarts, H. (2007). Effects of priming and perception on social behaviour and goal pursuit. In J. A. Bargh (Ed.), *Social perception and the unconscious. The automaticity of higher mental processes* (pp. 51–131). New York, NY: Psychology Press.

Eplov, L. F., Davidsen, A. S., Christensen, K. S., Mikkelsen, J. H., Lau, M., Nielsen, J. N., & Licht, R. (2014). *Project collabri. The effect of a Danish model of collaborative care for people with anxiety and depression in general practice*. Retrieved from http://www.psykiatri-regionh.dk/cgi-bin/MsmGo.exe?grab_id=0&page_id=97962&query=collabri&hiword=collabri%20

Finset, A. (2010). Emotions, narratives and empathy in clinical communication. *International Journal of Integrated Care, 10*, 53–56.

Fischer-Kern, M., Fonagy, P., Kapusta, N. D., Luyten, P., Boss, S., Naderer, A., & Bluml, V. (2013). Mentalizing in female inpatients with major depressive disorder. *The Journal of Nervous and Mental Disease, 201*, 202–207.

Fonagy, P. (2003). Epilogue. *Bulletin of the menninger clinic, 67*, 271–280.

Fonagy, P., & Luyten, P. (2009). A developmental, mentalization-based approach to the understanding and treatment of borderline personality disorder. *Development and Psychopathology, 21*, 1355–1381.

Gardner, R. (2001). *When listeners talk. Response tokens and listener stance*. Amsterdam: John Benjamins Publishing.

Gask, L., Klinkman, M., Fortes, S., & Dowrick, C. (2008). Capturing complexity: The case for a new classification system for mental disorders in primary care. *European Psychiatry, 23*, 469–476.

Goodwin, C. (1995). Co-constructing meaning in conversations with an aphasic man. *Research on Language and Social Interaction, 28*, 233–260.

Husserl, E. (1983). *Ideas pertaining to a pure phenomenology and to a phenomenological philosophy*. Dordrecht: Kluwer.

Kennedy, S. H., Lam, R. W., Parikh, S. V., Patten, S. B., & Ravindran, A. V. (2009). Canadian network for mood and anxiety treatments (CANMAT) clinical guidelines for the management of major depressive disorder in adults. *Journal of Affective Disorders, 117*, S1–S2.

Lakin, J. L., & Chartrand, T. L. (2003). Using nonconscious behavioral mimicry to create affiliation and rapport. *Psychological Science, 14*, 334–339.

Luyten, P., Fonagy, P., Lemma, A., & Target, M. (2012). Depression. In A. Bateman & P. Fonagy (Eds.), *Handbook of mentalizing in mental health practice* (pp. 385–417). Washington, DC: American Psychiatric Publishing.

Luyten, P., van Houdenhove, B., Lemma, A., Target, M., & Fonagy, P. (2013). Vulnerability for functional somatic disorders: A contemporary psychodynamic approach. *Journal of Psychotherapy Integration, 23*, 250–262.

May, C. (2013). Towards a general theory of implementation. *Implementation Science, 8*(18), 1–14.

Merleau-Ponty, M. (2012). *Phenomenology of perception.* London: Routledge.

Mondada, L. (2011). Understanding as an embodied, situated and sequential achievement in interaction. *Journal of Pragmatics, 43*, 542–552.

National Institute for Health and Clinical Excellence. (2009). NICE. Depression in adults: Full guidance. Retrieved from http://guidance.nice.org.uk/CG90/Guidance/pdf/English

Norcross, J. C. (2010). The therapeutic relationship. In B. L. Duncan, S. D. Miller, B. E., Wampold, & M. A. Hubble (Eds.), *The heart & soul of change. Delivering what works in therapy* (2nd ed., pp. 113–141). Washington, DC: American Psychological Association.

Pardo, J. S. (2006). On phonetic convergence during conversational interaction. *The Journal of the Acoustical Society of America, 119*, 2382–2393.

Peräkylä, A., Antaki, C., Vehviläinen, S., & Leudar, I. (2008). *Conversation analysis and psychotherapy.* Cambridge: Cambridge University Press.

Pilgrim, D., & Bentall, R. (1999). The medicalisation of misery: A critical realist analysis of the concept of depression. *Journal of Mental Health, 8*, 261–274.

Pomerantz, A. M. (1984). Giving a source or basis: The practice in conversation of telling 'how i know'. *Journal of Pragmatics, 8*, 607–625.

Ramseyer, F., & Tschacher, W. (2011). Nonverbal synchrony in psychotherapy: coordinated body movement reflects relationship quality and outcome. *Journal of Consulting and Clinical Psychology, 79*, 284–295.

Richards, D. A., Hill, J. J., Gask, L., Lovell, K., Chew-Graham, C., Bower, P., et al. (2013). Clinical effectiveness of collaborative care for depression in UK primary care (CADET): Cluster randomised controlled trial. *British Medical Journal, 347* (f4913), 1–10.

Rudebeck, C. E. (2001). Grasping the existential anatomy: The role of bodily empathy in clinical communication. In K. S. Toombs (Ed.), *Handbook of phenomenology and medicine* (pp. 297–316). Norwell: Kluwer Academic.

Ruusuvuori, J. (2001). Looking means listening: Coordinating displays of engagement in doctor–patient interaction. *Social Science & Medicine, 52*, 1093–1108.

Sacks, H., & Schegloff, E. A., Jefferson, G. (1974). Simplest systematics for organization of turn-taking for conversation. *Language, 50*, 696–735.

Schegloff, E. A. (1988). On an actual virtual servo-mechanism for guessing bad news – A single case conjecture. *Social Problems, 35*, 442–457.

Schegloff, E. A. (1992). Repair after next turn – The last structurally provided defense of intersubjectivity in conversation. *American Journal of Sociology, 97*, 1295–1345.

Shai, D., & Belsky, J. (2011). When words just won't do: Introducing parental embodied mentalizing. *Child Development Perspectives, 5*, 173–180.

Stivers, T. (2008). Stance, alignment, and affiliation during storytelling: When nodding is a token of affiliation. *Research on Language and Social Interaction, 41*, 31–57.

Stivers, T., & Sidnell, J. (2005). Introduction: Multimodal interaction. *Semiotica, 156*(1–4), 1–20.

ten Have, P. (1989). The consultation as a genre. In B. Torode (Ed.), *Text and talk as social practice* (pp. 115–135). Dordrecht: Foris.

ten Have, P. (2007). *Doing conversation analysis: A practical guide* (2nd ed.). London: Sage.

Toma, C. L. (2014). Towards conceptual convergence: An examination of interpersonal adaptation. *Communication Quarterly, 62*, 155–178.

Weiste, E., & Peräkylä, A. (2014). Prosody and empathic communication in psychotherapy interaction. *Psychotherapy Research, 24*, 687–701.

Zahavi, D. (2010). Empathy, embodiment and interpersonal understanding: From Lipps to Schutz. *Inquiry-An Interdisciplinary Journal of Philosophy, 53*, 285–306.

The person-centred approach as an ideological discourse: a discourse analysis of person-centred counsellors' accounts on their way of being

Sophia Sflakidou and Maria Kefalopoulou

In accord with humanistic psychology, the person-centred approach (PCA) highlights individuality and is characterised by subjectivity and freedom vs. objectivity and determination. This study endeavoured to define how person-centred counsellors position themselves within PCA. In order to employ a critical frame of mind, analysis focused on identifying constructions, contradictions and functions of language that pointed to power relations. This study revealed a power relation between PCA and the counsellors, displaying five discourses: the philosophical discourse, the discourse of freedom, the discourse of religion/spirituality, the discourse of militarism and the discourse of eros (love). PCA is thought to empower the client in relation to its respectful and non-directive, therapeutic framework. Analysis suggests that despite rhetorical endorsement of PCA as enabling, the approach has implications for subjectivity and practice regarding the counsellor him/herself. Adhesive attachments closely resembling religious and erotic ones seem responsible for dogmatic and militaristic phenomena as described by participants. Strong emotions such as pride and guilt are indicative of this adhesive investment. Furthermore, the analysis shows that as the discourse of freedom becomes embedded in the philosophical discourse of PCA, it has connotations of truth. Lastly, the discourse of religion/spirituality seems to organise PCA in terms of meaning coherence.

In Übereinstimmung mit der humanistisch-psychologischen Tradition betont der „Personenzentrierte Ansatz" (PZA) die Individualität des Einzelnen und ist gekennzeichnet durch die Dualismen Subjektivität vs. Objektivität und Freiheit vs. Determiniertheit. Die vorliegende Studie unternimmt den Versuch, näher zu konkretisieren, wie sich personenzentriert arbeitende Berater innerhalb des eigenen PZAs verorten. Um hierfür eine kritische Haltung einnehmen zu können, nimmt die Studie ihren Ausgangspunkt bei Parkers diskursanalytischer Methode (2004, 1990), die wiederum mit dem, sechs Stufen umfassenden, Analyseleitfaden von Willig (2001) in Beziehung gebracht wurde. Die Untersuchung legt dabei ein Machtverhältnis zwischen PZA und Beratern offen, die sich anhand von fünf Diskursen nachzeichnen lassen: den philosophischen Diskurs, den Freiheitsdiskurs, den religiösen/spirituellen Diskurs, den militaristischen Diskurs und den Diskurs des Eros (Liebe). Mithilfe der PZA sollen Klienten durch einen respektvollen und nichtdirektiven therapeutischen Rahmen befähigt werden (Rogers, 1978). Die Untersuchung hingegen legt nahe, dass die rhetorische Bekräftigung der PZA als einem befähigenden Ansatz, dieser vielmehr Folgen für die Subjektivität und Praxis der Beraterin/des Beraters hat. Zudringliche Bindungen, ähnlich den religiösen oder erotischen, scheinen, so die Teilnehmer, für dogmatische und militaristische Vorgänge verantwortlich zu sein. Starke Emotionen wie Stolz und Schuld sind bezeichnend für solch ein bindendes Investment. Darüber hinaus kann durch die Untersuchung gezeigt werden, dass, wenn der freiheitliche Diskurs in den philosophischen Diskurs der PZA eingeschlossen wird, dieser Wahrheitsansprüche besitzt. Der religiöse/spirituelle Diskurs scheint, so das letzte Ergebnis, die PZA im Sinne eines zusammenhängenden Ganzen zu strukturieren.

De acuerdo con la psicología humanística, el modelo de tratamiento centrado en la persona destaca la individualidad y se caracteriza por la subjetividad y libertad versus objetividad y determinación. Este estudio se propone definir cómo el orientador se posiciona dentro del modelo. Para utilizar un marco de trabajo crítico, el análisis se basó en el marco teórico del discurso de Parker (1990, 2001) y empleó la guía de seis estadios de Willig (2001). El estudio reveló una relación de poder entre el método y los orientadores, mostrando cinco discursos: filosófico, de libertad, de religión/espiritualidad, militarismo y el de eros (amor). Se piensa que el método da poder al cliente en relación con su marco de trabajo respetuoso y no-directivo (Rogers, 1978). El análisis sugiere que a pesar de la aprobación del método como habilitante, tiene implicaciones de subjetividad y práctica profesional en relación con el orientador mismo. Se establecen apegos adhesivos que hacen recordar adicciones religiosas y eróticas responsables por fenómenos dogmáticos y militaristas, según han descrito algunos participantes. Emociones fuertes como orgullo y culpa son indicativas de este tipo de apego. Además el análisis muestra que como el discurso de libertad se inserta en el discurso filosófico adquiere connotaciones verdaderas. Finalmente el discurso de religión/espiritualidad parece organizar el método en términos de coherencia significativa.

In accordo con la psicologia umanistica, l'approccio centrato sulla persona (PCA) sottolinea l'individualità ed è caratterizzato da soggettività e libertà in contrapposizione all'obiettività e alla determinazione. Questo contributo cerca di definire come i counsellor centrati sulla persona posizionano se stessi entro il PCA. Al fine di utilizzare una struttura critica della mente, l'analisi si è basata sulla struttura teorica del discorso di Parker (2004, 1990) ed è stata utilizzata la guida in sei fasi di Willig (2001). Questo studio ha evidenziato una relazione rilevante tra PCA e i counsellor, mettendo in evidenza cinque tipologie di discorso: il discorso filosofico, quello della libertà, il discorso della religione/spiritualità, quello relativo alla partecipazione e il discorso sull'eros (amore). Il PCA è preso in considerazione per rafforzare il cliente in relazione alla struttura terapeutica rispettosa e non direttiva (Rogers, 1978). L'analisi suggerisce che, al di là dell'aspetto retorico dell'abilitazione al PCA, l'approccio presenta implicazioni che riguardano il counsellor stesso, nella sua oggettività e nella pratica. Attaccamenti adesivi molto somiglianti a quelli religiosi ed erotici sembrano all'origine di atteggiamenti dogmatici e militanti, in linea con quanto descritto dai partecipanti. Sentimenti forti come l'orgoglio e il senso di colpa sono indicativi di questo investimento adesivo. Inoltre, l'analisi mostra come nelle situazioni in cui il discorso della libertà si incorpora in un discorso filosofico relativo al PCA, esso presenti connotazioni di verità. Infine, il discorso della religione/spiritualità sembra organizzare il PCA in termini di significato di coerenza.

En accord avec la psychologie humaniste, l'approche centrée sur la personne (PCA) met en avant l'individualité et se caractérise par la subjectivité et la liberté en opposition avec l'objectivité et la détermination. Cette étude avait pour objectif de définir comment les thérapeutes centrés sur la personne se positionnent eux-mêmes au sein de la PCA. Dans un souci d'esprit critique, l'analyse s'appuie sur le cadre théorique de Parker (2004, 1990) concernant le 'discours' et a suivi le modèle en six étapes de Willig (2001). Cette étude a révélé une relation de pouvoir entre PCA et les thérapeutes illustrée au travers de cinq discours : le discours philosophique, le discours de la liberté, le discours de la religion/spiritualité, le discours du militarisme et le discours de l'éros (amour). PCA est censé responsabiliser les clients grâce à son cadre thérapeutique respectueux et non-directif (Rogers, 1978). L'analyse suggère que malgré l'approbation rhétorique de PCA considérée comme aidante, l'approche a des implications en ce qui concerne la subjectivité et la pratique des thérapeutes eux-mêmes. Des attachements adhésifs, à rapprocher d'émotions religieuses et érotiques, apparaissent comme responsables de phénomènes dogmatiques et militaristes tels que décrits par les participants. Des émotions fortes comme la fierté et la culpabilité constituent les indicateurs de cet investissement adhésif. Par ailleurs, l'analyse montre que plus le discours de la liberté est ancré dans le discours philosophique de PCA, plus il a des accents de vérité. Enfin, le discours de la religion/spiritualité apparait comme organisant PCA lui fournissant une cohérence signifiante.

Σε συμφωνία με την ανθρωπιστική ψυχολογία, η προσωποκεντρική προσέγγιση τονίζει την ατομικότητα και χαρακτηρίζεται από υποκειμενικότητα και ελευθερία έναντι της αντικειμενικότητας και του καθορισμού. Η παρούσα έρευνα προσπάθησε να ορίσει τον τρόπο με τον οποίο οι προσωποκεντρικοί σύμβουλοι τοποθετούνται στο πλαίσιο της προσωποκεντρικής προσέγγισης. Προκειμένου να χρησιμοποιήσει ένα κριτικό πλαίσιο σκέψης, η ανάλυση βασίστηκε στο θεωρητικό πλαίσιο του Parker για το «σύστημα λόγου» (2004, 1990) και χρησιμοποίησε για την ανάλυση τον οδηγό των έξη σταδίων της Willig (2001). Η μελέτη αποκάλυψε μια σχέση εξουσίας μεταξύ της προσωποκεντρικής προσέγγισης και των συμβούλων, παρουσιάζοντας πέντε συστήματα λόγου: το φιλοσοφικό λόγο, το λόγο της ελευθερίας, το λόγο της θρησκείας / πνευματικότητας, το λόγο του μιλιταρισμού και του λόγου του Έρωτα (αγάπη). Η προσωποκεντρική προσέγγιση θεωρείται ότι ενδυναμώνει τον πελάτη μέσα σε ένα θεραπευτικό πλαίσιο που βασίζεται στο σεβασμό και τη μη-κατευθυντικότητα (Rogers, 1978). Η ανάλυση δείχνει ότι, παρά τη δέσμευση, σε επίπεδο θεωρίας, της προσωποκεντρικής προσέγγισης με μια στάση ενδυνάμωσης, η ίδια η προσέγγιση έχει επιπτώσεις στην υποκειμενικότητα και στην πρακτική του ίδιου του συμβούλου. Η στενή προσκόλληση που μοιάζει με θρησκευτική και ερωτική προσκόλληση φαίνεται υπεύθυνη για φαινόμενα δογματισμού και μιλιταρισμού, σύμφωνα με τις περιγραφές των συμμετεχόντων. Ισχυρά συναισθήματα, όπως η υπερηφάνεια και η ενοχή, είναι ενδεικτικά αυτής της υπερβολικής προσήλωσης. Επιπλέον, η ανάλυση δείχνει ότι καθώς ο λόγος της ελευθερίας ενσωματώνεται στο φιλοσοφικό λόγο της προσωποκεντρικής προσέγγισης, αποκτά συνδηλώσεις της αλήθειας. Τέλος, ο λόγος της θρησκείας / πνευματικότητας φαίνεται να οργανώνει την προσωποκεντρική προσέγγιση όσον αφορά τη σχετικότητα του νοήματος.

Introduction

The construct of ideology

Ideology could be generally defined as a set of values, beliefs and aspirations that informs us about the ultimate reason and purpose of life (Deurzen, 2011). According to post-structuralism, ideology controls, first, what passes as knowledge in any society and it constructs, secondly, human beings as ideological subjects (Alcorn, 2009). Respectively, it is used to stabilise certain versions of the world through wider procedures of social legitimisation, while it 'provides the language' (Berlin, 1992 cited in Alcorn, 2009, p. 333) to define the subject, its relation to other subjects and its position within the material and social world.

In this context, people cannot invent the words and phrases being appropriate to each mental, situational or emotional occasion, but rather they use existing sets of meaning in order to describe the world and their position within it (Parker, 1997). Subsequently, the person through his/her talk constructs certain versions of the world and rejects others. These discursive practices have social consequences that refer, firstly, to a direct interpersonal accounting and the building of a moral profile and, secondly, to a wider political meaning. Consequently, whether we view ideology as 'false consciousness' or 'status of truth', as 'felt experience' or 'dilemmatic', ideology has to do with knowledge and power (Burr, 1995).

What Foucault (1977, cited in Hook, 2003) suggests regarding disciplinary power is that it not only objectifies individuals in the sense of making them objects of forms of categorical knowledge, but it subjectifies them also by generating individualities based on such object categories. In this framework, the 'subject' is presented as being both subject to control and direction and bound up to her/his own identity through self-knowledge and conscience (Foucault, 1982 cited in Hook, 2003).

In the light of the aforementioned, what is suggested is that psychology/ psychotherapy like any discipline is not neutral or value free. For instance, critical psychologists argue that personality theories tend to reinstate the normal function of people within their ideological chains. In this context, normality is equated with ideologically fixed concepts of personality while it is presented as scientifically sustained (Fox & Prilleltensky, 2003).

The construct of person-centred approach

Person-centred approach (PCA) is claimed to be in conflict with the dominant ideology of 'evidence' which originates in the medicalisation of distress (Sanders, 2006). At the time, Rogers formed his theory; PCA came to be committed to self-authority and self-responsibility placing the client in charge of the therapeutic relationship, the decision-making and the effects of these decisions. Consequently, PCA was thought to be politically centred to the client – a concept that reversed the power relations between persons (Rogers, 1978).

From a critical view point, what PCA claims to expostulate, the therapist's power and expertise, is neglected as a prime concern in order to promote the person-centred version of growth (Rogers, 2004). In the light of this account, the therapeutic conditions are provided in order for the client to engage in PCA's value framework and not in the belief of them as expressions of respect. This tendency is described as instrumental non-directivity and addresses the reproduction of a person-centred professional ideology rather than a trustful attitude of the counsellor towards the client.

According to Elkins (2009), our profession seems so dominated by the medical discourse from the moment that 'one's professional competence is judged by one's ability to speak medical jargon' (p. 6). Thus, it seems that PCA, in order to gain validity, moved towards professionalisation (House, 2003 cited in Rogers, 2004) through the construct of a theoretical narrative accordant with the mainstream individualistic notions of the Western culture and nowadays, is becoming further entrenched in medical model assumptions and practices, failing to feature the social causes of human distress. As Proctor (2006a) argues, using individual experience to campaign for social change neglects the structures of power implicated in whose experiences are heard.

In conclusion, although humanism is required in order to do progressive work in or against the discipline, interpretation is necessary in understanding both of ourselves and the vision for which we find ourselves working (Parker, 1999).

The following study aimed to explore how person-centred counsellors position themselves within PCA. A Foucauldian approach to discourse analysis was used in order to define PCA's ideological impact on the participants: how PCA enables or constrains counsellors, and what are its implications for subjectivity and practice.

According to Parker (1994), discourse is defined as 'sets of statements that construct objects and an array of subject positions' (p. 245), and what is explored is how one particular object came to be as it is. From the moment that an object is constructed by discourses, it is difficult not to be treated as if it were real, in the sense that discourses provide frameworks for debating versions of reality (Parker, 1990). Respectively, this study endeavoured to define in which way discourses construct PCA, how they reform it through time, and how they make it seem as real according to the participants' subjective experience (Fox & Prilleltensky, 2003).

Method

Participants and data collection

Six person-centred counsellors were interviewed for this research. They (a) had completed the diploma-level training in person-centred counselling and their training as facilitators, (b) had at least 7 years of experience and (c) at the time of the interview they were practicing person-centred counselling. The partici-pants were recruited through an announcement in the staff meeting of the Insti-tute of Counselling and Psychological Studies (ICPS). During this meeting, an information sheet relevant to the rationale of this research was issued.

Interviews were semi-structured including six questions that explored the thoughts, the feelings and the meaning of being a person-centred counsellor. For instance, the participants were asked how they understand PCA as a way of being or how they feel about this way of being. Interviews-transcripts constituted the basis of the subsequent data analysis.

Data analysis

In the first phase of analysis, the transcripts were read several times in order to identify constructions, contradictions and functions of language. Subsequently, these discursive practices were mapped into patterns according to common dis-cursive constructs that draw on cultural networks and through reconstructing pre-supposed rights and duties of the subjects specified in the texts (Parker, 2004). These patterns of language constituted the emerging discourses of the texts.

Subsequently, the six-stage guide of Willig (2001) was employed and the accounts of the counsellors were analysed according to the following six stages: (1) Discursive constructions, (2) Discourses, (3) Action orientation, (4) Positioning, (5) Practice and (6) Subjectivity.

Ethical issues

Ethical issues were highlighted as well as the right to withdraw from research whenever someone wished.

Analysis

Five major embedded discourses were identified as follows: the philosophical discourse, the discourse of freedom, the discourse of religion/spirituality, the dis-course of militarism and the discourse of eros (love). These discourses were employed in order to construct the discursive objects of the text: PCA, the counsellor, the way of being and other approaches in counselling and psychotherapy.

The discourses are described using quotes from interviews while the participants are numbered (Participant A, B ...) for reasons of anonymity.

The philosophical discourse

Philosophy refers to a process of mental exploration of the human being and his/her relation to the world resulting in an integration of values with the form of assumptions and postulates or principles (Patterson, 1959). It reflects a truth about the human being and the world, while, by definition, it is not available for critique (Dussel, 2009). Philosophies originate in myths: although these are organised through rational processes, their transition to philosophical categories is based on 'the possibility of abstraction in modes of analysis' (Dussel, 2009, p. 502).

PCA was found to be constructed as 'an open platform, a philosophical one which allows flexibility' (Participant B). Furthermore, it is described as a 'democratic' and 'humanistic' approach that 'expresses the trust to the person's potential' (Participant F). Thus, PCA is presented as a philosophical system which in turn draws upon the discourse of humanism and the discourse of phenomenology in order to define its context.

Subsequently, the way of being is conceptualised as meeting the other in his/her humanity. Embracing the person-centred way of being means to 'be able to identify the existence of the other, to meet the others as persons that are important to be met' (Participant E). The main ideas of that kind of encounter are of 'being equal to and respecting the other' (Participant B).

Taking into account that assertions in discourse, also pose an opposing, implicit position (Billig et al., 1988 cited in Parker, 1990), other approaches were found to be constructed as lacking in philosophical perspective. Thus, other approaches are constructed as 'much more technocratic' (Participant F). 'The cognitive-behavioral approach, for instance, has a much more mechanistic way of understanding' (Participant B).

Subsequently, while other approaches are presented as having a limited framework of positivism and technocracy, PCA is described as 'an alternative paradigm, having a philosophical base' (Participant C). According to Patterson (1959), a philosophy is an integration of values that have a connotation of 'right' or 'should' in that sense of addressing the desirable. Thus, by locating PCA within a philosophical discourse, PCA is implied to be something good, being 'defined by its values' (Participant D).

In conclusion, the employment of the philosophical discourse positions the counsellor within a moral sphere while the embedded discourses of humanism and phenomenology specify his/her rights and duties: that of the trust and the respect of human beings. In the level of practice, that location could generate passivity because to diverge from it would mean to violate PCA's ethical code, a probability that makes the counsellor feel confusion and ambivalence:

For instance, I watch the politicians. How may I accept them with what they are doing and afterwards I am thinking that I don't like the fact that there are many people who blame them and swear at them because we don't really know what they pass through and what actually happens. All these create a system of values which constantly changes. (Participant E)

The discourse of freedom

The construction of PCA as a philosophical system is gradually converted to a way of being defining the life of the participants, their selfhood and their way to be related to the others. Thus, PCA becomes 'a life attitude' (Participant B), 'an essential experience' (Participant D) that 'permits someone to be what he is' (Participant F).

Phenomenology focuses on the idea of the human being as the sole creator of reality, in the sense that reality exists, only in terms of individual perception and interpretation at a given time (Hjelle & Ziegler, 1981). In particular, freedom is innate to human beings in terms of an inborn capability. In this context, the human being is thought to, naturally and inevitably, move towards greater differentiation, autonomy and maturity (Hjelle & Ziegler, 1981).

Respectively, PCA was found to be constructed as an 'ideology of change'. It is about an approach that 'changes and evolves' and 'has openness' (Participant C). Words like 'change' and 'openness' recruit the discourse of freedom that, in turn, constructs the counsellor as a person. Thus, the counsellor renounces a professional identity as he/she 'is not a psychoanalytic mask. He/she is a person with all his/her "being" there' (Participant B). Being released from requirements and specifications, the counsellor 'does not expect perfection from him/herself' (Participant C) and provides a pure and honest selfhood within the therapeutic relationship 'with the personality he/she has' (Participant F) endeavouring 'to be truly related to the other' (Participant F).

Consequently, the discourse of freedom functions as an axiom defining the rights and duties of the counsellor. The counsellor is free to be him/herself and has the duty to act accordingly in the therapeutic setting. On the opposing pole of discourse, other approaches are constructed as being directive and having power where 'the therapist is in the position of the decision-maker, in the position of the authority' (Participant B). In combination with the presentation of them as lacking in philosophical context, there is an implied construction of other approaches as being unethical. Thus, unlike other counsellors, the person-centred counsellor 'won't violate the client', and 'won't try to push him anywhere' (Participant E).

Constructing PCA as a way of being accomplishes its validation. PCA is presented as an ontological truth about human beings, as something real and natural, attuned with life. Thus, the counsellor feels 'satisfied' in the sense that 'he/she gains that learning about him/herself, about relationships, about life' (Participant F). Subsequently, by locating PCA within the discourse of freedom, PCA is presented as enabling and liberating offering to the counsellor 'that sense of free existence' (Participant E). In this context, being a counsellor gives the impression of a natural quality: 'The personal part is inextricable from the professional one' (Participant D).

The construction of the counsellor as a person positions him as an active, reflective and independent agent. The constructions of PCA as a way of being and as an ideology of change reinforce this active positioning. Therefore, the counsellor represents a free agent, oriented towards an understanding of its own being, a procedure through which he/she can freely choose and change.

Positioning the counsellor as a free agent having the power legitimises individualism while constructing him/her as a person certifies this notion as the substantive essence of the self. Thus, the counsellor 'is not scared of the PCA being bedded down in him/her, because it is not an ideology, it is an essential experience' (Participant D). Consequently and in combination with the pre-sentation of PCA as a way of being, the practice of the counsellor is prescribed by the individualistic concept and its accompanying vision of good life.

Therefore, the counsellor could engage in the practice of instrumental non-directivity floundering to comply with that vision: 'My intention to be equal with my client is clear, but I know more, for sure! I can't erase my knowledge nor my experience' (Participant A).

In some cases, the frailty to conform to PCA's value context seems to lead to feelings of shame and guilt: 'I feel guilty for my anger, many times, as I'm saying to myself that I wasn't able to understand the other … where does my empathy go in these cases?' (Participant E).

The discourse of religion/spirituality

Fromm (1950 cited in Ed de St. Aubin, 1999) has described two types of religion: the humanistic and the authoritarian. The former acknowledges a divine potential within all human beings, while the second refers to obedience practices presupposing the surrender to a superior power. On the other hand, Proctor (2006b) describes therapy as the new opium of the masses in the sense that it provides a meaning and a purpose in life in terms of self-fulfilment, self-awareness and similar goals. Additionally, as with religion, she claims that therapy makes people believe that they have more control and power over their lives, than they often have in reality. Both of these descriptions of religious-ness were found to be echoed in the participants' accounts, while that delusion of power was found to frame up their subjective experience.

Thus, PCA is constructed as a dogma which the counsellor 'has to deeply believe in, to represent, to embody, to be inspired by' (Participant A). It is also, about an approach that 'has a spiritual dimension, a transcending one' (Participant E), while in some cases its implementation 'creates dogmatic per-sons, for instance, the Christians and the non Christians' (Participant C). Subsequently, engaging in the person-centred way of being is presented as a gradual, working process of escaping the secular. Thus, through the therapeutic practice, the counsellor 'really feels like breaking on through to another world' and 'being found at last in the core of the client's soul' (Participant F).

The construction of the way of being as a working process implies that it does not constitute the thoughtless embracing of a theory, but on the contrary one challenging, working process. Furthermore, in combination with its presentation as an experience of transition, the person-centred way of being gives the impression of initiation to a divine truth: 'if we could really experience that as a process of incorporation and become a body within it, for me, it has a spiritual and a transcending dimension in which I deeply believe' (Participant E).

Thus, the counsellor is positioned as being on a mission. In order for the counsellor to perform his/her mission has to possess a divine potential: 'The route from "I" to "We" connects the soul giving it qualities beyond the secular ones …' (Participant E).

Positioning the counsellor as being on a mission combined with the construction of PCA as a dogma could lead to dogmatism: 'It seems like any of us being threatened by change, by evolution, by different perspective' (Participant B). Furthermore, the positioning of the counsellor as having an unearthly potential with its entailing vocabulary could complicate the communication of the approach: '… just because of the way it (the approach) is communicated, it may be very easily distorted … On account of its openness everyone may conceive it as he wishes' (Participant E).

Lastly, being positioned as being on a mission may make some counsellors feel proud and blessed. According to participant A's subjective experience, 'it is about a way of being that contains compassion, but in general richness, with all these within, the joy and the sadness, the pride'. Additionally, being positioned as having a divine potential may elicit a feeling of gratitude: 'I am really grateful for, by any aspect, for this contact with PCA' (Participant A). Consequently, PCA emerges as a given truth while the counsellor is captivated by this generosity: 'it feels like knowledge … because I consider the person-centered way of being as a gift' (Participant F).

The discourse of militarism

Words like 'polemical' and 'defensive' identified in the texts recruit the discourse of militarism that in turn constructs the counsellor as a soldier of PCA. With respect to a 'must' faith, Hoose (2010) argues that it can lead, at best, to a smug feeling of unity and, at worst, to loathing towards anyone or any idea that threatens this unity. Moreover, the practice of extrinsic religiousness has been empirically linked with extremism such as dogmatism and ethnocentrism (Wulff, 1991 cited in Ed de St. Aubin, 1999). Respectively, the counsellor is conceptualised as constituting a nation (Participant C: 'the Greeks and the Barbarians') or as incarnating 'a Hitleric conviction' (Participant B).

From one aspect, the discourse of militarism and its embedded discourses of nationalism, fascism and cannibalism are employed in order to signify the bad implementation of the approach (Participant B: 'what I would like is to stop eating each other'), from another it is used in order to describe the experience of the counsellor (as a believer) in terms of an internal fight: 'Because I may talk about unconditional positive regard and in my personal relationships, it may be hard for me to act accordingly and need to fight for it' (Participant F). Consequently, the use of the military discourse highlights the difficulty of being a person-centred counsellor – a hardly accessed quality in the light of its high moral background (PCA as a dogma).

Consequently, the construction of the counsellor as a soldier positions him/her as being in a battle, having 'the mission to protect the purity of the tribe' (Participant B) while the discourse of religion positions him/her, in turn, as a soldier of faith. Thus, the counsellor from being a believer slips into being a soldier of faith and dogmatism leads to fanaticism: 'I'm afraid that in many cases, particularly, the implementation of the approach creates dogmatic persons ... for instance, the Christians and the non Christians, the Greeks and the barbarians, the person-centered and the non person-centered' (Participant C). In this context, the construction of the counsellor as a soldier was found to have implications for insecurity, fear and hostility: 'economy demands efficiency and PCA doesn't conform nor repair quickly ... that sometimes makes us feel insecure as person-centered counsellors and we become very defensive or polemical concerning what is directive or not' (Participant D).

In the preceding example, defensiveness could be understood in terms of trying to preserve PCA's theoretical system intact and the necessity of this kind of resistance is well explained by Althusser's view of the subject as an ideological effect. According to Althusser, ideology provides an 'imaginary relationship of individuals to their real conditions of existence (Alcorn, 2009, p. 6). Consequently, the maintenance of the subject's ideological identity becomes a matter of life and death, a condition that justifies, in turn, feelings of insecurity, fear, even hostility. Concisely, the use of the military discourse highlights the battle for ideological survival.

The discourse of eros

Psychoanalysis describes ideological impact in terms of libidinal attachments and defensive subject positions in the case of an outer discourse invasion (Alcorn, 2009). According to it, the adhesive investments that subjects have to discourses work ceaselessly to represent identity, providing a temporal stability to it (Alcorn, 2009). In this framework, 'ideology is, in fact, the condition of being an individual' (Alcorn, 2009, p. 7).

What has been observed within the texts is an emotionally charged thinking – indicative of the libidinal power of discourse (Alcorn, 2009). In particular, PCA was found to be identified as the meaning of life, an identification which indicates its overwhelming impact on the participants. In these contexts, the person-centred way of being is constructed as giving meaning to life. Thus, it is about a way of being that makes the counsellor 'feeling so very rich' (Participant A) and that keeps someone living his/her life 'deliberately, with purpose, with direction' (Participant D).

Subsequently, the discourse of eros in combination with the discourse of freedom constructs the counsellor as a helper. Thus, the counsellor is permitted 'to be and at the same time to become what is helpful for the other, to become the other's tool within his trip, within his existence' (Participant E). Being a helper means to 'allow other people to find their own way of living' (Participant D) and to 'proceed with the intention to respect the other and his needs' (Participant F).

Consequently, the counsellor is presented as compassionate and trustful while that presentation subtly locates him/her in the position of a non-possessive lover. In this context, the discourse of freedom outlines the legitimate boundaries of acting while the discourse of eros specifies the nature of this acting. Thus, being a person-centred counsellor constitutes an attitude of love, while to love means to respect the other's integrity and not to exert power: 'I help people to find a more complete way, a happier one … without imposing or wanting to impose, that is to say, having the intention to do it, my own way' (Participant D).

In conclusion, the participants were found to be positioned as lovers. Experiencing PCA is conceptualised as a condition of connection and affection (Participant B: 'Through PCA, I feel like being connected to the whole – to life, to other human beings, to myself – in a way that is very open, that is "hug"…') while practicing PCA is described in terms of an erotic contact (Participant F: 'PCA enables me to approach so very close to the other. I feel like experiencing on my skin his/her gooseflesh …').

Positioning the counsellor as a lover could make the questioning or criticising of PCA's legitimacy difficult. As Morin (1997) claims, we need to be polluted by the other's truth in order to be in love. Love is like a myth that from the moment it is identified as such ceases being so. Respectively, the participants' enthralment identified in the texts designated their adhesive attachment on PCA: 'It (PCA) bewitches me and it excites me, it gives me joy and it lets me feel the sorrow. I am alive through this. It justifies my reason to be. It is a meaning of life' (Participant B).

Discussion

The present study endeavoured to display the discourses of PCA in order to offer an understanding of how discourses may influence the counsellors' behaviour and what implications they may have for subjectivity and practice.

PCA was found to constitute a powerful ideological discourse while its most obscuring version could lead to militarism. The analysis revealed adhesive attachments of the participants closely resembling religious and erotic ones, while the discourse of freedom was found to be embedded in the person-centred philosophy in axiomatic terms empowering this adhesive investment.

Dussel (2009) describes philosophies as 'unintentional, underlying ideologies' (p. 508) that provide a framework of interpretation and ethical guidance. With respect to phenomenology, the focus on freedom and rationality as innate qualities in human beings constructs the individual in accord with the traditional, humanist fantasy of an absolutely self-determined agency (Burr, 1995). In the same vein, contemporary psychology is committed to the 'unified image of the self' which, in fact, is no more than that, an image (Parker, 2004, p. 167). Examining contradictions in people's talk reveals the conflicting and divided nature of the self being subjected by discourse (Parker, 2004). Respectively, Althusser claims that ideology is not something that individuals deliberately choose (Alcorn, 2009). In this context, the subject is a product of discourse where some discourses are characteristic, working ceaselessly and defensively to represent identity (Alcorn, 2009).

In this study, being free and self-directed is what characterised PCA as a way of being in the counsellors' accounts. Thus, the participants were found to be 'principle of their own subjection' through procedures of subjectification as described by Foucault (Foucault, 1977 cited in Hook, 2003, p. 613), and the counsellor was found to be positioned as a free person, no longer paradoxically 'always through this ideological determination' (Participant A). The retention of contradictory subject positions by the participants, in turn, indicated their resistance to 'ideological death' (Alcorn, 2009), while positioning the counsellor as being in a battle and as a soldier of faith illustrated this kind of existential anxiety.

Consequently, PCA emerged as an undisputable truth while the discourse of religion achieved its moral consolidation. As Deurzen (2011) claims, western thought has been dominated by Christian narratives for many years. A shift was observed at the end of the nineteenth century where the religious ideology was replaced by scientific explanations of human activity and evolution. Nevertheless, it seems that PCA is constructed in accord with the Christian rationale while the remainders of this rationale – such as the concepts of connectedness and love – define its context.

Respectively, it could be claimed that what Hook (2003) describes as professionalised forms of love and kindness with respect to psychotherapy in clinical practice are also detected in PCA in relation to its moral context being defined by the love for the human being. As Morin (1997) argues, the concept of love is shaped in the terrain of an encounter between the holy and the secular, the mythological and the sexual. Whatever comes from religion may now be performed in an individual, as the subject of the love adhesion.

With respect to methodological limitations, it needs to be highlighted that this study constitutes itself a discursive construction based on a sample of just six participants. The basic discourses that emerged – named by the researchers – are of great breadth and there could be more, even different interpretations of the findings. The authors' expectations or frustrations as them being members of the person-centred 'community' could also have influenced the analysis. As Parker (1999) suggests, there is always an interpretive gap between what is observed and how it is interpreted in the sense that the researcher is him/herself subject to discourse.

According to Foucault (1977, cited in Hook, 2003), 'power and knowledge imply one another' (p. 6) where power is considered as a production of particular knowledge that constructs and legitimises, in turn, certain versions of social reality. This study could serve as a form of reflexivity indicating possible value commitments and entailing power relations that underwrite our professional work. Moreover, deconstructing our experience seems promising in introducing new perspectives in relation to clinical practice, training and supervision. In this framework where our basic beliefs are challenged, knowledge alters and permits different living spaces for negotiation and action (Parker, 1994).

Conclusion

It could be argued that the person-centred philosophy grasps the Christian narrative in the form of one's own, authentic and unique experience. The concept of a pure agency (Parker, 1994), being highlighted by the phenomenological and humanistic approach, seems to be responsible for this corollary. Moreover, the notion of freedom, being constructed as an innate quality on an axiom basis, subtly vindicates individualism. The right to self-determination presupposes a self absolutely responsible for life choices while this responsibility is restricted by the available meaning and practice resources in specific societal structures of power.

Disclosure statement

No potential conflict of interest was reported by the authors.

References

Alcorn, M. W. (2009). Changing the subject of postmodernist theory: Discourse, ideology, and therapy in the classroom. *Rhetoric Review, 13*, 331–349.

Burr, V. (1995). *An introduction to social constructionism.* London: Routledge.

de St. Aubin, E. (1999). Personal ideology: The Intersection of personality and religious beliefs. *Journal of Personality, 67*, 1106–1139.

Deurzen, E. (2011). *Psychotherapy and the quest for happiness.* Athens: Kondyli.

Dussel, E. (2009). A new age in the history of philosophy: The world dialogue between philosophical traditions. *Philosophy and Social Criticism, 35*, 499–516.

Elkins, D. N. (2009). *Humanistic psychology: A clinical manifesto. A critique of clinical psychology and the need for progressive alternatives.* Colorado Springs, CO: University of the Rockies Press.

Fox, D., & Prilleltensky, I. (2003). *Critical psychology: An introduction.* Athens: Ellinika Grammata.

Hjelle, L. A., & Ziegler, D. J. (1981). *Personality theories: Basic assumptions, research and applications.* Singapore: Mc Graw.

Hook, D. (2003). Analogues of power: Reading psychotherapy through the sovereignty discipline-government complex. *Theory & Psychology, 13*, 605–628.

Hoose, B. (2010). Religion, truth, mystery and morality. *Irish Theological Quarterly, 75*, 144–156.

Morin, E. (1997). *Love, poetry, wisdom.* Athens: Twenty first.

Parker, I. (1990). Discourse: Definitions and contradictions. *Philosophical Psychology, 3*, 187–204.

Parker, I. (1994). Reflexive research and the grounding of analysis: Social psychology and the psy-complex. *Journal of Community and Applied Social Psychology, 4*, 239–252.

Parker, I. (1997). Discourse analysis and psychoanalysis. *British Journal of Social Psychology, 36*, 473–495.

Parker, I. (1999). Critical reflexive humanism and critical constructionist psychology. In D. J. Nightingale & J. Cromby (Eds.), *Social constructionist* (pp. 23–26). Buckingham: Open University Press.

Parker, I. (2004). Discursive practice: Analysis, context and action in critical research. *International Journal of Critical Psychology, 10*, 150–173.

Patterson, C. H. (1959). *Counselling and psychotherapy. Theory and practice.* New York, NY: Harper & Row.

Proctor, G. (2006a). Opening remarks. In G. Proctor, M. Cooper, P. Sanders, & B. Malcolm (Eds.), *Politicizing the person centered approach. An agenda for social change* (pp. 1–4). Ross-on-Wye: PCCS Books.

Proctor, G. (2006b). Therapy: Opium of the masses or help for those who least need it? In G. Proctor, M. Cooper, P. Sanders, & B. Malcolm (Eds.), *Politicizing the person centered approach. An agenda for social change* (pp. 66–79). Ross-on-Wye: PCCS Books.

Rogers, C. R. (1978). *Carl Rogers on personal power inner strength and its revolutionary impact* (1. Delta print Ed.). New York, NY: Dell.

Rogers, A. (2004). What kind of 'counsellor' am I? *David Smail's Website.* Retrieved November 11, 2011, from http://davidsmail.info/rogers.htm

Sanders, P. (2006). Politics and therapy: Mapping areas for consideration. In G. Proctor, M. Cooper, P. Sanders, & B. Malcolm (Eds.), *Politicizing the person centered approach. An agenda for social change* (pp. 5–16). Ross-on-Wye: PCCS Books.

Willig, C. (2001). *Introducing qualitative research in psychology: Adventures in theory and method.* Buckingham: Open University Press.

Reading qualitative research

John McLeod

In recent years, qualitative research has emerged as an increasingly significant source of evidence for counselling and psychotherapy policy and practice. As a result, it is important for readers of qualitative studies to develop an appreciation of what kind of knowledge is made available, and not available, through this form of inquiry. The present paper offers a critical reflection on a series of qualitative studies published in the current issue of this journal. From a reader perspective, it is possible to identify a set of key themes: the capacity of qualitative research to address major issues within the field; contrasts between professional knowledge and other sources of evidence; the positionality of the author; the challenges associated with the accomplishment of contextuality; and, the struggle to determine the credibility and reliability of findings. The paper concludes by suggesting a shift in publication practice that might enhance the value and readability of qualitative articles.

In den letzten Jahren hat sich innerhalb von Beratung und Psychotherapie der qualitative Forschungszweig hinsichtlich praktischen wie auch politisch-inhaltlichen Aspekten zu einem wesentlichen Pfeiler wissenschaftlicher Evidenz entwickelt. In Anbetracht dessen ist es für Rezipienten qualitativer Studien wichtig, ein Verständnis dafür zu entwickeln, welches Art von Wissen durch diese Form der Erkenntnisgewinnung verfügbar gemacht wird – und welches nicht. Der vorliegende Artikel richtet demgemäß einen kritischen Blick auf eine Reihe der in dieser Ausgabe veröffentlichten qualitativen Studien. Aus Sicht des Lesers sind einige Schlüsselthemen identifizierbar: Das Vermögen qualitativer Studien, (problematische) Kernthemen innerhalb eines Feldes zu adressieren; Vergleiche zwischen Expertenwissen und anderen Erfahrungsquellen; der Verortung des Autors; der Herausforderung im Hinblick auf deren Kontextualität; und dem Problem, die Glaubwürdigkeit und Reliabilität der Ergebnisse eindeutig bestimmen zu können. Zum Abschluss macht der Artikel den Vorschlag, durch eine veränderte Publikationspraxis den Nutzen und die Lesbarkeit qualitativer Studien zu verbessern.

La investigación cualitativa ha surgido en años recientes como una evidencia creciente y significativa en las políticas y práctica de la orientación psicológica y la psicoterapia. Como resultado es importante que los lectores de estudios cualitativos desarrollen una apreciación de la clase de conocimientos disponibles o no disponibles a través de esta forma de investigación. El presente artículo ofrece una reflexión crítica en una serie de estudios publicados en el presente número de esta revista. Desde la perspectiva del lector es posible identificar un conjunto de temas clave: la capacidad de la investigación cualitativa para tratar temas importantes dentro del campo; contrastes entre conocimiento profesional y otras fuentes de evidencia; la posición del autor; los retos asociados con el logro de contextualidad; y por último la lucha para determinar la credibilidad y confiabilidad de los resultados. El artículo concluye sugiriendo un cambio en la manera en que se hacen las publicaciones, lo cual puede aumentar el valor y la legibilidad de los artículos sobre este tema.

Negli ultimi anni, la ricerca qualitativa si è andata costituendo come fonte di sempre maggior rilievo per verifiche relative al metodo e alla pratica del counselling e della psicoterapia. Come conseguenza, è divenuto importante che quanti si rifanno a questi studi qualitativi abbiano la possibilità di esprimere una valutazione sul tipo di conoscenza disponibile, oppure non disponibile a questo riguardo. Il presente contributo propone una riflessione critica su alcuni studi qualitativi pubblicati nel presente numero di questa rivista. Dal punto di vista del lettore, è possibile individuare una serie di temi chiave: l'idoneità della ricerca qualitativa ad affrontare le questioni principali in questo campo; la contrapposizione tra la conoscenza professionale e altre fonti di evidenza; il posizionamento dell'autore; le sfide connesse con la contestualizzazione; infine, la battaglia per definire la credibilità e l'affidabilità dei risultati. L'articolo si conclude suggerendo un cambiamento nell'attività di pubblicazione che potrebbe accrescere il valore e la chiarezza di articoli relativi alla ricerca qualitativa.

Récemment, la recherche qualitative a émergé comme source importante d'éléments concrets pour la pratique et les politiques qui concernent la psychothérapie et le counselling. Il est donc important que les lecteurs d'études qualitatives puissent développer une appréciation du type de savoir qui est disponible mais également de ce qui n'est pas disponible, dans ce genre d'investigation. Cet article propose une réflexion critique sur une série d'études qualitatives publiées dans ce numéro spécial du journal. D'un point de vue du lecteur, il est possible d'identifier une série de thèmes : la capacité de la recherche qualitative à adresser les problèmes majeurs de son champ d'investigation ; les contrastes entre le savoir professionnel et les autres sources fournissant des preuves; la position prise par l'auteur ; les défis associés à l'accomplissement de la contextualité et le combat pour déterminer crédibilité et fiabilité des résultats. Cet article conclut en suggérant un changement des pratiques de publication qui permettrait de mettre en valeur la valeur et la lisibilité des articles qualitatifs.

Τα τελευταία χρόνια, η ποιοτική έρευνα έχει αναδειχθεί ως μια ολοένα και πιο σημαντική πηγή δεδομένων για την συμβουλευτική και την ψυχοθεραπευτική πολιτική και πρακτική. Ως εκ τούτου, κρίνεται σημαντικό για τους αναγνώστες ποιοτικών ερευνών να μπορούν να εκτιμήσουν το είδος της γνώσης που είναι διαθέσιμη ή όχι, μέσω αυτής της μορφής διερεύνησης. Το παρόν άρθρο παρέχει έναν γόνιμο αναστοχασμό σχετικά με μια σειρά από ποιοτικές μελέτες που δημοσιεύονται στο τρέχον τεύχος του περιοδικού. Από την οπτική του αναγνώστη, είναι δυνατό να προσδιοριστούν μια σειρά από βασικά θέματα: η ικανότητα της ποιοτικής έρευνας νε μελετήσει σημαντικά ζητήματα στο πεδίο αυτό, οι αντιπαραθέσεις ανάμεσα στην επαγγελματική γνώση και σε άλλες πηγές δεδομένων, η τοποθέτηση του συγγραφέα, οι προκλήσεις που συνδέονται με την αναγνώριση του ρόλου του πλαισίου και η προσπάθεια να καθοριστούν η ακρίβεια και η αξιοπιστία των ευρημάτων. Το άρθρο καταλήγει προτείνοντας μια αλλαγή στην πρακτική της δημοσίευσης που θα μπορούσε να ενισχύσει την αξία και την αναγνωσιμότητα των ποιοτικών άρθρων.

Within the field of research in counselling and psychotherapy, one of the most important developments in recent years has been the gradual increase in the proportion of published research articles that make use of qualitative methodologies. After a period in which qualitative researchers struggled to get their work into journals, there is a growing acceptance of the value of this form of inquiry. Partly this enhanced level of acceptance is due to development of robust, widely understood qualitative methodologies (Hill, 2012; Smith, Flowers, & Larkin, 2009). It can also be partly attributed to the way in which qualitative researchers have become better at identifying research questions that are amenable to this type of investigation (McLeod, 2013) and have been able to use qualitative meta-synthesis to capitalise on the accumulation of studies within some areas (Hill, Knox, & Hess, 2012; Timulak, 2009; Timulak & Creaner, 2013).

Quantitative research can be regarded as a largely top-down, theory-driven enterprise that privileges the voice of the expert. By contrast, qualitative research can be characterised as a largely bottom-up, grounded and descriptive approach to inquiry that privileges the voice of the client or the worker. The papers in the current edition of this journal seek, one way or another, to describe and make sense of the experience of therapy (and related activities, such as assessment) from the perspective of front-line participants. The aim of this paper is to explore the ideas that if therapy research is to achieve its potential as a means of informing policy and practice, it also needs to take account of the experience of the reader.

Little is known about the requirements of readers of counselling and psychotherapy research articles or what it is like for them/us to navigate the literature as a whole, and then particular articles within that literature. From as far back as Morrow-Bradley and Elliott (1986), surveys of therapy practitioners have found that experienced therapists regard most research articles as lacking in clinical relevance, do not read such papers on a regular basis, and tend not to use them as a source of guidance in respect of their work with clients.

My aim in this paper is to offer some reflections on the articles in this issue of the present journal, as a means of opening a discussion around the nature of the experience of reading qualitative research. This discussion is framed in terms of a series of issues that are typically faced by readers: reconciling the tension between ambition and achievement, coming to terms with the nature of professional knowledge, the struggle to develop an appreciation of the position of the researcher/author, the contextuality dilemma and the problem of partial reporting. The final section of the paper makes some suggestions about how these issues might be addressed in order to enable readers to gain more value from this type of research report.

Ambition

The studies included in the current edition of this journal are typical of contemporary qualitative research, in their willingness to address major issues of theory and practice:

- Díaz Martínez, Solano Pinto, Solbes Canales, and Calderón López (2015) use life story interviews with therapy clients and others who have experience of eating disorders, as a means of exploring and elaborating one of the most widely applied models within the field of therapy practice – the Prochaska and DiClemente (1983) transtheoretical model of stages of change;
- Dreier (2015) reports on the findings from a series of qualitative studies carried out on the relationship between what happens in psychotherapy and the everyday life of the client. This research asks fundamental questions about current assumptions about the process and mechanisms of change of therapy, and invites consideration of new forms of therapeutic intervention;
- Roxburgh and Roe (2015) interviewed therapists around their experience of meaningful coincidences (synchronicity) in their work with clients. This study examines a rare phenomenon, but one that has the potential to be both personally highly significant and memorable, as well as puzzling;
- Sflakidou and Kefalopoulou (2015) investigate the underlying assumptions that shape the professional identity of person-centred counsellors and psychotherapists. This study uses an innovative methodology, centred on analysis of metaphor and discourse, to look more closely at issues that are central to how to make sense of the tension between 'purist' and 'integrative' approaches to therapy;
- Davidsen and Fogtmann Fosgerau (2015) explore the ways in which institutional context and professional role shape the ways in which different practitioners interact with their clients. This study represents an example of how qualitative methodology can be used to develop an understanding of processes that are outside of the conscious awareness of participants.

These are big questions that touch on issues of substantial theoretical and practical significance. The ambition reflected in the work of these researchers is no doubt welcomed by many readers – these are papers that are worth reading. This kind of work also raises expectations, and opens up the possibility of disappointment. What we are reading does not appear to resemble what the philosopher of science Kuhn (1962) characterised as 'normal science' – the painstaking detailed working out of sub-questions parcelled-off from within an overall guiding paradigm. Instead, these are more like pictures at an exhibition, each one striving to be sufficient in itself.

Professional knowledge

Most of the time, people who carry out qualitative research (or any research) in counselling and psychotherapy are therapists. The people who read these studies are also mainly therapists or those in training to become therapists. As a result, while the knowledge that is being both produced and consumed is certainly 'academic' knowledge, in the sense of being part of an academic discipline, it is also 'professional' knowledge, in the sense of being embedded within professional practice. The qualitative studies in this journal issue represent a range of forms of engagement with the task of developing professional knowledge. The studies by Diaz et al. Dreier and Davidsen and Fogtmann Fosgerau can be viewed as contributing to a general background level of knowledge, reflected in a capacity to conceptualise the work that is being done. The study by Sflakidou and Kefalopoulou represents a contrasting perspective on professional knowledge. Here, the practitioner-reader is invited to look at himself or herself: do these themes refer to me? If they do not, do they allow me to understand the stances taken by some of my colleagues? The study into meaningful coincidences (Roxburgh et al.) comes even closer to practice, by offering framework for making sense of events that may occur in specific therapy relationships. The paper by Roxburgh et al. goes further: not only do the findings of the study provide a resource for professional practice, but the literature review at the start of the article offers a succinct and lucid guide to current thinking on the topic being explored.

An important dimension of the experience of reading a qualitative research paper arises from the challenge of integrating the formal, research-based knowledge, that is on offer, with the reader's personal knowledge of the same topic. I believe that it is valuable to acknowledge the coexistence of different 'knowledges' that we draw on in our work with clients: practical knowledge arising from doing therapy; personal knowledge generated by life experience and personal therapy; theoretical knowledge; and cultural knowledge. For the reader, the formal knowledge provided in a research article is evaluated in relation to the pre-existing structure of the reader's personal knowledge, in the form of two key questions: (i) Does what I am reading seem credible in relation to my personal knowledge? (ii) In what ways does this article move my personal knowledge forward? Sometimes, it is necessary to be willing to conclude that what is being read is not sufficiently plausible, as an account of a phenomenon or process: just because it is a piece of 'research' does not mean that it is a valid guide to action. But it is also necessary to be open to the possibility that a research study may function as a catalyst for a new level of understanding and practice, even when set against the accumulated weight of personal knowing.

Reflexivity

Within all research, there is an understanding that it is essential for the reader to be informed about the background and interests of the researcher. For example, studies of medical interventions routinely include information about the links between the researcher and pharmaceutical companies or other relevant groups. In qualitative research, the role of the researcher in the co-construction of knowledge has been widely recognised. In most qualitative studies, the researcher interacts in person with informants, and has the potential to influence their responses in many ways. The analysis of qualitative data involves interpretation of the meaning of statements and actions, and the selection of specific examples that are highlighted in an article or report. Again, the person of the researcher inevitably influences this process. The issue of researcher reflexivity has been discussed at length within the qualitative research literature (see, for example, Finlay & Gough, 2003). Strategies for incorporating awareness of reflexivity into qualitative research design and reporting have been included in guidelines for enhancing the validity of qualitative studies (Elliott, Fischer, & Rennie, 1999). For readers of qualitative studies, there are two ways in which it can be important to know about the identity and experience of the researcher. On the one hand, when reading a study, there is always some level of concern that the researcher is trying to persuade, to 'sell' an approach to therapy or use the research process to verify or reinforce their pre-existing ideas. On the other hand, knowing that a researcher has positively used their previous experience to drive knowledge forward, and has been engaged in a genuine process of discovery, can help a reader to trust the account that is being offered. In either case, it is necessary for the researcher to let the reader know who they are. This is not an easy thing to do. Too much researcher reflexivity can end up with a situation where the actual topic of inquiry gets lost. In other situations, more limited reflexive self-description may not answer the questions that are of concern to the reader. This is likely to be a particular problem for practitioner readers, who are more likely to be willing to make use of researcher findings if they come from a 'trusted source'.

Contextuality

Any single research study, no matter how expertly conducted, is of limited value in itself. Research knowledge exists in the form of the 'literature' – a massive, interconnected, evolving body of studies. It is therefore important, in any research article, to help the reader to make connections between the findings of that study, and the broader knowledge context within which it sites. This is usually accomplished in three ways. In the introduction of the article, the author explains how the study represents a logical and necessary next step in relation to previous research on the topic under investigation. In the method section of an article, the author explains the provenance of the study in relation to the methods of data collection and analysis that were utilised. Finally, the discussion section of the paper looks at how the findings of the study confirm, refute or extend existing knowledge of the topic. The issue of contextuality presents a challenge for qualitative research researchers. On the whole, quantitative research is organised around a linear strategy of knowledge-construction, in which hypotheses are derived from previous theory and research, and then tested in some manner. By contrast, because of its open-ended, inductive nature, qualitative research is not an entirely linear process. The discovery-oriented aspect of qualitative research means that there may be dimensions of the findings, or the implications that could be drawn from the findings, that do not easily fit within the original formulation or plan of the research. This issue can be illustrated through reflection on the findings reported by Davidsen and Fogtmann Fosgerau (2015) into how psychiatrists and GPs interact with patients who have received a diagnosis of depression. The findings of this study are mainly discussed in relation to the theory of mentalisation and the ways in which practitioners may attune themselves to the inner worlds of their clients. However, the findings of this study are equally interesting within the context of research into the ways in which health professionals respond to expressions of emotion by their patients (see, for example, Blanch-Hartigan, 2012). The lack of discussion, by Davidsen and Fogtmann Fosgerau (2015) on the literature on responsiveness to emotion in doctors and nurses, is not intended as a criticism. It is merely that their study illustrates particularly clearly the difficulties faced by all qualitative researchers – the accomplishment of sufficient contextuality within the limits of a research paper. Readers of other papers in this journal issue, or indeed any qualitative papers, often ask themselves 'this is a fascinating study, but how does it relate to my interest in X ...?'

Credibility

Qualitative research needs to strike a balance between obviousness and discovery. Qualitative studies investigate aspects of lived experience of which the reader will already possess some degree of personal knowledge, even if it is only second-hand or third-hand knowledge. Research findings therefore need to map onto that existing knowledge. At least to some extent, findings need to be 'obvious', through being an expression of what is already known or taken-for-granted. However, reading about what you already know is not all that interesting. Good research therefore goes beyond what is known. It clears a space within which new understandings and insights are made available. But are these new insights actually, in some sense, 'true'. The issues around how to establish the validity, credibility or plausibility of qualitative research are complex (Stiles, 1993). Nevertheless, from the point of the reader, the credibility of a study represents a central concern. Basically, readers want to know the extent to which the conclusions arise from the research process or whether the researcher already believed or knew these things, and is merely using the structure of a research paper for the purpose of presenting their ideas in a maximally persuasive manner.

When reading a qualitative paper, a reader is searching for indicators of credibility. One of the main indicators is that the author(s) are willing to acknowledge that readers will be interested in this set of issues, and have made a good-faith attempt to explain what they did and how they did it, in terms of recruitment of participants, data presentation and data analysis. A further, more specific, indicator relates to the number of unanswered questions that accumulate for the reader, as they work their way through a paper. Qualitative researchers tend to be mainly focused on the meaning of what they have found, and rather less good at providing detailed information about the participants, what was done with them, how long it took, where it took place, how many participants contributed to each theme and so on. A further credibility indictor relates to the degree of externality with which emerging themes and findings were scrutinised. Did anyone else look at the data and the conclusions? How fully did the researchers open themselves up to alternative interpretations of the material?

Reading qualitative research

What do we think about when we read a qualitative research article? The issues discussed in the earlier sections of this paper can be condensed into a set of questions:

- What is this paper aiming to achieve?
- How does this help me when I am in the therapy room with a client?
- What made this person/these people want to carry out this study? What is their angle? Do I trust them?
- Where does what I am reading fit into the rest of what I know?
- Is it true? How credible is it? How much of it do I believe?

These questions highlight some important differences between what an author is thinking when he or she writes a qualitative paper, and the subsequent experience and interests of the reader. An author seeks to present the knowledge that he or she has generated, within the format of a research paper. By contrast, a reader arrives at the paper with a broad set of purposes that reflect his or her life experience and professional role. There is an inevitable gap between what the author can offer, and what the reader is looking for.

Conclusion: alternative ways of engaging with the findings of qualitative research

When reading any research paper, it is essential to keep in mind that the article that has been published is not the same as the process of inquiry that was carried out. There are always many stories that can be told about any research study. A research paper represents an effort on the part of the researcher(s) to communicate their aims, methods, findings and understanding within the journal format that is available to them. I have outlined some ways in which the experience of reading a qualitative research paper can be problematic, particularly from the standpoint of practitioners. I would like to use this closing section to explore the possibility that there may be alternative publication formats that may have a role to play in addressing these issues.

Traditionally, it has been the job of the journal editor and reviewers to do their best to close the gap between the author and the reader. Reviewers fulfil a complex set of tasks, which include evaluating papers in accordance with established criteria of good practice in science, while at the same time pointing out ways in which the article might be augmented or altered in order to communicate more effectively to readers. This can be a valuable process; anyone involved in academic journal editing and reviewing will be able to describe occasions when articles have been hugely improved due to the contribution of reviewers. However, it is essential to recognise that, usually, no more than two or three reviewers will read a paper. As a result, it is certain that there would be many questions of potential interest to readers that would just never occur to them, and as a result would not be presented to the author. It is also important to accept that certainty is not attainable in any type of research, and certainly not in qualitative research. No matter how expert and committed journal reviewers and editors might be, it is inevitable that the article that is finally published will represent a good-enough version of the study that was carried out, rather than a perfect one.

The implication here is that it is unlikely that even the most searching and thorough review process will yield an article that answers all the questions that might be of interest to readers. It may be worthwhile, therefore, to consider alternative ways of conveying the findings of qualitative research. Within the current landscape of research dissemination, there are two options that are being actively pursued by various groups: using creative media and using online open access platforms.

In recent years, some qualitative researchers have used creative media as an alternative or adjunct to conventional journal publishing. For example, Haines (2013) interviewed people about work and employment experiences that had been meaningful to them and made them feel happy. This material was presented in a written journal article, and also in a video. Rouse, Armstrong, and McLeod (in press) interviewed therapists about the meaning of creativity in their practice. These participants were also invited to make artworks that conveyed these meanings in a material form, which were disseminated through a book and art exhibition. Other qualitative researchers have communicated their findings through poetry, drama and performance. These forms of research dissemination are generally well received by audiences because they are effective in expressing emotional, felt dimensions of a topic that can get lost in written reports. They also provide a means of communication that that is in tune with the learning and problem-solving style of some research consumers. However, expressive and creative media do not, in themselves, address the questions that may be in the forefront of the minds of therapy practitioners who wish to use qualitative research findings to inform their practice. These modes of research dissemination may be more appropriately regarded as existing within a long tradition of using the arts as a means of promoting public awareness of science. Indeed, within a democratic society, it is necessary and desirable to use all possible means of allowing as wide a proportion of the population as possible to engage constructively with outcomes of scientific research that will affect their lives.

A parallel set of developments within research dissemination has involved the use of online information technology to enable different forms of access to research reports. Open access online journals allow anyone with access to the internet to read research findings. This speeds up the flow of information, opens up research to disadvantaged groups and communities and makes it much easier for practitioners to read research papers. However, removing paywalls and other barriers that restrict readership to those affiliated to universities has been only a first step. Some journals have started to employ open reviewing practices, in which signed reviews are published alongside journal articles. Other journals have adopted review software similar to those used in commercial sites such as Tripadvisor or Amazon, and in many newspapers, which allow anyone to post a review of an article (and allow the author to reply). A useful and comprehensive account of why this is a good idea, and how it can work, can be found in a paper by Nosek and Bar-Anan (2012).

In conclusion, it has been suggested in this paper that qualitative research has a great deal to offer, in relation to building an evidence base that is relevant to the needs and interests of practising counsellors and psychotherapists. However, it would be helpful if those involved in the construction of this kind of research product (researchers, authors, reviewers and editors) could adopt a more dialogical approach to the process of communicating findings. The experience of reading a qualitative paper typically generates many questions that are not answered by the paper itself. If readers could ask these questions, it would give authors the possibility of replying, and also the possibility of learning how to write papers that were more reader-friendly from the start. This kind of dialogue has the potential to allow practitioners to see the value of research through a more active form of involvement. Finally, and of central importance, a key advantage of a more dialogical approach to research writing and reading is that it allows more learning to accrue from each study that is carried out. Authors and researchers may spend many months, or years, carrying out a study. Yet, no matter how immersed they are in the topic, there will always be aspects of their findings and methods that they themselves have not considered, but which have unfolded and been explicated through a later stage of reflection within a broader community or practice. And of course, this could be highly motivating for authors and researchers who, within the present system, typically receive very little reader feedback.

Disclosure statement

No potential conflict of interest was reported by the author.

References

Blanch-Hartigan, D. (2012). An effective training to increase accurate recognition of patient emotion cues. *Patient Education and Counseling, 89*, 274–280. doi:10.1016/j.pec.2012.08.002

Davidsen, A., & Fogtmann Fosgerau, C. (2015). Mirroring patients – Or not. A study of general practitioners and psychiatrists and their interactions with patients with depression. *European Journal of Psychotherapy & Counselling, 17*(2).

Díaz Martínez, F., Solano Pinto, N., Solbes Canales, I., & Calderón López, S. (2015). Eating disorders in the course of life: A qualitative approach to vital change. *European Journal of Psychotherapy & Counselling, 17*(2).

Dreier, O. (2015). Interventions in everyday lives: How clients use psychotherapy outside their sessions. *European Journal of Psychotherapy & Counselling, 17*(2).

Elliott, R., Fischer, C. T., & Rennie, D. L. (1999). Evolving guidelines for the publication of qualitative research studies in psychology and related fields. *British Journal of Clinical Psychology, 38*, 215–229. doi:10.1348/014466599162782

Finlay, L., & Gough, B. (Eds.). (2003). *Reflexivity: A practical guide for researchers in health and social sciences*. Oxford: Blackwell.

Haines, G. (2013). Using documentary to explore the interwoven strands of self-concept and happiness through work: Findings and reflections. *Australian Journal of Career Development, 22*, 36–44. doi:10.1177/1038416213481684

Hill, C. E. (Ed.). (2012). *Consensual qualitative research: A practical resource for investigating social science phenomena*. Washington, DC: American Psychological Association.

Hill, C. E., Knox, S., & Hess, S. A. (2012). Qualitative meta-analyses of consensual qualitative research studies. In C. E. Hill (Ed.), *Consensual qualitative research: A practical resource for investigating social science phenomena* (pp. 159–171). Washington, DC: American Psychological Association.

Kuhn, T. S. (1962). *The structure of scientific revolutions*. Chicago, IL: University of Chicago Press.

McLeod, J. (2013). Qualitative research: Methods and contributions. In M. J. Lambert (Ed.), *Bergin and Garfield's handbook of psychotherapy and behavior change* (5th ed., pp. 49–84). New York, NY: Wiley.

Morrow-Bradley, C., & Elliott, R. (1986). Utilization of psychotherapy research by practicing psychotherapists. *American Psychologist, 41*, 188–197. doi:10.1037/0003-066X.41.2.188

Nosek, B. A., & Bar-Anan, Y. (2012). Scientific Utopia: I. Opening scientific communication. *Psychological Inquiry, 23*, 217–243. doi:10.1080/1047840X.2012.692215

Prochaska, J. O., & DiClemente, C. C. (1983). Stages and processes of self-change of smoking: Toward an integrative model of change. *Journal of Consulting and Clinical Psychology, 51*, 390–395. doi:10.1037/0022-006X.51.3.390

Rouse, A., Armstrong, J., & McLeod, J. (in press). Enabling connections: Counsellor creativity and therapeutic practice. *Counselling and Psychotherapy Research,* doi:10.1002/capr.12019

Roxburgh, E., & Roe, C. (2015). Exploring the meaning in meaningful coincidences: An interpretative phenomenological analysis of synchronicity in therapy. *European Journal of Psychotherapy & Counselling, 17*(2).

Sflakidou, S., & Kefalopoulou, M. (2015). The person centered approach as an ideological discourse: A discourse analysis of person-centered counsellors' accounts on their way of being. *European Journal of Psychotherapy & Counselling, 17*(2).

Smith, J. A., Flowers, P., & Larkin, M. (2009). *Interpretative phenomenological analysis: Theory, method and research.* London: Sage.

Stiles, W. B. (1993). Quality control in qualitative research. *Clinical Psychology Review, 13*, 593–618.

Timulak, L. (2009). Meta-analysis of qualitative studies: A tool for reviewing qualitative research findings in psychotherapy. *Psychotherapy Research, 19,* 591–600. doi:10.1080/10503300802477989

Timulak, L., & Creaner, M. (2013). Experiences of conducting qualitative meta-analysis. *Counselling Psychology Review, 28*, 94–104.

Whose voice are we hearing, really?

Rachel Waddingham

This article, written from the position of someone who has lived experience of therapy for 'psychosis' and an interest in participation, explores the degree to which qualitative research truly conveys the voice and perspective of research participants. By exploring five papers focused on diverse experiences of psychotherapy, from the perspective of clients and therapists, it draws out some of the tensions inherent in making interpretations and connections within research papers and the impact this may have on the quality of any conclusions drawn. Finally, it makes some suggestions for ways of meaningfully involving research participants in the process and argues for an ongoing dialogue to prevent our own assumptions and theoretical frameworks from obscuring the importance of this involvement to improve the quality of future research.

Der Artikel untersucht, inwieweit qualitative Forschung versucht ist, die Sprache und Perspektive von Forschungsteilnehmern wahrheitsgemäß zu transportieren. Hierzu werden fünf Artikel näher betrachtet, die sich mit der Praxis der Psychotherapie aus der Sicht von Klienten und Psychotherapeuten beschäftigen. Auf diesem Hintergrund werden schließlich immanente Spannungen innerhalb der Publikationen offengelegt, die durch das Interpretieren und in Beziehung setzen entstehen und so Auswirkungen auf die Qualität der Ergebnisse haben können. Abschließend werden Vorschläge dahingehend gemacht, wie sich Teilnehmer in einer aussagekräftigeren Art und Weise in den Forschungsprozess einbinden lassen. Darüber hinaus wird für ein permanentes Zwiegespräch mit den Forschungsteilnehmern optiert, um unsere eigenen Prämissen und den verwendeten theoretischen Rahmen davor zu bewahren, dem Moment der Beteiligung keine entscheidende Bedeutung beizumessen. Damit soll schlussendlich die Qualität zukünftiger Forschung verbessert werden.

Este artículo explora el grado en el cual la investigación cualitativa transmite la voz y la perspectiva de los participantes en ella.explorando cinco artículos enfocados en diversas experiencias de psicoterapia, desde la perspecitva de los clientes y los terapeutas, pone de manifiesto algunas de las tensiones inherentes en dar interpretaciones y establecer conexiones en los artículos, acerca de las investigaciones y el impacto que ésto pueda tener en la calidad de las conclusiones. Finalmente, se hacen algunas sugerencias para una participación más significativa de los participantes en el proceso y propone un diálogo continuo para prevenir que nuestras propias suposiciones y marco teórico obscurezcan la importancia de esta participación para mejorar la calidad de las investigaciones futuras.

Il presente contributo intende esplorare quanto la ricerca qualitativa sia davvero in grado di dare voce e di interpretare la prospettiva di coloro che partecipano alla ricerca. Attraverso l'esplorazione dei cinque contributi presenti in questo special issue, basati su diverse esperienze di psicoterapia, considerate sia dal punto di vista dei clienti che dei terapeuti, ci si focalizza su alcuni temi cruciali insiti nell'attività di interpretazione, sugli elementi di contatto presenti nei diversi contributi e sull'impatto che tutto ciò potrebbe avere sulla qualità delle conclusioni della ricerca. Infine, il contributo propone suggerimenti per l'attuazione di strategie di coinvolgimento partecipato nel processo di significazione della ricerca e sostiene la necessità di un dialogo continuo affinché sia evitata l'assunzione di ipotesi e di modelli teorici che potrebbero tacitare l'importanza di tale coinvolgimento, necessario per migliorare la qualità delle ricerche future.

Cet article explore dans quelle mesure la recherche qualitative fait réellement une place à la voix et aux perspectives des participants. L'exploration des cinq articles de ce numéro spécial qui décrivent différentes expériences de la psychothérapie, selon les perspectives des clients ainsi que celles des thérapeutes, permet de mettre l'accent sur les tensions inhérentes aux interprétations et connexions faites entre des articles de recherche et l'impact que cela peut avoir sur la qualité des conclusions tirées. Cet article fait également des suggestions quant à une implication plus significative des participants dans le processus de recherche. Enfin, il plaide en faveur d'un dialogue constant qui nous permettrait d'éviter que nos propres présuppositions et cadres théoriques viennent obscurcir l'importance de notre contribution à l'amélioration de la qualité de futures recherches.

Το παρόν άρθρο διερευνά το βαθμό στον οποίο η ποιοτική έρευνα αποδίδει πραγματικά τη φωνή και την οπτική των συμμετεχόντων στην έρευνα. Μέσα από τη διερεύνηση πέντε άρθρων που εστιάζουν σε διαφορετικές εμπειρίες της ψυχοθεραπείας, από τη σκοπιά των πελατών και των θεραπευτών, σε αυτή την εργασία αναδεικνύονται ορισμένα από τα σημεία έντασης στις ερμηνείες και στις συνδέσεις που γίνονται στις ερευνητικές μελέτες και οι επιπτώσεις που μπορεί αυτό να έχει για την ποιότητα των συμπερασμάτων που εξάγονται. Τέλος, αναφέρονται ορισμένες προτάσεις για τους τρόπους με τους οποίους θα μπορούσαν να εμπλακούν ουσιαστικά οι συμμετέχοντες στην ερευνητική διαδικασία και υποστηρίζεται ότι είναι σημαντικό να υπάρξει συνεχής διάλογος με στόχο να αποτραπεί η πιθανότητα οι δικές μας παραδοχές και θεωρητικά πλαίσια να επισκιάσουν τη σημασία της συμμετοχής αυτής για τη βελτίωση της ποιότητας της μελλοντικής έρευνας.

On first glance, these articles sit uneasily together in a collection exploring people's experience of therapy. The differences between them are huge – in terms of focus, scope, methodology and style. Whereas one article immerses itself in therapists' experiences of synchronistic experiences (Roxburgh, Ridgway, & Roe, 2015) another turns a narrow analytical gaze at the conversations between patients and their doctors (Davidsen & Fogtmann Fosgerau, 2015), eschewing content for structure. So, in preparing my commentary, I found myself treating the articles individually as I struggled to say anything coherent about them as a whole. When the links aren't so obvious it is, perhaps, easier to explore contributions as if they are separate bubbles of information that exist in isolation, disconnected from the whole. To do more than this, to draw links between the bubbles, involves a risk. I must imbue them with my own meaning, my own perspective, to weave the threads that connect them. As such, this response says much more about me than the authors and participants we find between these pages. As someone who has personal experience of therapy (both helpful and unhelpful) and a string of psychiatric diagnoses that I have since confined to the dustbin (including 'schizophrenia') I must also admit to a vague concern gnawing at the edges of my awareness. Will you, the reader, hear my words as I intend them – or will you analyse and interpret my interpretations? This concern was, for a time, a block to forming the words to write this commentary. But, what is life without risk? I, like the participants in the research papers that form this collection, have a voice. After years of struggling to find it – and even more years struggling to be heard – I welcome the opportunity to use it. In this vein, what follows are my personal reflections and engagement with these papers – not academic theory or analysis. This is, perhaps, a departure from 'the norm' – but I hope it will enrich your own exploration of this journal.

Despite the obvious differences between these articles, I see one coloured thread woven into the fabric of each of them – their exploration of connections. Whilst this connectivity is explored in the context of therapy, it goes far beyond this. It shows itself in the connection therapists have with their lived experience of synchronicity experiences (SEs) and the way they weave this into their understanding of the person they are working with. It appears in Díaz Martínez, Solano Pinto, Solbes Canales and Calderón López's (2015) exploration of the way people diagnosed with an eating disorder integrate their life experiences into a pattern that accounts for their journey's twists and turns.

Within the PCA article (Sflakidou & Kefalopoulou, 2015), we read about the connections therapists have with their modality and what this means to them on a deeper level – as well as the connections they intuit or experience with their clients. In the 'Interventions in Everyday Lives' article (Dreier, 2015), the author shares their beliefs about how families connect therapy with their outside lives in all their complexity. Finally, in exploring mirroring in doctor–patient relationships (Davidsen & Fogtmann Fosgerau, 2015), we are encouraged to question the depth and quality of the connections made in specific circumstances. On reflection, it makes sense that this thread appears repeatedly in this tapestry of articles. After all, our connections with our sense of selves, our narrative and those around us are not just the bread and butter of therapeutic relationships – they are the bedrock of the way we experience and talk about our worlds.

In this commentary, I am going to focus on one specific aspect of this theme of connection – our connection with the research participants found within these pages.

Proponents of qualitative research, including myself, often emphasise the power of these methodologies to 'give voice' to the experiences of the participants. Reading a qualitative paper can be engaging. It can paint a vivid and powerful picture that leaves us with a real sense of the people who took part in the study and the perspectives and experiences they chose to share with the researchers. In the field of mental health, this is a welcome antidote to more abstract statistical analyses that sacrifice the complex depth of personal meaning in their search for generalisable 'truths' on which to build clinical practice and channel limited resources. As someone who has had my story analysed, squashed into ill-fitting diagnostic boxes and handed back to me with a bow, I want to believe that the qualitative researcher is well placed to treat people's experiences with respect. When reading qualitative papers, I seek evidence that the researcher can carefully attend to the complex meanings wrapped in our words, phrasing and tone. Ultimately, I want the research participant to feel that they still have ownership of their words and meanings and that any interpretation given by the authors is tentative and recognises the subjectivity inherent in all interpretations. In a field where many have felt their meanings to be stolen, warped or colonised by those with socially legitimised professional 'expertise', this sense of ownership of our own stories feels essential.

As I read through these papers, I found myself entering into an imaginary dialogue with the authors. I was left searching for the perspectives and viewpoints of the research participants, unconvinced that I always knew where to find them. Given that some of these articles feature lengthy, and rich, quotes from participants that arguably give lived experience centre stage – why is it that I was left questioning whose voice I was really hearing?

To illustrate this, I will begin by exploring Díaz Martínez et al. (2015) engaging article on the experiences of people diagnosed with an eating disorder and the change processes they go through throughout their journey. In this article ('Eating Disorders in the course of life'), the authors share some beautiful and rich excerpts from their qualitative interviews. These excerpts tell stories that are familiar to me, on a personal level as well as through my work.

They speak to me, at least, of identity, ownership (over ourselves, our lives and our bodies), trauma and the complexity of our relationships with others. I love that they didn't restrict their gaze purely to the 'defined problem' of an eating 'disorder', but allowed it to flow into the very real issues people have in their lives. Such issues can only be artificially removed from these narratives, stripping them of their meaning and sense. However, despite its many strengths, I found myself wondering – as I often do – what was this experience like for those who took part in the research?

To their credit, the authors explicitly identified a key critique of the trans-theoretical model of change (TMC) and the assumptions that it is built upon. The categorisation of one's situation as problematic 'behaviours' is, at its core, judgemental when the person defining this so-called problem is the one with the power. Yet, in looking specifically for categories of change and exploring how this might map on to the TMC model, I sometimes felt like the authors were sifting through a complex landscape looking for their version of Gold. It was as if intensely personal and meaningful narratives just fell through the net, unheard and unexplored. This feeling weighed heavily on me and relates to an issue I often question when considering research.

I am curious as to whether, on reading this paper, the participants would have felt that their stories had been truly respected and communicated within it. I wonder whether they would have recognised the change processes identified by the authors. I'm curious if they found the themes valuable, or whether reading them left the participants feeling as if their narratives had been stripped of their meaning and utilised for the authors' own academic benefit. Or, more worryingly, I'm wondering if it occurred to the participants, authors and reviewers to ask these questions. Does it feel important to researchers to develop themes in partnership with participants, or even to check them – or do we sometimes assume that once we have the data the process rests in the hands of the 'experts'? Do we write papers with the belief that the participants should have the opportunity to read them and, if we do, would it change the way we write? Specific to this paper and others where therapists are involved in interviewing their own clients for research, how much attention do we give to the power dynamics within the research process – and how honest are we in exploring these when writing them up in a word count that forces us to prioritise the parts of our studies that we believe will be important to those who will read and review them? These are difficult questions, and I'm not the first to ask them, yet they feel important to consider when conducting and reporting research with people.

There is a tension inherent in qualitative research when we ask open questions that elicit a rich narrative yet – to answer our research question – need to restrict our analysis to a narrow aspect of it. When we are looking to identify or explore a process that we are not explicitly asking about, this tension is perhaps more obvious. In doing research such as this, we are looking for underlying processes and themes, and perhaps assuming that if we were to ask the person openly about these processes they would not necessarily give us the answer we seek. Why? We may believe that they are unaware of the 'real' processes that are going on underneath the surfaces. It is as if we – as researchers

– must look for the ripples in an opaque pond to infer the existence of a fish underneath that is making the waves. More than this, some may feel that if we explicitly ask about the matter at hand the very act of asking the direct question will alter the answer that is provided. Instead, we may feel it safer to ask more general questions and then carefully steal sideways glances to view the issue that we are truly interested in. Whilst there is merit to this perspective and it can be argued that few of us are aware of our own 'fish', when we notice the ripples in our own experience. Still, our failure to explicitly engage research participants in our sense-making (either during data collection or analysis) might intrinsically alter the quality of the data we collect and our interpretations of it. The very human challenges we have around recognising the degrees to which we truly hear another's narrative are bound up in this. The more layers we have between what someone says and what we write about – layers of focus, interpretation, thematic analysis and theory generation – the more opportunity we have to obscure the stories of those who generously place their experiences in our hands. The less direct we are about what we are looking for, arguably the more layers we place in between the person and the themes we construct.

The above critique explores the degree to which we change or colonise someone else's story when we draw out themes – and questions how aware we can, or can't, be about doing this. In these cases, the voices of participants were in the article, yet I felt disconnected from them. Later, towards the end of the article, something strange happened. I felt as if the voice of the participants left the room entirely, leaving their parents to take the floor. Whilst the wider study interviewed parents as well as those diagnosed with eating disorders, in this article the authors restricted their focus to those with the diagnosis themselves and the changes they go through. Given the complexity and diversity of the different stories they would have collected, this restriction makes sense to me. However, in explaining their theme of 'pre-contemplation in retrospect', the authors only give us examples of parents who describe times when they struggled to recognise the difficulties faced by their loved one. As valid and engaging as these excerpts are, in an article focusing on the lived experience of people with an eating disorder diagnosis they felt jarring and out of place. I asked – where is *their* voice? As sensible as the theme sounds, based on my own experiences, I was left wondering why the authors made this stark choice that stands out from the rest of their article. I was left wondering whether the participants who had the diagnosis related to this theme at all and, if they did, why their words were not included? If they didn't, then how valid is a theme that needs quotes from parents to justify it – is there another theme that better describes what the participants voiced?

Given the authors' earlier acknowledgement of the difficulties surrounding someone in a position of power identifying the 'problem' and imposing this framework on the individual it concerns, this leap of focus feels very confusing to me. As valid and important as the voices of parents and clinicians are, it feels interesting that the only time we hear their voices is when they identify a problem in the person defined as 'ill'. Are we simply echoing a situation that we see often in the mental health system, where when the person themselves does not agree with our idea of a problem we switch our attention to someone who does? How often do we make these leaps in research or practice, or observe them being made within our teams or organisations? Staying fully present with a person's story, even if it does not fit in to the framework we are hoping for, is a challenge that is harder to meet than one might initially think.

From what was reported, neither of the two papers focusing on the experiences of clients in therapy involved clients in the study's development, implementation or analysis. Without such involvement, there is the danger that those studies that seek to develop theories and interpretations that are grounded in the lived experience of the participants, rather than shaped by pre-existing theories, may be ultimately flawed. It is hard for any of us, myself included, to bracket off structures of knowledge that we have worked so hard to develop and approach interview data with a fresh and open mind. Even if we manage this, this is no guarantee that we are hearing what the participant is trying to communicate to us. If we come from an orientation that places much emphasis on what is not explicitly said, this potential for a disconnect may be even greater. There is no easy resolution to this – yet I would ask that all researchers consider their reasons for not involving participants at all stages of the process. Perhaps, we can make changes if we, together, make a concerted effort to involve more diverse voices into the research arena and support one another by respectfully questioning our assumptions in order to increase our awareness of what possibilities we open and close through the choices we make.

At this juncture, it is perhaps wise to draw my attention to the way in which the papers in this collection dealt with the lived experience of therapists and other clinicians. A natural comparator with the paper described above would be the Interpretative Phenomenological Analysis of synchronicity in therapy (Roxburgh et al., 2015). From what I understand, SEs are experiences that stand out from the crowd – they have an intense felt quality to them that a qualitative interview can elicit and explore openly. As such, it's unsurprising that I felt much more connected to the voices of participants more strongly in this paper. The quotes provided were rich and felt more directly linked to the interpretations and themes provided.

Whilst the different methodologies used by the researchers may account for much of this, I'm curious if there are any other layers to this. How might the position of the researchers and the participants impact on the process? I think it's striking that, for me, the first two themes ('a sense of connectedness' and 'therapeutic process') were the ones that I felt more strongly connected to. They jumped off the page at me and I found myself nodding along, seeing the links the authors made in the quotes they provided. Why is this striking? The one theme I felt less connected to was 'professional issues'. Such a title seems rather distant and cold in comparison to the descriptive nature of the others. This seemed even more disjointed when I read how the authors described the often profound impact of SEs on the therapists involved – even to the extent of 'challenging their reality'. I am curious as to why such deep and personal material is allocated such a stark and unemotive title. This theme was the only one that dealt, purely, with therapists' perspectives whereas the others more heavily featured their beliefs about the utility of SEs for client work and therapeutic relationships. I do not know if this difference is as significant as it feels to me – nor what may account for it – but it makes me curious to know more. I am left wondering whether it relates, at all, to the position of the researchers and their relationship to the subject matter. Or, perhaps, that for a therapist the term 'professional issues' is imbued with meaning that I am unable to see. After all, our profession can be central to our sense of self and our place in the world. Perhaps, my position as a non-therapist means that I am simply reading it differently than the authors intended.

The Davidsen and Fogtmann Fosgerau's paper takes a different approach, entirely. Rather than asking participants about their experiences outright, they used conversational analysis to explore the interactions of doctors and patients in minute detail. As someone who has seen more than their fair share of doctors, I found this paper fascinating and imbued it with all of my own meaning and experiences. Yet, when considering the issues of connection and 'voice', I began to feel uneasy once more. Whilst it is, perhaps, easiest for me to fill this paper with my own experience and sense-making, I began to feel a heavy absence and became curious once more. I wanted to speak to the doctors and patients and ask them what they felt about participating in this study.

On my first reading I had made the assumption that the GPs, showing evidence of what the authors suggest is 'implicit mentalisation' are creating a more human relationship with their patients. I had also felt some annoyance at the behaviour of the psychiatrists who seemed uninvolved and unresponsive to their patient's distress. I connected with my version of what these patients needed/wanted based on what I, as a human and an ex-patient, needed and wanted. My interpretation, as always, said more about me than the participants. But, when stepping back and really trying to listen for the voice of the participants I began to shift. I wondered what would have happened if we had asked the patients, and the doctors, what their experience of the interaction had been. Whilst we might assume the GP interactions with their non-verbal, tonal and expressed connection would feel more validating to someone in distress. Is this the case, or did it – sometimes – feel patronising or as if the participant was getting a surface-level response that sounded empathic but didn't feel it? Whilst we might assume the less responsive psychiatrist response may feel cold and uncomfortable, did it in fact leave some patients feeling like they had a respectful space from which to experience and communicate their own feelings in their own way. After all, the same set of behaviours, recorded on video, may feel validating to one and oppressive to another. This is a point I never imagined I'd make in a paper, and it's one I think that may leave my previous psychiatrists to sit down. I myself prefer someone to be expressive – but that's the point. Despite my lived experience of psychiatry, I am not in a position to be able to infer meaning in the bubble of a conversation by looking in on it from the outside. I need to be able to talk with people, engage with them in an open and respectful manner in order to collaboratively form a story about it. Yet, when we read papers, we are reliant on the authors to have done this for us – and for them to be able to communicate their process as fully as possible so we can understand how they came to their conclusions. Analysing specific aspects interactions or narratives without paying some attention to the complexity of the whole invites a disconnect that we must work consciously to mitigate.

So, what are we to do? Despite these challenges, qualitative research remains, for me, a step forward from more positivist assumptions of knowledge and objectivity. This is far from simple, however. On the one hand, we understand that people's lived experience of the world is nuanced, complex and intrinsically bound up with millions of different stories, factors and ideas (with are, in turn, tied to an array of other stories, factors and ideas). On the other, we feel the need to analyse, draw conclusions and develop theories to understand the worlds of ourselves and others. As such, we attempt to filter out some of the parts of experience that seem extraneous to the matter in hand, whilst retaining a sense of the context that makes these methodologies so powerful. As we have seen, the line between that is essential and what feels extraneous is difficult to draw. More than this, if researchers are conducting their research from a position of privilege their perception of where this line should be drawn – and the decisions they make because of it – may be a world away from the perspective of the people participating in their study. How are we, as readers, to make sense of whose voice we are hearing within the pages?

I don't come to this commentary with concrete solutions. If I did, I would perhaps be much richer than I am and have a whole host of books under my belt. As it is, I come with some ideas – but more importantly I come inviting a continued dialogue. It is not as simple as asking direct and explicit questions to participants, nor being transparent about whether we check out our interpretations with participants and record points of difference. The answer is not a participation checklist, nor is it relying on individual researchers to bracket off their own assumptions or expecting readers to hold on to the tentativeness of interpretations and how deeply they are embedded in the researcher's experience of their connection with the participant. It feels, to me, like the answer is something we need to develop in conversation – with each of us inviting opposing and different viewpoints to enable us to more readily question our own. One of the issues, I think, is that we have accepted a certain way of conducting research without fully feeling able to critique ourselves, and it, in the process. The pressures of funding, the peer review process and the expectations of readers sometimes lead us into making unfortunate shortcuts that speak volumes to those of us who have been on the receiving end of research. Proper involvement needs planning, funding and – most of all – space to think. It can happen, but it is not yet the norm. However, it is something I would like us to commit to developing to increase the quality of the research we are conducting. Qualitative research, and the papers in this collection, all provide some interesting and engaging insights into therapeutic relationships. What more could we accomplish if we worked together in a more collaborative way?

Disclosure statement

No potential conflict of interest was reported by the author.

References

Davidsen, A., & Fogtmann Fosgerau, C. (2015). Mirroring patients – Or not. A study of general practitioners and psychiatrists and their interactions with patients with depression. *European Journal of Psychotherapy & Counselling, 17*(2). doi: 10.1080/13642537.2015.1027785

Díaz Martínez, F., Solano Pinto, N., Solbes Canales, I., & Calderón López, S. (2015). Eating disorders in the course of life: A qualitative approach to vital change. *European Journal of Psychotherapy & Counselling, 17*(2). doi: 10.1080/13642537. 2015.1027782

Dreier, O. (2015). Interventions in everyday lives: How clients use psychotherapy outside their sessions. *European Journal of Psychotherapy & Counselling, 17*(2). doi: 10.1080/13642537.2015.1027781

Roxburgh, E., Ridgway, S., & Roe, C. (2015). Exploring the meaning in meaningful coincidences: An interpretative phenomenological analysis of synchronicity in therapy. *European Journal of Psychotherapy & Counselling, 17*(2). doi: 10.1080/ 13642537.2015.1027784

Sflakidou, S., & Kefalopoulou, M. (2015). The person centered approach as an ideological discourse: A discourse analysis of person-centered counsellors' accounts on their way of being. *European Journal of Psychotherapy & Counselling, 17*(2). doi: 10.1080/13642537.2015.1027783

Therapeutic community for children with diagnosis of psychosis: What place for parents? The relation between subject and the institutional 'Other'

Katia Romelli and Giuseppe Oreste Pozzi

ABSTRACT
This contribution explores the perspective of a group of parents whose children are hosted in a residential community in Northern Italy. This community hosts children with diagnosis of psychosis, separated from their families by medical decision or by judgement. This compulsory separation leads to a relationship between the institutional network and parents characterised by a struggle for power. In Hegelian terms, there is a creation of an imaginary relation between *master* and *slave*. In this situation, three main questions emerged: (1) What can be done with the parental suffering, anguish and aggression caused by this separation? (2) Where placing these affections inside the institutional work with children? (3) What effect will produce this situation, on the institutional transference? A place named 'Parents' place' was created. During these meetings, parents were invited to speak about their own children with the professionals of the community. Using a theory-driven conceptual framework, Imaginary and Symbolic registers of Lacan, the transcripts of this meeting group were analysed. Analysis highlights how this work with parents allows elaborating in a symbolic way this separation, producing a symbolic adjustment of the imaginary relationship between the network of institutions and parents with consequences on the clinical practice with children.

COMUNIDAD TERAPEUTICA PARA NiñOS CON DIAGNOSTICO DE PSICOSIS: el lugar de los padres. La relación entre el sujeto y el 'otro' institucional

Este artículo explora la perspectiva de un grupo de padres cuyos niños son huéspedes en una comunidad residencial en el Norte de Italia, la cual ha sido destinada a niños con diagnóstico de psicosis y han sido separados de sus padres por decisión médica o dictamen jurídico. Esta separación obligatoria conduce a una relación entre la red institucional y los padres que se caracteriza por una lucha de poder. En términos hegelianos existe la creación de una relación imaginaria entre amo y esclavo. En esta situación emergen tres preguntas: 1. Qué se puede hacer por el sufrimiento parental, la angustia y la agresión causadas por la separación? 2. Dónde colocar estos afectos dentro del trabajo institucional con losniños? 3. Qué efecto tundra esta situación en la transferencia con la institución? Se creó un espacio llamado "el lugar de lospadres".Durante las reunions se invitó a los padres a conversar acerca de sus niños con los profesionales de la comunidad. Se analizaron las transcripciones de las reunions de los grupos utilizando el marco conceptual de la teoría de los instintos y los registros imaginario y simbólico de Lacan. Se destacó cómo este trabajo con los padres, les permitió elaborar la separación de una manera simbólica, produciendo un ajuste también simbólico de la imaginaria relación entre la red de instituciones y los padres, el cual dejó consecuencias en la práctica clínica con los niños.

Comunità Terapeutica per i bambini con diagnosi di psicosi: quale posto per i genitori? La relazione tra soggetto e istituzionale 'Altro'

Questo contributo esplora il punto di vista di un gruppo di genitori i cui figli sono ospitati in una comunità terapeutica residenziale nel Nord Italia. Questa comunità ospita i bambini con diagnosi di psicosi, separati dalle loro famiglie per una decisione medica o a causa di una sentenza. Questa separazione obbligatoria comporta un rapporto tra genitori e rete istituzionale caratterizzato da una lotta di potere. In termini hegeliani, si crea una relazione immaginaria tra padrone e schiavo. In questa situazione emergono tre questioni fondamentali: 1) cosa si può fare con la sofferenza dei genitori, l'angoscia e l'aggressività causata da questa separazione? 2) dove collocare questi sentimenti entro il lavoro istituzionale con i bambini? 3) Quali effetti produrrà questa situazione, sul transfert istituzionale? È stato creato un luogo chiamato "spazio genitori". Durante gli incontri i genitori sono stati invitati a parlare dei propri figli con i professionisti della comunità. Le trascrizioni di questi incontri di gruppo sono state analizzate utilizzando un quadro concettuale guidato dalla teoria che fa refereimnto al registro Immaginario e al registro Simbolico di Lacan. L'analisi evidenzia come questo lavoro con i genitori consenta di elaborare in modo simbolico la separazione, producendo una regolazione simbolica della relazione immaginaria tra la rete istituzionale e i genitori con ricadute sulla pratica clinica con i minori.

Communauté thérapeutique pour les enfants avec un diagnostic de psychose : quelle place pour les parents ? La relation entre le sujet et l'Autre institutionnel

Cette contribution explore la perspective d'un groupe de parents dont les enfants sont accueillis dans une communauté résidentielle du nord de l'Italie. Cette communauté accueille les enfants avec un diagnostic de psychose séparés de leur famille soit par une décision médicale soit par une décision de justice. Cette séparation obligatoire entraîne une relation entre le réseau institutionnel et les parents se caractérisant par une lutte de pouvoir. En terme hégélien c'est la création d'une relation imaginaire entre le maître et l'esclave. Dans cette situation trois questions principales ont émergé : 1) que peut-on faire pour les parents qui ressentent angoisse et agression du fait de la séparation? 2) où situer ces problèmes dans le cadre du travail institutionnel avec les enfants? 3) quels sont les effets d'une telle situation sur le transfert institutionnel ? Un lieu nommé « le lieu des parents » a été créé. Lors de ces réunions les parents étaient invités à parler de leurs enfants avec les professionnels de la communauté. En faisant référence à un cadre théorique et conceptuel, les registres imaginaire et symbolique de Lacan, les retranscriptions de ces réunions ont été analysées. L'analyse montre comment ce travail avec les parents permet l'élaboration symbolique de la séparation, produit un ajustement symbolique de la relation imaginaire entre le réseau des institutions et les parents avec des conséquences sur la pratique clinique auprès des enfants.

Θεραπευτικές κοινότητες για παιδιά με διάγνωση ψύχωσης: Υπάρχει χώρος για τους γονείς; Η σχέση ανάμεσα στο υποκείμενο και στο έγκλειστο «άλλο»

ΠΕΡΙΛΗΨΗ

Αυτό το άρθρο διερευνά τις απόψεις μιας ομάδας γονέων των οποίων τα παιδιά φιλοξενούνται σε έναν κοινοτικό ξενώνα στη Βόρεια Ιταλία. Αυτή η κοινότητα φιλοξενεί παιδιά με διάγνωση ψύχωσης, που μένουν μακριά από τις οικογένειες τους μετά από ιατρική ή δικαστική απόφαση. Αυτός ο υποχρεωτικός χωρισμός οδηγεί στη διαμόρφωση μιας σχέσης ανάμεσα στο δίκτυο και στους γονείς η οποία χαρακτηρίζεται από μια πάλη για τη δύναμη. Με όρους του Hegel δημιουργείται μια φαντασιακή σχέση ανάμεσα σε ένα αφέντη και σε ένα δούλο. Σε αυτή την κατάσταση εγείρονται τρεις βασικές ερωτήσεις: 1) τι μπορεί να γίνει με το «πάσχειν» των γονέων και την επιθετικότητα που προκαλείται από τον χωρισμό; 2) Που μπορούν να εισαχθούν αυτά τα συναισθήματα στη δουλειά με τα παιδιά στο ίδρυμα; 3) τι επίδραση μπορεί να έχει αυτή η κατάσταση στην ιδρυματική μεταβίβαση; Δημιουργήθηκε ένας χώρος ο οποίος ονομάστηκε «Ο χώρος των γονέων». Κατά τη διάρκεια αυτών των συναντήσεων οι γονείς προσκλήθηκαν να μιλήσουν για τα παιδιά τους με τους επαγγελματίες του Κέντρου. Οι συνομιλίες αυτής της συνάντησης αναλύθηκαν με τη χρήση του θεωρητικού εννοιολογικού πλαισίου του Lacan για το Φαντασιακό και το Συμβολικό. Η ανάλυση τονίζει πως η εργασία με τους γονείς επιτρέπει να εμπλουτιστεί συμβολικά αυτός ο χωρισμός, παράγοντας μια συμβολική προσαρμογή της φαντασιακής σχέσης ανάμεσα στο δίκτυο των ιδρυμάτων και των γονέων με συνέπειες στην κλινική πράξη με τα παιδιά.

Background

Working in a therapeutic community (TC) for children means taking care of children and, at the same time, taking care of their families' problems (Baio, 2004; De Halleux, 2010). Indeed, in a TC, treatment is oriented not only toward the problems that brought the children into the residential community but also toward helping the family's system to manage and continue to work on those problems, so that the children can return home from residential treatment. In the last decades, several studies have shown how parental involvement reduces the stress related to the separation of children from families and is associated with shorter lengths of stay in foster care (that is, Frensch & Cameron, 2002; Merritts, 2016; Tam & Ho, 1996). In this vein, working with parents appears, on the one hand, to be a sine qua non condition for managing and developing a possible therapeutic project but, on the other hand, introduces peculiar difficulties and moments of deadlock (Baker, Heller, Blacher, & Pfeiffer, 1995; McDonald, Owen, & McDonald, 1993) for mental health professionals that they must be able to manage. For the family, transitioning to a residential community is associated with high levels of stress and a sense of failure and guilt (Frensch & Cameron, 2002; Goldberg, 1991). Moreover, as argued by Frensch and Cameron (2002), 'placing a child in residential treatment can leave a family feeling vulnerable and fearful due to a perceived threat to a family's autonomy, coupled with the exposure of family idiosyncrasies during treatment' (p. 308). This is especially true, considering that residential communities admit children and adolescents who have been separated from their families through decisions made by public mental health agencies or juvenile justice authorities, after hospital stays, or, sometimes, by parents who are no longer able to cope with the behaviour of their own children. As a consequence, the parents' perspectives of and relationships with the institutions involved in moving their children into treatment are negative and often characterised by claims, conflicts, and frustration (De Halleux, 2010). Hence, the presence of the TC indicates to the family the crisis moment experienced by one of its members and the difficulty of the other members in helping and supporting him/her, or the dysfunctional models that characterised the familiar dynamics. These circumstances may affect clinical practice with young patients and the development of treatment projects.

Considering the ambivalence that characterises the relations between parents and institutional network in moving children to residential care, this study presents a way of working with parents to make their relations with the TC less problematic. This method is rooted in Lacanian psychoanalysis, which provides a theoretical conceptualisation through which the dynamics characterising the emerging relationship between parents and the TC can be analysed. In particular, the methodology introduced with this work is influenced by Lacanian reflections about the concepts of psychosis and otherness (Lacan, 1949/2002, 1953/2002, 1959/2006), while strongly influenced by the reading of Hegel's (1807/1976) dialectic of master and slave as well as the tradition of Lacanian psychoanalytic practice for children with psychosis and autistic spectrum disorders, which began in Belgium at the beginning of the 1970s (Baio, 1993; De Halleux, 2010; Di Ciaccia, 2005).

Intersubjective relations and struggle of power: Hegel with Lacan

Drawing on Hegelian reflections, Lacan suggests a conception of human subjectivity rooted in mutuality and based on the development of self-consciousness in encounters with another subject. Inspired by Hegel's texts, Lacan argued that the master–slave dialectic is most informative for mapping this logic. Inside the relation between master and slave, the master's satisfaction is met through the subordination of others. In this vein, the slave only exists to affirm the master's superiority of the master and to take care of the master and the master's desires. The master is regarded as an oppressor and a frustrating authority who deprives his or her slave of freedom and is the cause of the slave's discomfort. Moreover, the realisation of mutuality is doomed to failure, because the subject can be satisfied by recognition from one whom the subject recognises as being worthy of recognising him. The slave unsatisfied with his condition craves and attempts to realise a world in which his value will finally be recognised and his own desires satisfied. However, the result of this struggle of power, expressive of autonomy, is an impasse as not a mutual recognition because this restoring the master and slave dialectic. Thus, adequate recognition can only be achieved within an institutionalised order that secures truly mutual recognition – in other words, through the introduction of a third element: the guarantee of the intersubjective relation. Beyond this condition, we do not have recognition but a dialectic characterised by inequality, division and subordination.

Otherness in the Lacanian perspective: Imaginary and symbolic registers

Throughout his teachings, Lacan (1949/2002, 1953/2002) distinguishes two different forms of otherness which differentiate between imaginary and symbolic modes of relating: the *other*, with a lowercase 'o', and the *Other*, with an uppercase 'O'. The first case of otherness emerges through the narrative of the *mirror stage*, as an explanation of the genesis and functions of the Freudian psychic agency of the *ego* (Lacan, 1949). This reflection relies on empirical observation of infants and their ability to identify their own images in a mirror, which is matched with feelings of rejoicing and fascination. Due to a biological lack of sensory and motor coordination, infants' self-experience is fragmented and only gradually becomes organised through this recognition of a self-image. In the Lacanian vein, the other, with a lowercase 'o', designates the imaginary ego and its accompanying alter ego (Vanheule & Verhaeghe, 2009). Indeed, infants discern their self-image from images of the others through this perception; consequently, it is in the outside world that the ego is constituted and one's sense of identity is established. Furthermore, identity is acquired by ascribing characteristics in a relational matrix through the positioning with someone else. In other words, humans gain a sense of unity by assuming characteristics to someone else and relating with this assumptions. For this reason, imaginary identification is accompanied by a tendency towards misrecognition and, at the same time, inaugurates aggressive rivals and conflicts (Lacan, 1948). This is why the imaginary relations appear as a dyadic world characterised by a permanent fluctuation between the image of the ego-ideal and the effects of antagonism and aggression. Still, the human world is not limited to this imaginary fluctuation because it is immersed in language.

From the Lacanian point of view, the subject is an effect of the language, and the Other, with an uppercase 'O', is a place of language (Lacan, 1953). Thus, if the other represents a relation with a similar someone with whom I might identify, by contrast, the Other is a code and stands beyond the realm of imaginary identifications. For this reason, the imaginary fluctuations are subordinate to a symbolic order. Indeed, the Other is defined as a set of communicative rules and symbolic codes which forms the ground of all meaning-making. According to Hook (2008), 'the Other remains always radically exterior, beyond the horizon of any conceivable intersubjectivity' (p. 55). It entails the Other being a kind of 'supra-agency' (Hook, 2008, p. 55) that envelops the subject even before he or she was born and determines it. As Lacan claims, speaking means asking to be heard. In other words, it means asking to be recognised as a subject. The symbolic Other responds to this need for recognition by guaranteeing the grounds for relationships among people: the Other ensures membership inside an order that makes affiliations and exchanges within society both possible and intelligible. In closing, we can affirm that the Other gives place to a subject, fixes the imaginary fluctuation, and allows the relationship between subject and society.

Psychosis and otherness in the Lacanian perspective

The meeting mode that occurs with the otherness structures the subject's psychic reality, in terms of neurosis, psychosis, or perversion (Lacan, 1946). Although it could be possible to highlight different stages in Lacanian reflections about psychosis, the core of these conceptualisations was always the subject–Other relationship. As Vanheule (2011) suggests, psychosis could be read through a 'mirror-and-meaning paradigm' (p. 16); with psychosis, the subject is captured in a dual dimension which excludes the third: the symbolic Other. In this perspective, the psychotic structure concerns the radical exclusion of the bond with the Other as well as the closure of the subject in an imaginary dyadic relation;

in this way, the imaginary fluctuations are not subordinate and are oriented by symbolic order. As a consequence, the psychotic structure implies a relation with others in term of similarity. Also, the differentiation between self and other is weak, with affections of confusion, ambivalence, and intrusion, since with psychosis, the subject is not guaranteed due to the absence of symbolic limits and is at the mercy of the other. Indeed, what characterises psychosis is the subject's position in relation to language, since with psychosis, the subject is outside of the dialectic of recognition. Hence, the subject shows a peculiar relation with the Other, who appears as the Other of deprivation. In this vein, this structural reflection about psychosis clarifies that the basic structure of psychosis is present as functioning before and beyond the triggering of psychosis because it concerns a mode of identification in social relationships. The weakness of the symbolic order deletes the possibility of social bonds; indeed, language is a cultural product which aims to create rules of social coexistence.

The identificatory structure characterising psychosis affects treatment because the withdrawal or rejection that children and youth with a psychotic structure present in front of the other suggests a relationship experienced as threatening. This observation imposes that treatment must be oriented to the pacification of this relation, first of all, in sweeping away any pedagogical, adaptive, and normalising therapeutic motives and obligations destined to increase the rejection of the relation with the other (Baio, 1993; Di Ciaccia, 2005). The treatment, on the one hand, concerns putting a range of 'possibilities' at the residents' disposition, in terms of distractions, occupations or creativity inside and outside of the institution, so that the residents might use the possibilities as they wish, if it pleases them. This disposition is a possible path to an identificatory ideal, through which to treat the Other and –accept a possible social bond. Thus, it does not concern therapeutic activities to which the subject must submit, but a series of possibilities offered to the 'spontaneous work of psychosis' (Zenoni, 2002, p. 8). On the other hand, the treatment implies work with the Other by the hosts, both institutional and familiar. In treatment, it is important not to occupy the position of the third, of the Other, but rather for the therapist to be placed on the same side as the subject facing this Other. In treatment, staff is involved both as witness and support for the solutions that the subjects themselves pose as a guarantee of order and a limit facing the intrusive Other, introducing the limit that the imaginary dyadic relations preclude. The treatment of psychosis is the treatment of the Other and not of the subject.

Method

Setting: The TC

For this study, we worked with a TC in a small town located in Northern Italy that provides accommodations for eight residents. The TC was created to accommodate children and adolescents until the age of 18 with diagnoses of psychosis and autistic spectrum disorders. The residents stay in the TC for an average of 24 months. The working principles of the community are informed by Lacanian psychoanalysis. However, therapeutic interventions are based on a bio–psycho–social approach; for this reason, the professional team is multidisciplinary and made up of psychotherapists, psychiatrists, nurses and educators. The therapeutic projects consist of activities outside of the community, such as schools, gymnasiums, and centres of aggregation; frequent internal activities, such as workshops and group and individual support; and periodical stays with resident's family.

Instrument

Creation of the Parents' Place meeting group

The compulsory separation introduced by admission to a TC creates two groups, at an imaginary level: the institution group vs. the family group. The institution group is assembled by experts who have knowledge, exercise parental responsibility and take decisions. The family group is assembled by parents who have been evaluated as not being able, lacking resources and being in a helplessness position. In other words, an imaginary relation is created between master and slave. In the TC presented in this paper, a meeting group named Parents' Place (PP) was created to manage this circumstance and its imaginary effects. During these meetings, parents were invited to speak with the community staff about their own children. The hypothesis that led to the creation of the PP meeting group was to produce a symbolic adjustment of the imaginary relationship established between the network of institutions and parents through the introduction of a symbolic order that both the TC and parents underwent.

This decision instituted a new clinical practice with parents in the TC and, at the same time, a longitudinal research aimed at monitoring and evaluating the clinical effects of this decision.

Structure and functioning of Parents' Place

Some points were set to create a symbolic framework for the PP:

(1) All parents are invited every 15 days to speak about their own sons/daughters. Every time a new parent or family participates in a PP session, the group's facilitator reads a message about the goal of the meetings:

Good evening. Let me introduce myself. I'm a psychologist and the facilitator of this meeting group. The PP is aimed at creating a place to speak about the knowledge that parents have about their own sons and daughters. The transcript of this meeting will be read by a panel of professionals, and the panel will provide a 'receipt' about the topics that emerged in the meeting. This receipt will be read at the beginning of the following meeting.

(2) One facilitator – a psychologist member of the TC's professional team – and one recorder will attend the meeting.

(3)   Every meeting will be transcribed verbatim, and the excerpts will be read by a panel formed by psychotherapists trained in Lacanian psychoanalysis. The reading of these excerpts provides a 'receipt' which highlights the themes that emerged among the parents during PP but does not contain explanations, comments or interpretations. The receipt would be the sign of the presence of someone who has heard and recognised what the parents said. The receipt starts with this sentence: 'Good evening. We will start with the receipt. We are here to verify if we understood what you said during the last meeting. In the last meeting, it emerged that ...'

Analysis and corpus

Patterns within the data were identified in a theoretical or 'top-down' way (Braun & Clarke, 2006), bearing upon the Lacanian concept of discourse. As Parker (2005) suggests:

> A Lacanian approach to discourse has consequences for the way we think of 'criteria' for research. It sets itself against attempts to arrive at a richer, more complete understanding of a text. Lacanian discourse analysis would require a quite different perspective on the reading of texts, a perspective that focused on deadlocks of perspective. (p. 175)

Indeed, although the human subject is defined by the act of speaking, and although psychoanalysis is an attempt to highlight the effects of speech on the subject, Lacanian analysis forgoes a form of interpretation that aims to reveal 'signifieds' submerged in the text or the internal world of speakers (Parker & Pavón Cuéllar, 2013; Pavón Cuéllar, 2010). At the core of a Lacanian discourse analysis is the identification of blockage points around which the text is constructed and revolves. These anchoring points – named *quilting points* – are linked to certain signifiers or metaphorical substitutes; they keep the signifying system in place and show something about the structure of the discourse and the position of the subject within it (Parker, 2005). These quilting points are the foundation of speech because they have a predominant role in subjectivity and society; we can identify as anchoring points all signifiers around which the subject and the culture organise their own identities (Laclau & Mouffe, 2001). That is, these quilting points provide stability to the signifying system but, at the same time, are the way through which the imaginary identifications emerge. In this vein, each description is not merely a description but an attempt to provide the quilting point that anchors the others. Hence, the delimiting of these rhetorical strategies shows how the subject shapes social bonds through language; in other words, they show the subject–Other relationship.

Within this theoretical perspective, members of the panel and the authors read the excerpts of the PP session. The transcripts were subdivided into fragments, each covering a different idea that was brought up in the PP group meetings. Both the members of the panel and the authors separately studied the transcripts to identify patterns and recurring structures. Consequently, they consulted each other to discuss these patterns. This resulted in the identification of five specific patterns. Pattern 1 is related to arguments about relations with the institutional network. For Pattern 2, we gathered opinions, perceptions and affects towards the TC. Pattern 3 includes definitions, viewpoints and ideas that the parents expressed about the mental illness of their own sons and daughters. Pattern 4 was related to negative feelings, such as the shame that parents could feel towards their friends, neighbours or colleagues. Pattern 5 included fantasies, fears, expectations and desires about the future.

Based on the focus of this paper, we only present the results related to Patterns 1 and 2 because they are the patterns in which emerged the relations among the institutional network, TC and parents. We present and discuss these patterns to check and investigate the switches from imaginary identification to symbolic recognition.

The corpus constitutes all of the transcripts of the PP meetings conducted in 2015. The families involved in the present study signed an informed consent form giving their approval for the use of the material.

Findings

Pattern 1: Relations with institutional network

We present two extracts taken from the first session attended by parents of a young boy aged 9, 10 days after his admission in the residential community. The mother is identified by the code M1, the father as F1 and the facilitator as by PSY.

Extract 1:

M1: I don't know what to say … I feel lost.

PSY: How many days has your son been in TC?

M1: He's been there for ten days. I feel lost; without him, my life has no sense. We have arrived … my husband and I used to quarrel quite often, and the social worker decided to send us to a mother–infant community. I called her horrible names. It was hard for me; it was like being in jail. Now, I'm being treated by a psychiatrist, but I have no psychopathologies. I have anxiety with depressive traits; for this reason, I drink wine. But I've never hit my son – not a slap, not a scream.

F1: The worst is over. He is quiet now.

M1: No, the judge was cruel to me. The things they said about me were wrong!

Extract 2:

PSY: The residential staff will learn to know him and will provide the necessary treatment project.

F1: That's okay to me; I just want him to be okay. I do not want a doll stuffed with drugs.

M1:   He is a little boy. You can work with him. I trust in you. You are my hope.

F1:   He was to come here immediately; moreover, the TC is closer to home ... I can't accept my son not improving.

In the first part of the session, the mother described experiences with the institutional network – composed of social services, the juvenile court, and a previous educational community for mothers and child – while the second part, the parents spoke about the TC. The signifiers that appeared in the texts are related to two different semantic areas: in the first extract, the mother used the signifiers 'jail' and 'cruel', through which an image emerged of the other as harsh and malevolent; in the second extract, the signifiers were linked to 'hope' and trust, and on the imaginary level, the community emerged as *the right place* because it was an idealised place. Although feeling hopeful at the beginning of a new treatment may be understandable, this situation again proposed two separate groups. The group of professionals was identified as experts who have knowledge, in Lacanian words, and identified with the position of *tout savoir* (Lacan, Lacan, 1969–1970/2007). Hence, this is another form of the imaginary relation between master and slave.

During a PP meeting, the mother (M2) of a boy aged 13 talked about the institutional network:

M2:   I call the lawyer. The court doesn't want to show me the files ... they want to hide something. At the beginning, my son was treated by the psychiatric department of V. (town in Northern Italy). In the psychiatric department, four cops had to stop me; otherwise, I would have killed everyone! The district should have had to help us, and instead, it took away our son. I can't take it anymore. There are people who raped, and look at it, look what they did to us!

Even though the meeting from which this extract was drawn occurred one year after the boy's admission into the community, the text presents a high level of frustration and aggression. The mother presents all of the social actors who played a role in the decision to separate the boy from his family: the juvenile court, social services and the psychiatric department. The mother did not provide an explicit description of the institutional network, and it was not easy to identify peculiar signifiers linked to these social actors; however, the public institutions clearly appeared as malevolent and persecutory. Considering that identity is acquired by assuming characteristics through positioning with someone else, this negative image of the institutional network emerged through the parent's positioning, related to sadness ('I can't take it anymore'), frustration and helplessness ('look what they did to us!'), and aggression ('I would killed everyone!'). Furthermore, from our point of view, it is interesting to highlight how all of these institutions overlapped and were condensed into a single image. All of the differences in their roles and positions were erased, and all that was unfamiliar – in this case, because of the public institutions – became one.

Pattern 2 – relations with the TC

In this paragraph, we present extracts related to the relationship between the parents and the TC. In the first extract, the parents (M3 and F3) of a boy aged 14 who arrived at the TC 2 years beforehand described the meeting that they had with a district social worker and complained about the head of the professional team at the TC (HPT). This boy is the youngest of four brothers; all of them were separated from their parents and admitted to educational or therapeutic communities; for this reason, the family had been involved with several public agencies for many years.

F3:   I wanted to start saying one thing … the last meeting I had with the social worker went badly … HPT wasn't a man of his word. He said that he would call after the team's meeting on Friday, and on the contrary, he moved forward with the issue of the community meeting. So, you should ask HPT if he is afraid of the social workers of G. (town in Northern Italy). He must tell the social worker that we want our own child back home.

M3:   No! They must not say that he has dumb parents! We are not dumb! They have killed me; suddenly, they took my son, and he never came back home. And now, they are reducing the visiting time from 2 hours to 1; you have to prove to them that we are able to stand 2 hours with our son. And, why now should we have you as a watchdog?

PSY: Listen, we read the decree and have to conform to it. I understand your position. Maybe it is too strong … I don't know … but we have to respect it; we have no choice.

F3:   You have to overstep it! Come on!

PSY: Well, I understand your point of view and your suffering, but if we don't adhere to the conditions, we make the situation worse, and they could have more reasons to act in an even more severe way. HPT will speak with the social worker – it is the procedure – but there are technical times to respect. Moreover, the social worker will read our report. Maybe there will be a change, but we can't say anything now. Unfortunately, you have to be patient …

M3:   Well, that's fine. This thing scared us. The previous HPT made us feel like 'parents'; we felt that we were not the parents described in the decree. This is a nightmare to me. I cry. I'm feeling bad … and then when we arrived in the TC, we didn't find the previous HPT, but a new one, new professionals … I'm an aggressive person but … well, now you (referred to PSY) reassured me and that's fine. Now, I'm quiet, and so I will stop complaining.

In the parents' narrative about the TC, we identified expressions related to suspicion, such as 'watchdog', and disrepute, such as 'he wasn't a man of his word', associated with claim However, their image of the TC was not solely linked to these signifiers. Indeed, in the text, it was possible to isolate another semantic area related to reassurance ('reassured') and recognition ('made feel parents'). This shift emerged in response to a peculiar intervention by the facilitator aimed at, first, accepting and containing the anger; second, allowing questioning about the clinical practices in the TC without feeling threatened; and third, bringing out differences in the roles, positions and borders among the different agencies involved. For instance, the facilitator highlighted how professionals have to respect procedures or judge's decisions, exactly like the parents do. By assuming this position, the facilitator made present the existence of a third element – the symbolic order – to which he is subjected.

During a PP meeting which took place several months before the conclusion of the therapeutic project, the parents (M4 and F4) of a young girl aged 16 spoke about a fight that occurred in the TC which upset her daughter.

M4:   Has TC insurance, especially for glasses?

PSY: I have no idea about insurance; I can ask … What about the fight?

F4:   I do not know; someone touched a boy's privates.

M4:   One educator was speaking with her, and she unwittingly gave him a kick, and then another girl touched his privates. The educator said something to her, and she started to shout. She called me and shouted, and I do not know, but you have to find some ways to calm her, so she doesn't reach these levels. F4: Our daughter is just here because you have to take care of her. If you are not able, we will take her away and go somewhere else!

PSY: In your opinion, what would help your daughter to calm down?

M4:   yeah … well … to be honest, it's difficult to calm her in certain moments. Finally, she just relaxed because another educator had spoken with her, maybe you could do it before, but I don't know.

In our opinion, this extract shows the breaking point in the idealised position where families could place residential staff, at which professionals are called by parents not only to take care of their children, but also to solve or erase their children's suffering. The *mirror stage* illustrates how the narcissistic function of love is closely connected with aggression; hence, this imaginary identification is subjugated to fluctuations between the ideal and aggression. Speaking about their daughter's distress and angst while living in the TC, the parents questioned the clinical expertise of the residential staff ('you are not able'; 'you have to find some way'). Even though the parents questioned the professionals' expertise, the facilitator did not reply by justifying or explaining the reason why their daughter's moment of distress was managed in that peculiar way; instead, he explicitly consulted the parents for knowledge about what would help their daughter to calm down. In other words, the facilitator consulted the parents on their own knowledge about their daughter – he treated the parents as 'experts on their child' (Jinvjee, Friesen, Kruzich, Robinson, & Pullmann, 2002, p. 2). As suggested by Lacan, the psychoanalyst does not answer on the side of the ideal, because that would close the relationship inside the imaginary fluctuations, but must highlight differences and subjective peculiarities. The analyst's act is done 'to obtain absolute difference' (Lacan, 1964, p. 276).

Discussion

In the prior literature, many studies (that is, Jenson & Whittaker, 1987; Frensch & Cameron, 2002; Tam & Ho, 1996) highlighted how family participation in foster care, such as residential treatment and hospital stays, improved post-treatment outcomes and well-being; moreover, it reduced the length of stay of out-of-home placements. However, besides these positive effects, the literature showed that work with families presents relevant moments of difficulties and deadlocks (Baker et al.,1995; McDonald et al.,1993), in which barriers aimed to exclude parents could emerge (Jinvjee et al., 2002). Indeed, having a child in a TC is often related to increased sense of guilt and failure as well as instability in family relationships, and may generate strong fears of exclusion (Frensch & Cameron, 2002; Goldberg, 1991). Moreover, it is important to recall that this kind of separation may exacerbate family situations that were already characterised by difficulties due to the children's conditions. Parents of children with psychosis or autistic spectrum disorders are more likely to experience serious psychological distress – which is often associated with diagnoses of affective disorders or traits such as impulsivity, oversensitivity and aloofness (Murphy et al., 2000) – than parents of children with other developmental disabilities (Sivberg, 2002).

In the light of these reflections, we aimed to present and describe a way of working with families oriented by Lacanian psychoanalysis. Indeed, as a new master, the institutional network is regarded as an oppressor by parents, and as a frustrating authority that deprives the slave of freedom and causes discomfort. Additionally, the TC is a member of the institutional network; hence, this imaginary identification, due to the high level of aggression and conflicts entailed, becomes an obstacle to the therapeutic project.

The PP meeting had no therapeutic aims for parents; indeed, the main effect of these meetings was on the positioning of the professionals themselves, who moved from the imaginary position of master to the establishment of a third element – the symbolic Other – which guaranteed order and intersubjective relations. This movement was possible after following a symbolic recognition that occurred, on the one hand, through the formal device that was designed, on the other hand, through the facilitator's responses. Regarding the device, an important role was assigned to the practice of 'receipt', which is rooted in the Lacanian concept of *act*. In this perspective, the analyst's act was not related to doing, but is associated with the language. In the analytic act, the language is not aimed at providing or constructing a meaning; rather, it is achieved to highlight and support a process of subjective knowledge. The receipt has as its goal to support parents' subjective knowledge about their children's suffering. Indeed, during the PP meetings, parents are invited to speak about their own children and to express questions and doubts about the clinical practice within the TC. In this way, the professionals presented themselves as people who have expertise about mental illness but at same time required parents to understand the peculiarities of their own children. This did not mean transforming parents into co-therapists, but it did mean that the professionals did not hold all of the knowledge about these children.

Finally, we suggested some reflections about the staff's answers. Our analysis underlined that the staff members' responses were sharper and more frequent when the parents' discourse specifically 'threatened' the TC. On the contrary, when feelings of anger and frustration were explicitly pointed towards other institutions, or when the parents' positions, at first glance, did not appear problematic for the TC, such as an idealised position, the staff abstained from replying. In our opinion, in the last case, the silence can be interpreted as confirming a peculiar master and slave relationship, in which mastery is associated with the position of *tout savoir*. Indeed, according to Foucault (1972), knowledge entails effects of power. Although it was impossible to eliminate the negative affections and aggression among the parents, moving from an imaginary identification to a symbolic recognition made it possible to manage these kinds of affections and to introduce a gap in the parents' perceptions among the institutional network and the TC. The image of the institutional network was always negative and cruel, whereas the image of the TC appeared variable and floating. We believe that these conditions are essential to realise the therapeutic project and support the reintegration of patients into their family and society.

Disclosure statement

No potential conflict of interest was reported by the authors.

References

Baio, V. (1993). L'autiste: un psychotique au travail. *Préliminaire, 5*, 33–38.
Baio, V. (2004). Partenaires d'une énonciation originale. *Préliminaire, 14*, 15–22.
Baker, B., Heller, T., Blacher, J., & Pfeiffer, S. (1995). Staff attitudes toward family involvement in residential treatment centers for children. *Psychiatric Services, 46*, 60–65.

Braun, V., & Clarke, V. (2006). Using thematic analysis in psychology. *Qualitative Research in Psychology, 3*, 77–101.

De Halleux, B. (Ed.). (2010). *«Quelques chose à dire» à l'enfant autiste*. Paris: Éditions Michèle.

Di Ciaccia, A. (2005). La pratique à plusieurs. *Préliminaire, 12*, 107–118.

Foucault, M. (1972). *The archaeology of knowledge*. (A. M. Sheridan Smith, Ed.). New York, NY: Pantheon Books.

Frensch, K. M., & Cameron, G. (2002). Treatment of choice or a last resort? A review of residential mental health placements for children and youth. *Child & Youth Care Forum, 31*, 307–339.

Goldberg, K. (1991). Family experiences of residential treatment. *Journal of Child and Youth Care, 6*(4), 1–6.

Hegel, G. W. F. (1807/1976). *Phenomenology of spirit*. (A. V. Miller, Ed.). Oxford: Oxford University Press.

Hook, D. (2008). Absolute other: Lacan's 'Big Other' as adjunct to critical social psychological analysis? *Social and Personality Psychology Compass, 2*, 51–73.

Jenson, J M., & Whittaker, J. K. (1987). Parental involvement in children's residential treatment: From preplacement to aftercare. *Children and Youth Services Review, 9*, 81–100.

Jinvjee, P., Friesen, B. J., Kruzich, J. M., Robinson, A., & Pullmann, M. (2002). Family participation in system of care: Frequently asked questions (and some answers). *Series on Family and Professional Partnerships, 5*(1), 1–8.

Lacan, J. (1946/2002). Presentation on psychical causality. In B. Fink (Ed.), *Écrits* (pp. 123–160). New York, NY: WW Norton.

Lacan, J. (1948/2002). Aggressiveness in psychoanalysis. In B. Fink (Ed.), *Écrits* (pp. 101–124). New York, NY: WW Norton.

Lacan, J. (1949/2002). The mirror stage as formative of the I functions as revealed in the psychoanalytic experience. In B. Fink (Ed.), *Écrits* (pp. 75–81). New York, NY: WW Norton.

Lacan, J. (1953/2002). The function and field of speech and language in psychoanalysis. In B. Fink (Ed.), *Écrits* (pp. 237–322). New York, NY: WW Norton.

Lacan, J. (1959/2006). On a question prior to any possible treatment of psychosis. In B. Fink (Ed.), *Écrits* (pp. 445–488). New York, NY: WW Norton.

Lacan, J. (1964/1979). *The four fundamental concepts of psycho-analysis*. (A. Sheridan Ed.). Harmondsworth: Penguin.

Lacan, J. (1969–1970/2007). *The seminar of Jacques Lacan: The other side of psychoanalysis. Book XVII*. (R. Grigg, Ed.). New York, NY: WW Norton.

Laclau, E., & Mouffe, C. (2001). *Hegemony and socialist strategy*. London: Verso.

McDonald, L., Owen, M., & McDonald, S. (1993). Quality care in residential placement for children and youth with developmental disabilities. *Behavioral Residential Treatment, 8*, 187–202.

Merritts, A. (2016). A Review of Family Therapy in Residential Settings. *Contemporary Family Therapy, 38*, 75–85.

Murphy, M., Bolton, P. F., Pickles, A., Fombonne, E., Piven, J., & Rutter, M. (2000). Personality traits of the relatives of autistic probands. *Psychological Medicine, 30*, 1411–1424.

Parker, I. (2005). Lacanian discourse analysis in psychology: Seven theoretical elements. *Theory & Psychology, 15*, 163–182.

Parker, I., & Pavón Cuéllar, D. (Eds.). (2013). *Lacan, discourse, event: New psychoanalytical approaches to textual indeterminacy*. Oxford: Routledge.

Pavón Cuéllar, D. (2010). *From the conscious interior to an exterior unconscious: Lacan, discourse analysis, and social psychology*. New York, NY: Karnac Books Publisher.

Sivberg, B. (2002). Family system and coping behaviors. A comparison between parents of children with autistic spectrum disorders and parents with non-autistic children. *Autism, 6*, 397–409.

Tam, T. S. K., & Ho, M. K. W. (1996). Factors influencing the prospect of children returning to their parents from out-of-home care. *Child Welfare, 75*, 253–268.

Vanheule, S. (2011). *The subject of psychosis: A Lacanian perspective*. London: Palgrave Macmillian.

Vanheule, S., & Verhaeghe, P. (2009). Identity through a psychoanalytic looking glass. *Theory & Psychology, 19*, 391–411.

Zenoni, A. (2002). The psychoanalytic clinic in institution: Psychosis. *Courtil Papers*. Retrieved from http://www.ch-freudien-be.org/Papers/

Hurting and healing in therapeutic environments: How can we understand the role of the relational context?

Simon P. Clarke, Jenelle M. Clarke, Ruth Brown and Hugh Middleton

ABSTRACT

It has long been recognised that relationships are key to good mental health service delivery and yet the quality of the relational context remains poorly understood. This article brings together three studies that utilize very different methodologies to explore the various ways in which a process of therapeutic change can be aided or prevented by relational factors. All three studies took place within the context of therapeutic communities. The first study uses narrative ethnography and interaction ritual theory to explain how the mechanisms of everyday encounters in two therapeutic communities transform negative feeling into a sense of belonging and positive emotions such as confidence. The second study uses grounded theory to explore how the relational setting and the altered context of the researcher in a therapeutic faith community environment induces either a positive or negative quality of relationships. The final study uses a novel autoethnographic methodology to inform understanding of the relational experience of mental health treatment by comparing and contrasting multiple perspectives of different treatment environments. The paper concludes by identifying the expression and containment of affect in a congruent environment, belonging and hope, and fluid hierarchies of relational structures as key aspects of the relational context informing change.

SUFRIMIENTO Y SANACION EN AMBIENTES TERAPEUTICOS: cómo podemos entender el papel del contexto relacional?

Desde hace mucho tiempo se ha reconocido que las relaciones interpersonales son la clave para suministrar buen servicio en salud mental, sin embargo, la importancia de la calidad del contexto relacional permanence pobremente explorada. Este artículo reúne tres estudios que utilizan diferentes metodologías para explorar las diversas maneras en las cuales un proceso de cambio terapéutico puede ser asistido o impedido por factores relacionales. Los tres estudios tuvieron lugar en el contexto de comunidades terapéuticas. El primero utiliza etnografía narrativa y teoría de integración ritual para explicar cómo los mecanismos de encuentros de cada dia, en dos comunidades terapeuticas, transforman sentimientos negativos en sentimientos de pertenencia y emociones positivas tales como la confianza. El segundo estudio utiliza "grounded theory" para explorar cómo el escenario relacional y el contexto modificado del investigador, en el ambiente de una comunidad basada en la fé, inducen cualidades positivas o negativas en las relaciones. El estudio final utiliza una nueva metodología auto-etnográfica para comprender la experiencia relacional en tratamientos de salud mental, comparando y contrastando multiples perspectivas en diferentes ambientes de tratamiento. En conclusion se identifican: la expresión y la capacidd para contener afectos en un ambiente congruente, el sentido de pertenencia y esperanza, así como también jerarquías fluidas de estructuras relacionales como aspectos clave del contexto relacional que facilita el cambio.

Ferire e curare entro I contesti terapeutici: Come possiamo comprendere il ruolo del contesto relazionale?

È stato da tempo riconosciuto che gli aspetti relazionali sono fondamentali per l'erogazione di un buon servizio sanitario mentale, tuttavia la qualità del contesto relazionale rimane poco analizzata. Questo articolo unisce tre studi che utilizzano metodologie molto diverse per esplorare i possibili modi in cui un processo di cambiamento terapeutico può essere aiutato o ostacolato da fattori relazionali. Tutti e tre gli studi sono stati condotti in comunità terapeutiche. Il primo studio si basa sull'approccio etnografico/narrativo e sulla teoria dei rituali dell'interazione per spiegare come le dinamiche degli incontri quotidiani entro due comunità terapeutiche possano trasformare sentimenti negativi in senso di appartenenza ed emozioni positive come la fiducia. Il secondo studio utilizza la grounded theory per esplorare come il setting relazionale e le alterazioni di contesto del ricercatore in una comunità terapeutica produca relazioni sia con qualità positive sia negative. Lo studio finale utilizza una innovativa metodologia autoetnografica per innovare la comprensione dell'esperienza relazionale nel trattamento della patologia mentale attraverso il confronto e la contrapposizione delle molteplici prospettive dei diversi ambienti di trattamento. L'articolo si conclude identificando l'estrinsecazione e il controllo delle dinamiche affettive in un ambiente simile, il senso di appartenenza e la speranza, oltre che gerarchie fluide delle strutture relazionali come aspetti chiave del cambiamento entro i contesti relazionali

Souffrance et guérison en milieu thérapeutique: comment comprendre le rôle du contexte relationnel?

Il est depuis longtemps reconnu que les relations sont en élément clé dans la dispensation de bons soins en santé mentale. Pourtant la qualité du contexte relationnel est mal comprise. Cet article rassemble trois études utilisant des méthodologies très différentes qui explorent de façons diverses comment le processus thérapeutique de changement peut être facilité ou empêché par des facteurs relationnels. Ces trois études ont été réalisées dans un contexte de communautés thérapeutiques. La première étude utilise une méthodologie ethnographique pourtant sur le récit ainsi que la théorie de l'interaction rituelle pour expliquer comment les mécanismes des rencontres quotidiennes au sein de deux communautés thérapeutiques transforment les sentiments négatifs en sentiment d'appartenance et en émotions positives telles que la confiance. La seconde étude utilise la méthode de la théorie ancrée (grounded theory) pour explorer comment le contexte relationnel et le contexte altéré du chercheur dans une communauté thérapeutique spirituelle induisent soit une qualité de relation positive soit négative. Pour finir, la dernière étude utilise une méthodologie auto-ethnographique novatrice aidant à la compréhension de l'expérience relationnelle du traitement en santé mentale en comparant et contrastant des perspectives multiples sur les différents lieux de soins. Cet article se conclut par l'identification de l'expression et la maitrise de l'affect dans un environnement congruent, appartenance et espoir, et l'identification de hiérarchies fluides de structures relationnelles en tant qu'aspects clés du contexte relationnel sous-tendant le processus de changement.

Επιβλαβή και επουλωτικά θεραπευτικά περιβάλλοντα: Πώς μπορούμε να κατανοήσουμε το ρόλο του σχεσιακού πλαισίου;

Εδώ και χρόνια αναγνωρίζεται ότι οι σχέσεις αποτελούν κομβικό στοιχείο στην παροχή ποιοτικών υπηρεσιών ψυχικής υγείας, αλλά παρόλα αυτά η ποιότητα του σχεσιακού πλαισίου παραμένει ελάχιστα κατανοητή. Το παρόν άρθρο παρουσιάζει τρεις μελέτες που χρησιμοποίησαν πολύ διαφορετικές μεθοδολογίες, με στόχο να διερευνηθούν οι ποικίλοι τρόποι, με τους οποίους η εργασία της θεραπευτικής αλλαγής μπορεί να διευκολυνθεί ή να παρεμποδιστεί από σχεσιακούς παράγοντες. Και οι τρεις μελέτες πραγματοποιήθηκαν στο πλαίσιο θεραπευτικών κοινοτήτων. Η πρώτη μελέτη χρησιμοποιεί την εθνογραφική αφήγηση και τη θεωρία των τελετουργικών αλληλεπίδρασης για να εξηγήσει τον τρόπο με τον οποίο οι μηχανισμοί της καθημερινής συνάντησης σε δύο θεραπευτικές κοινότητες μπορούν να μετατρέψουν το αρνητικό συναίσθημα σε μια αίσθηση του «ανήκειν» και σε θετικά συναισθήματα, όπως η αυτοπεποίθηση. Η δεύτερη μελέτη χρησιμοποιεί τη θεμελιωμένη θεωρία για να διερευνήσει τον τρόπο με τον οποίο το σχεσιακό πλαίσιο και η παρουσία του ερευνητή σε ένα θεραπευτικό κοινοτικό πλαίσιο που βασίζεται στην πίστη επηρεάζει θετικά ή αρνητικά την ποιότητα των σχέσεων. Η τελευταία μελέτη χρησιμοποιεί μια πρωτότυπη αυτοεθνογραφική μεθοδολογία για να διευρύνει την κατανόηση της σχεσιακής εμπειρίας της θεραπείας στην ψυχική υγεία, συγκρίνοντας και αντιπαραθέτοντας πολλαπλές οπτικές διαφορετικών θεραπευτικών πλαισίων. Το άρθρο καταλήγει αναγνωρίζοντας ότι η έκφραση και η εμπερίεξη του συναισθήματος σε ένα συνεκτικό περιβάλλον, η αίσθηση του «ανήκειν» και η ελπίδα, και η ρευστή ιεραρχία των σχεσιακών δομών αποτελούν βασικές όψεις της επίδρασης που μπορεί να έχει το σχεσιακό πλαίσιο.

Introduction

Relationships are implicated in both 'the creation and amelioration of mental health problems' (Pilgrim, Rogers, & Bentall, 2009, p. 235). Or, as one member of a therapeutic community put it, 'it is people that hurt us and people that heal us'. These statements have found strong support in the research literature: from the role of attachment as both a significant predictor of psychological difficulties and as a resilience factor against stress (Ma, 2006), to the quality of the therapeutic alliance as the most consistently reliable predictor of psychotherapeutic outcome (Lambert & Barley, 2001). In these terms, relationships are not just an important aspect of any mental health intervention – they *are* the intervention (Middleton, 2015).

However, despite the evidence suggesting relationships are both the cause and solution of most mental health problems, surprisingly little has been written about the specific qualities of the relational 'climate' that are likely to contribute to positive or negative emotional effects. One of the exceptions to this is Carl Rogers. Rogers (1961) identified three core conditions that he believed needed to be present in the therapeutic relationship to establish 'contact' and provide the stimulus for positive behavioural change in a therapeutic setting. These interrelated factors included congruence (the willingness on the part of the therapist to be genuine and authentic), unconditional positive regard (the therapist's communication of total and complete acceptance of the client, without judgement) and empathy (the therapist's communication of their desire to understand and help the client). Rogers' theories have been highly influential in psychotherapy and have been supported by numerous empirical studies (Joseph & Murphy, 2013).

Foremost in Rogers' system was the role of the therapist as the principal creator of the relational climate necessary for personal change. However, in doing so it is possible that Rogers overstated whether these conditions were truly possible in therapy. In the celebrated dialogues between Rogers and other key thinkers of his time (Rogers, Kirschenbaum, & Henderson, 1989) the philosopher and theologian Martin Buber questioned whether a true sense of mutuality could really exist between therapist and client given the structural aspects of the therapeutic relationship and the obvious power differential between the two parties. In other words, it would be very difficult to conceive of a truly I-Thou relationship in Buber's (1937) terms when one person was seeking help from another person very different in status and role.

It is worth pointing out that Buber did not say that he believed contact was impossible between two people in therapy, only that there were limitations inherent in the therapeutic situation (Rogers et al., 1989). These limitations were also recognised by early pioneers of the therapeutic community (TC) movement (Winship, 2013). Working with traumatised veterans following Second World War, psychiatrists such as Wilfred Bion, Tom Main, Michael Foulkes and Maxwell Jones discovered that involving patients in all aspects of the running of the hospital led to vastly improved outcomes (Manning, 1989). Devolving the natural power structures between staff and patient (named 'flattened hierarchy' by Rapoport, 1960) became a key aspect of later TCs (Campling, 2001) along with the harnessing of peer relationships between members as a powerful therapeutic resource (Spandler, 2006). These innovations arguably anticipated the rise of several innovations in mental health services, including the recovery approach (Winship, 2016) and service user involvement (Haigh, 2004).

Whilst there are have been numerous studies focusing on treatment effectiveness and clinical outcomes (e.g. Capone, Schroder, Clarke, & Braham, 2016; Lees, Manning, & Rawlings, 2004), there have been relatively few studies that explore how the quality of interactions within TCs facilitates personal change. There have also been few studies that have looked at the influence of the relational context on the quality of the social interactions within TCs. Thus, whilst it is possible to point towards structural innovations in TCs such as democracy and peer support, the actual quality of the relational context in TCs, like in mental health generally, remains poorly understood.

This article presents three studies that attempt to address these issues using different qualitative methodologies. The three studies were selected because they each highlight different, yet interrelated, aspects of the quality of relationships in TCs. As far as the authors are aware, these are the only studies on TCs that have focussed on how the quality of relationships impact upon personal change.

The methods and results from each study are presented concurrently. A detailed analysis and discussion then brings together and examines the interrelated themes across all of the studies. These three studies together show a number of overarching themes. These include the importance of the everyday interaction between TC members, the role of context in determining the quality of the interactions, the communal dimension of hope, and the difference between professionalised and non-professionalised roles in TCs and psychiatric healthcare.

Study 1

Methods

J. M. Clarke's study investigated how everyday interactions supported personal change in two adult-democratic TCs for individuals with a diagnosis of personality disorder. Drawing on Interaction Ritual (IR) theory (Collins, 2004; Durkheim, 1912–2001; Goffman, 1967), the study explored the role of emotions, feelings of inclusion and how power is used during everyday interactions. An interaction ritual is a social encounter whereby individuals share their attention and emotion, generating feelings of group belonging, symbols of group membership and social expectations, or moral codes, for interaction (Collins, 2004). Social meanings that arise from interactions are fluid, reflective and continuously evolving. Key to IR theory is the role of emotions, as individuals will be drawn to repeat those interactions that provide the highest emotional reward (Collins, 2004). Additionally, Collins (2004) highlights that interaction rituals have a history and future and are linked together through 'chains'. These chains over time form social rules and expectations in groups and within individuals. How groups manage these social rules within interactions, and whether they mutually experience positive emotional feeling, indicates the relational quality between members. Summers-Effler (2004) distinguishes between 'power' rituals and 'solidarity' rituals. With power rituals, the positive emotional feeling is consolidated with the dominant members gaining positive feeling whilst the subordinates loose it and the relational dynamic is unequal. In contrast, in solidarity rituals all members, regardless of status, share the positive emotional feeling and the relational dynamic is mutual. Within a TC, examples of interaction rituals include mealtimes, smoking breaks, community meetings and grocery shopping. As IR theory explains social mechanisms of interactions, it is ideally placed to analyse the role of social encounters within TCs and provides a framework understanding issues of power.

The study used a narrative ethnographic approach to examine the mechanisms of social interactions outside of structured therapy and the relational dynamics between client members. Both TCs' therapy duration was 8–12 months and are anonymised in this article as 'Powell', a residential TC and 'Hawthorne', a day programme TC. Ethical approval for the study was granted by Nottingham Research Ethics Committee 1 in the UK. Specific methods of data collection included: over 700-h of participant observation; in-depth narrative interviews with 21 client members; semi-structured interviews with 7 selected staff members; and document analysis of community leaflets, list of social rules, forms for boundary or rule breaks, and excerpts of clients' reflective writing. The participant observation focused on times outside of structured therapy, such as community meetings, smoking breaks and meal times. At the residential community this included days, evenings, nights and weekends, and at the day community, times in between structured therapy groups. Interviews with clients explored their experiences being in the TCs, whilst interviews with staff members focused on contextualising information about their respective TCs and approach to overall therapy. Data analysis was interpretivist and thematic, with data being coded for key themes and interaction rituals chains. Fieldnotes were read in entirety for initial themes, particularly around inclusion, power and emotions, and then loaded into NVivo for further analysis and coding. Interviews were transcribed verbatim, forming the first stage of analysis (Langellier, 2001) and analysed holistically in order to closely analyse themes within a given narrative, and then cross-referenced with other interviews and fieldnote data.

Results

The research highlights that during everyday social interactions such as meal times, smoking breaks and informal times, maintaining solidarity between client members is important in the presence of negative emotions. It is through feelings of inclusion that negative emotions can be transformed into positive feeling, as the following extract from Powell illustrates:

> It is nearly 9 pm and I join some of the clients in the lounge. Julie, who is sitting with Anna on the sofa, is sobbing. Julie is explaining she wants to leave the unit but her mum will not come get her. Erica is colouring but clearly listening to the conversation. Julie says the only time her mum really seemed 'bothered' about her is when she jumped off the roof. Erica asks Julie about her urges and Julie says she does not feel safe and that is why she is in the lounge. Margaret (nurse) then comes in and joins the conversation. Talk revolves around Julie's eating disorder. Anna at times pats Julie's leg, and tells her she will get to the point where she can picture life without the disorder. She reminds Julie that the eating disorder is not her friend and does not help or protect her – it will kill her. Julie is crying and loudly sniffing. After a while the conversation moves on but every now and again someone will either gently pat Julie's shoulder or quickly check in with her.

Though there was anxiety surrounding Julie's distress, everyone stayed in the lounge, including Anna and Erica. Equally, Julie could have retreated to her room. Crucially, it seems individuals will tolerate negative emotions if over time they receive positive 'payoffs' from the interaction (Turner & Stets, 2005). Not only did Julie receive support and feelings of inclusivity from the group, but so too did those who remained in the lounge by giving their support. Moreover, the expression of negative emotions was often a motivator for community members to draw *together* rather than to isolate. Clients will still interact with one another, even if there are high levels of negative emotions, if group solidarity remains intact. This is akin to Collins's (2004) assertion that negative emotions can still generate long-term positive feeling if members come away with feelings of belonging.

Importantly, feelings of belonging and inclusion can help facilitate personal change. In total, 16 of 21 client members from both TCs explained their experience in working through negative emotions together had given them increased feelings of confidence and self-acceptance. Heather from Hawthorne said, 'They helped with my confidence, they helped me deal with facing things. […] I have this sense of feeling in myself that I know I'm going to be okay'. Echoing Heather's comments on confidence, Erika from Powell stated, 'I feel a lot more confident in that I don't have to act on urges'.

However, not all clients related feelings of positive changes or social inclusion through relationships. Robert from Hawthorne was consistently excluded from client member social interactions within the TC. During his interview, he explained:

> I've tried to join in more, I've tried to make more uh, give more feedback if you like. But … I still don't feel a part of the group. I feel like there's everybody else and me. So … that gets me down, that I'm not a part of it.

Robert's comment suggests social exclusion was sometimes present within client member relationships. He later went on to explain in his interview he felt there was a 'pecking order' and he was at the 'bottom'. Other clients also spoke of an invisible hierarchy based on things including length of time in the community, things they have in common, age and gender. Therefore, Robert's comments provide a challenge to traditional TC notions of a 'flattened' hierarchy (Rapoport, 1960; i.e. whereby all client and staff have equal status within the community). Instead, Clarke (2015) proposes a 'fluid' hierarchy, which is discussed in more detail in the discussion section.

Study 2

Method

Brown's study used a mixed methodological approach to investigate key factors involved in personal, positive change in the context of a therapeutic community. Data were collected over a two-year period from newcomers to Christ Church Deal (CCD), an open (i.e. non-residential) therapeutic faith community run by 'lay' members (Holmes & Williams, 2010). Throughout the study, Brown occupied numerous roles inside the community, including as a client member and a member of the Risk Management Team. Outside of the community, she worked as a specialist mental health pharmacist in the NHS and studied as a doctoral student. Brown adopted the perspective of 'the space between' (Dwyer & Buckle, 2009) both insider and outsider status. Standard psychiatric outcome measures were used at baseline and six-month intervals for those who joined the TC between 2007 and 2008. The qualitative method involved collecting data from questionnaires and in-depth interviews. Only the data from the in-depth interviews is discussed in this article. For the interview, participants were encouraged to tell their story about their previous experiences of mental health services and professionals, being interrupted by the interviewer only to ask clarifying questions or to offer encouragement. A total of nine participants were interviewed in total (eight female).

Results

At the 6-month interviews, all of the participants disclosed they had viewed Brown as someone with power to detain them under the UK Mental Health Act due to her status as a mental health pharmacist, and had thus provided inaccurate responses to the baseline outcome measures. As one participant admitted, 'the first time [I completed the forms] I was frightened of being locked up'. Once identified, the nature of this dissembling became the focus of the qualitative interviews. Participants began to tell their stories of experiences with mental health services and professionals, but also their experiences of being part of CCD. Participants admitted they had dissembled due to a fear of mental health services (including a fear of being sectioned), a fear of Brown's power as a mental health professional and also due to self-deception.

The interviews were analysed using Grounded Theory (Glaser & Strauss, 1967) to generate a theory of therapeutic change. The analysis generated an overarching theory of congruence, adapted from Rogers' (1961) definition cited in the introduction. In CCD, TC peer relationships were understood as congruent. However, a fundamental aspect of congruence in these terms was the initial recognition of *personal incongruence*. Personal incongruence was identified through participant interviews as a fragmented self, social isolation, a crisis of faith and a lack of environmental 'fit'. It was reinforced through *pathogenic*, or harmful, relationships characterised by 'unequal power relationships' resulting in a loss of trust, feeling judged, and experiencing shame and fear. The pathogenic relationships described in this study related to parents, healthcare professionals, church authorities and friendships. As one participant illustrated:

> I think as a patient you feel quite powerless. So if one doctor tells a nurse and the nurse tells so and so. The professionals listen to each other; they don't listen to you as a client.

Pathogenic relationships resulted in the participants adopting survival strategies in order to protect themselves from more shame and pain. These strategies included withholding information, dissembling or performing, which reinforced a fragmenting of self, loss of identity and social isolation:

> I would appear to be smiling at times when actually I was completely disorientated and quite often with these health professionals they would be amazed at what they saw as my rapid progress … It wasn't progress at all … I would manage to crack what I was being asked to do. … but I wasn't reaching [pointing inside her chest].

In contrast, becoming personally congruent was identified in two main areas: a personal self and a social self. The process of becoming congruent with a personal self began with external sources, namely with the participant's relationships within the social environment. These relationships, termed *salugenic* (or health-producing; Clinebell, 1984), were voluntary, volitional and mutual, characterised by mutuality, hope, openness, safety, freedom and trust. Mutual positive relationships developed through sharing stories of personal positive change, as one participant explained:

> When I first started seeing [another CCD member] she said, 'I tell you what I can do for you. I can give you true, hopeful stories, not kind of clap trap stuff and not my life's perfect now and whatever.' But I can authentically say that's where something has changed for me, that bit has changed. So I can share hope and I can do that with truth.

Clients identified that a congruent environment is where they feel they belong and where they can find hope, safety and freedom. The combination of congruent relationships and environment leads to the process of finding congruence with the self. As one participant framed the process:

> And the general ethos here is one of hope. Even though I actually don't have any hope at the moment I can see that other people have hope and because if I like it or not, I have got relationship with people here, I find it easier to not act on my self-harming and suicidal thoughts because out of relationship to them I don't want to hurt them.

In summary therefore, the theory of congruence proposes that individuals who have been socially isolated learn how to form salugenic relationships that facilitate personal, positive change through the expression of emotion. Congruent relationships positively impacts on clients' sense of self, leading to greater self-congruence.

Study 3

Method

S. P. Clarke's study used autoethnography to illustrate his experiences of the relational context of two treatment environments. As a methodology, autoethnography combines personal narrative ('auto') writing ('graphy') in order to reflect on, analyse and explore particular socio-cultural practices and institutions ('ethno'; Anderson, 2006). Autoethnography thus combines the conventions of autobiography in the retelling of 'epiphanies' with the explicit ethnographic goal of investigating the social world (Ellis, Adams, & Bochner, 2011). It is a 'methodology of the heart' (Sparkes, 2007) that employs the use of dramatic form in order to illustrate, challenge, educate and involve the reader (Ellis et al., 2011). It has also been used to illustrate the experiences of psychotherapy (Speedy, 2013) and mental health services (Short, Grant, & Clarke, 2007).

Results

In this article, two vignettes of S. P. Clarke's experiences of treatment environments are presented. The first account takes place in a psychiatric ward in 1994 and the second account describes an early visit in 2000 to an open TC where time was spent living in various types of community living, including with families (where the second vignette is set). These accounts were based upon a number of unpublished sources including Clarke's NHS clinical notes, his therapy notes, a carer's diary and interviews with his friends and family. The interviews were conducted in an unstructured format in order to gain background information regarding Clarke's experience. Each account represents an amalgam of these different impressions in a similar way to Sparkes (2007) methodology, and then told in the second person in order to 'induct' the reader into Clarke's experience. The two pieces are presented below and separated by three stars (***).

***

You are waiting for your first ward round. From the waiting room a cheerful nurse calls you in. She smiles pleasantly as she ushers you into a small room. The room is packed: there are at least seven people present. You weren't expecting this many people. Two middle-aged men in suits sit at the front introduce themselves as 'Consultants psychiatrists' and begin asking you questions.

Your anxiety rises. You sweat. You keep contradicting yourself. The two psychiatrists smile and seem to throw each other knowing glances. One of the nurses rolls her eyes – at you or at them? You don't know.

You have had enough. You mutter something in a quiet, barely audible, mumble. You walk out. The other doctor follows you out. You chat in a nearby room. The doctor asks why you left. He asks whether you will consider being an inpatient. No, you tell the doctor as you look through the barred windows that shimmer in the afternoon sun, I don't want to be an inpatient.

Suddenly and inexplicably the small doctor leaves the room. Was it something you said? You are not sure why he has left the room. What happens now? You open the door to the corridor and see the doctor running back to the ward round room. You don't know what to do. You are scared. There is a brief moment of hesitation and then you walk out of the hospital.

Outside, the warm September sun is all encompassing. You are in despair. All you have is this moment: the one, unfailing, unremitting sense of crushing despair, without hope of abatement or reprieve.

Slowly, like aspirin dissolving in water, your consciousness dissolves.

***

It is Easter and you are down for the week from London. The community has put you with this young family. The house is called Serendipity, which you are told means the occurrence and development of events by chance in a happy or beneficial way. The crash and suck of sea on shingle is heard in the background.

You are cleaning the ground story windows. The father tells you that it will keep the mind focussed and grounded. It's therapeutic, he says. And it is. You feel like you are offering something, giving something back.

Your consciousness is all broken up since the breakdown three months ago. Fragments of memories, occasional panicked thoughts, feelings, a phrase, a word, perhaps even fleeting desire; fear, hope, grief. The pieces slowly coalesce around the gentle intonation of a half-remembered poem:

Ah Sun-flower! weary of time,
Who countest the steps of the Sun:
Seeking after that sweet golden clime
Where the travellers journey is done.
Where the Youth pined away with desire,
And the pale Virgin shrouded in snow:
Arise from their graves and aspire,
Where my Sun-flower wishes to go.

You are that sunflower, you realise. The words hold both a promise and a certainty; there is hope in this grief. This is the trigger. The fragility breaks, finally. Things let go.

From inside the house you hear the distressed wail of the four-year old boy. Daddy, daddy, he cries, I've lost Simon! I've lost Simon! I can't find him! Daddy!

Around the corner they come, the little boy leading his father anxiously by the hand. They find you at the back window, bucket and wiper in hand. You are weeping uncontrollably, your body shuddering with sobs, tears streaming down your face into the bucket – salt water mixing with liquid detergent.

The father puts his hand on your shoulder and looks deep into your eyes. He takes the bucket from you.

Time to take a break, he says.

***

These two vignettes both portray psychological collapse. However, the 'affective resonance' of the two relational environments is very different. In the first vignette, which takes place in a psychiatric hospital, there are clear relational hierarchies and the tone is impersonal and intimidating, creating a sense of fear and shame in the patient. Paradoxically, the confusion created by the ward round leads to the patient's complete psychological collapse. The second vignette takes place in an open-style TC characterised by a sense of kindness and gentle, familial discipline, whereby the signification of hope (expressed by the memory of Blake's Sunflower poem) also leads to psychological collapse. However, in this second scenario the collapse represents breakthrough, not breakdown.

Discussion

This article presented the findings from three studies that examined the quality of the relational experience as a core component of a mental health intervention. Although the three studies employed very different methods and theoretical approaches, a number of core themes emerged that were present across all of the studies. These themes will be explored in the following discussion.

The first theme arising from these three studies is the role of emotion and the relational 'climate' in terms of whether an environment is able to facilitate the expression, and then transformation, of negative affect. The studies demonstrate that allowing for the expression of emotion authentically in community, or 'permissiveness' (Rapoport, 1960) is a crucial first step in providing the foundations through which a successful therapeutic process is built. Crucially this process can be recognised within everyday interactions rituals (such as supporting one another during informal times), whereby individuals express their emotions together, building a sense of belonging and hope (Collins, 2004). In terms of the three studies, Brown showed that the sharing of stories could be an important community ritual that facilitates trust and safety within the relationships. In

S. P. Clarke's study, everyday activities, such as washing windows in a safe family environment, can be the catalyst for the transformation of despair into hope. Finally, J. M. Clarke highlighted how the sharing of negative emotion in the lounge of a residential TC engendered a release of intense negative feelings that were transformed into feelings of belonging. In this sense, an effective relational context is one that both contains difficult emotions, but then goes further by transforming the negative experiences into positive experiences such as hope and wholeness through mutuality and feelings of inclusion.

The role of emotional expression within therapeutic relationships is, of course, not a new idea but has a long history in psychotherapy, from Freud's notion of 'catharsis', to behaviourist notions of emotional facilitation and exposure (Rachman, 1980) and the work of Carl Rogers (1961). However, the relational qualities described in these studies arguably go further. Instead, it is relationships formed out of mutual experiences of understanding on the basis of which Buber (1937) called I-Thou, rather than just the 'verstehen' of therapist empathy. Such 'expertise by experience' is more than simply a knowledge or awareness of distress, but an active expertise and experience of working through these experiences in relationships with like-minded peers that creates a group emotional IQ (Holmes & Williams, 2010) capable of facilitating a therapeutically congruent environment.

However, the authors would also argue that relational context and emotional expression are not enough by themselves to facilitate personal change. Two important factors identified in the three studies were belonging and hope. If there is no hope things can be different, then despair and inertia are likely to result. Conversely, when there is no sense of belonging in terms of the participant's identification with their social environment, in other words if the person is incongruent with their environment, then fear, inauthenticity and isolation are liable to result.

Hope is of course foundational to many spiritually informed psychotherapeutic approaches (Pargament, 2011). It has long been recognised by the Recovery movement as central to the experience of successful rehabilitation from severe mental illness, as well as a useful corrective against the overly pessimistic character of some psychiatric classification systems (Slade, 2009). However, many contemporary models of recovery miss the communal dimension and instead posit the recovery journal in entirely individualistic terms (Winship, 2016). The authors of these three studies would argue that hope is impossible without some notion of belonging to a community of like-minded individuals. In many ways, it is one's peers and community that are able to hold a vision of hope that is then transmitted to newer members, who may not have the capacity to generate hope on their own.

The final theme that arose from the three studies is whether the relational hierarchies of a mental health environment are able to facilitate emotional expression, hope and belonging. J. M. Clarke observed that TC relational structures can either be rigid and hierarchical, thus leading to exclusion and negative emotional expression, or they can be more 'fluid' and generate the positive emotional expression necessary for personal change. Similarly, Brown's and S. P. Clarke's studies the relational structures of the psychiatric system were contrasted negatively against the more egalitarian structures of an open TC whereby members felt able to be more authentic in their expression of negative affect without fear of institutional censure. For example, in Brown's study a fluid hierarchy can be observed even in a non-professionalised role, whereby more experienced TC members may take a guiding role (e.g. sharing personal stories and offering support to newer members). In S. P. Clarke's study, the family structure provides a safe, yet temporary, relational structure where both the expression of emotion and community responsibilities were held together.

Rather than a flattened hierarchy model advocated by many TC writers, a model of fluid hierarchy (Clarke, 2015) acknowledges clients at any one point might hold differing levels of power and social status. Furthermore, a fluid hierarchy model still allows for deliberate efforts to minimise power imbalances between staff and clients through shared responsibility and changing roles, whilst realistically acknowledging that at times, hierarchal components and power imbalances exist within the client cohort. This in itself is not problematic as long as positive feelings remain *shared* and clients do not become alienated, marginalised or isolated. What is central is whether these power roles become flexible or rigid resulting in emotional power imbalances. This follows Haigh (2013) who argues, '[a]uthority is fluid and questionable – not fixed but negotiated' (p. 13). Flexible social roles suggest that there is room for client members to change their social position and that the community allows for shifts in its hierarchy without power being consolidated in any one individual(s), staff or client.

The history of mental health services is often marked by a failure to adequately democratise and make use of patient expertise (Noorani, 2013). A notable exception to this are TCs who, from their earliest conception in the post-Second World War experiments of hospitals of Northfield and Mill Hill, attempted to subvert the natural order of staff/patients and create a genuinely patient-led therapeutic endeavour (Winship, 2013). These attempts were crystallised in the phrase 'flattened hierarchy', a concept which is considered to be one of the key components of a well-functioning TC (Manning, 1989). However, along with Bloor, McKeganey, and Fonkert (1988), we acknowledge 'the Foucauldian view of power as a strategic relationship, a routine fact of social life in therapeutic communities as elsewhere' (p. 190). Thus, the notion of a 'flattened hierarchy' does not adequately capture the complexities of relations in therapeutic environments. We would therefore suggest Clarke (2015) notion of a 'fluid' hierarchy as a more accurate depiction of the positions and roles different people may take at different times, and emphasises the importance of belonging and mutuality being shared by all clients.

In summary, this article presented three studies that, together, shed light on aspects of the relational context that can either afford positive psychological change, or hinder it. These factors include the expression and containment of affect in a congruent environment, belonging and hope, and fluid hierarchies of relational structures. We believe these factors provide the basis by which the relational context of all mental health interventions, and not just TCs, can be better understood.

Disclosure statement

No potential conflict of interest was reported by the authors.

References

Anderson, L. (2006). Analytic autoethnography. *Journal of Contemporary Ethnography, 35,* 373–395.

Bloor, M., McKeganey, N. P., & Fonkert, J. D. (1988). *One foot in eden sociological study of the range of therapeutic community practice*. London: Routledge.

Buber, M. (1937). *I and thou*. Mansfield Centre, CT: Martino Publishing.

Campling, P. (2001). Therapeutic communities. *Advances in Psychiatric Treatment, 7*, 365–372.

Capone, G., Schroder, T., Clarke, S. P., & Braham, L. (2016). Outcomes of therapeutic community treatment for personality disorder. *Therapeutic Communities: The International Journal of Therapeutic Communities, 37*, 84–100. doi:10.1108/TC-12-2015-0025

Clarke, J. M. (2015). *Where the change is: Everyday interaction rituals of therapeutic communities* (Unpublished PhD thesis). Nottingham: University of Nottingham.

Clinebell, H. (1984). *Basic types of pastoral care and counseling: Resources for the ministry of healing and growth*. Nashville, TN: Abingdon Press.

Collins, R. (2004). *Interaction ritual chains*. Princeton, NJ: Princeton University Press.

Durkheim, E. (1912/2001). The Elementary Forms of Religious Life. Oxford: Oxford University Press.

Dwyer, S. C., & Buckle, J. L. (2009). The space between: On being an insider-outsider in qualitative research. *International Journal of Qualitative Methods, 8*, 54–63.

Ellis, C., Adams, T. E., & Bochner, A. P. (2011). Autoethnography: An overview. *Forum: Qualitative Social Research, 12*, Art. 10. http://nbn-resolving.de/urn:nbn:de:0114-fqs1101108

Glaser, B. G., & Strauss, A. L. (1967). *The discovery of grounded theory: Strategies for qualitative research*. Mill Valley, CA: Sociology Press.

Goffman, E. (1967). *Interaction Ritual: Essays on Face-to-Face Behaviour*. New York, NY: Anchor Books.

Haigh, R. (2004). Charismatic ideas: Coming or going? *Therapeutic Communities: The International Journal of Therapeutic Communities, 26*, 367–382.

Haigh, R. (2013). The quintessence of a therapeutic environment. *Therapeutic Communities: The International Journal of Therapeutic Communities, 34*, 6–15.

Holmes, P. R., & Williams, S. B. (2010). The naked TC: Can a TC prosper without finance, buildings or staff? *Therapeutic Communities: The International Journal of Therapeutic Communities, 31*, 270–281.

Joseph, S., & Murphy, D. (2013). Person-centered approach, positive psychology, and relational helping: Building bridges. *Journal of Humanistic Psychology, 53*, 26–51. doi:10.1177/0022167812436426

Lambert, M. J., & Barley, D. E. (2001). Research summary on the therapeutic relationship and psychotherapy outcome. *Psychotherapy: Theory, Research, Practice, Training, 38*, 357–361. doi: 10.1037/0033-3204.38.4.357

Langellier, K. M. (2001). "You're Marked": Breast cancer, tattoo, and the narrative of performance identify. In J. Brockmeier & D. Carbaugh (Eds.), *Narrative and Identity: Studies in autobiography, self and culture* (pp. 145–184). Amsterdam: John Benjamins Publishing Company.

Lees, J., Manning, N., & Rawlings, B. (2004). A culture of enquiry: Research evidence and the therapeutic community. *Psychiatric Quarterly, 75*, 279–294.

Ma, K. (2006). Attachment theory in adult psychiatry. Part 1: Conceptualisations, measurement and clinical research findings. *Advances in Psychiatric Treatment, 12*, 440–449.

Manning, N. (1989). *The therapeutic community movement: Charisma and routinisation*. Oxford: Routledge.

Middleton, H. (2015). *Psychiatry reconsidered: From medical treatment to supportive understanding*. Basingstoke: Palgrave Macmillan.

Noorani, T. (2013). Service user involvement, authority and the 'expert-by-experience' in mental health. *Journal of Political Power, 6*, 49–68.

Pargament, K. I. (2011). *Spiritually integrated psychotherapy: Understanding and addressing the sacred*. New York: Guilford Press.

Pilgrim, D., Rogers, A., & Bentall, R. (2009). The centrality of personal relationships in the creation and amelioration of mental health problems: The current interdisciplinary case. *Health, 13*, 235–254. doi:10.1177/1363459308099686

Rachman, S. (1980). Emotional processing. *Behaviour Research and Therapy, 18*, 51–60.

Rapoport, R. N. (1960). *Community as doctor*. London: Tavistock Publications.

Rogers, C. R. (1961). *On becoming a person: A therapist's view of psychotherapy*. New York: Houghton Mifflin.

Rogers, C. R., Kirschenbaum, H., & Henderson, V. L. (1989). *Carl Rogers–dialogues: Conversations with Martin Buber, Paul Tillich, B.F. Skinner, Gregory Bateson, Michael Polanyi, Rollo May, and others*. Boston, MA: Houghton Mifflin.

Short, N. P., Grant, A., & Clarke, L. (2007). Living in the borderlands; writing in the margins: An autoethnographic tale. *Journal of Psychiatric and Mental Health Nursing, 14*, 771–782.

Slade, M. (2009). *Personal recovery & mental illness: A guide for mental health profession*. Cambridge: Cambridge University Press.

Spandler, H. (2006). *Asylum to action: Paddington day hospital, therapeutic communities and beyond*. London: Jessica Kingsley Publishers.

Sparkes, A. C. (2007). Embodiment, academics, and the audit culture: A story seeking consideration. *Qualitative Research, 7*, 521–550.

Speedy, J. (2013). Where the wild dreams are: Fragments from the spaces between research, writing, autoethnography, and psychotherapy. *Qualitative Inquiry, 19*, 27–34.

Summers-Effler, E. (2004). Defensive Strategies: the formation and social implications of patterned self-destructive behaviour. *Advances in Group Processes, 21*, 309–325.

Turner, J. H., & Stets, J. E. (2005). *The sociology of emotions*. New York: Cambridge University Press.

Winship, G. (2013). A genealogy of therapeutic community ideas: The influence of the Frankfurt School with a particular focus on Herbert Marcuse and Eric Fromm. *Therapeutic Communities: The International Journal of Therapeutic Communities, 34*, 60–70.

Winship, G. (2016). A meta-recovery framework: Positioning the 'New Recovery' movement and other recovery approaches. *Journal of Psychiatric and Mental Health Nursing, 23*, 66–73. doi:10.1111/jpm.12266

Mental health care and educational actions: From institutional exclusion to subjective development

Daniel Magalhães Goulart and Fernando González Rey

ABSTRACT

This paper is based on a qualitative research study within a Community Mental Health Centre in Brazil. It addresses professional actions within mental health services as a sensitive sphere in which to discuss deadlocks and critical strategies to expand practices towards deinstitutionalization. The idea of subjective development from a cultural-historical standpoint is discussed as a theoretical way to promote institutional practices which articulate education and mental health care. Subjective development is regarded as a non-universal, non-deterministic, and context-sensitive process, having the subject configuration as its unit. We argue that such discussion has heuristic value for understanding mental health as a living process, beyond hermetic diagnostic entities, overcoming the objectualization and hierarchical aspect which frequently characterize the relationship between service users and workers. Moreover, we discuss how professional actions geared toward subjective development could enhance dialogical relations capable of supporting individuals and groups to actively position themselves as subjects in their life pathways. From this point of view, individuals are not considered as an epiphenomenon of social forces, such as the result of the effects of power, but as a crucial moment of social experience.

ACCIONES EN EDUCACION Y ASISTENCIA A LA SALUD MENTAL: de la exclusión institucional al desarrollo subjetivo

Este artículo se basa en una investigación cualitativa realizada en un centro comunitario de salud mental en Brasil. Se refiere a las acciones profesionales dentro de los servicios de salud mental considerándolas como un campo sensitivo en el cual discutir impases y estrategias críticas para expandir prácticas hacia la des-institucionalización. Se discute la idea de un desarrollo subjetivo desde un punto de vista histórico-cultural, como una vía teórica para promover prácticas institucionales que articulen la educación y la asistencia a la salud mental. Se considera el desarrollo subjetivo como no-universal, no-determinista y como un proceso sensitivo en relación al contexto en el cual su unidad es la configuración del sujeto. Proponemos que tal discusión tiene un valor heurístico para comprender la salud mental como un proceso viviente, más allá de entidades diagnósticas herméticas, reduciendo la objetificación y el aspecto jerárquico que frecuentemente caracteriza la relación entre los usuarios de un servicio y los profesionales. Además, discutimos cómo acciones profesionales orientadas hacia el desarrollo subjetivo, podrían mejorar relaciones dilógicas capaces de dar apoyo a individuos y grupos en una toma de posición activa como sujetos en su sendero vital. Desde este punto de vista, los individuos no son considerados como epifenómenos de fuerzas sociales ni como resultado de efectos de poder.

Cura della salute mentale e azioni educative: dall'esclusione istituzionale allo sviluppo soggettivo

Questo contributo si basa su una ricerca qualitativa realizzata all'interno di una Comunità di un Centro di Salute Mentale in Brasile. Considera le azioni professionali entro i servizi di salute mentale come una complessa sfera in cui discutere immobilismi e strategie per implementare le prassi di deistituzionalizzazione. L'idea di sviluppo soggettivo da un punto di vista storico-culturale è discussa come una modalità teorica di promuovere pratiche istituzionali che organizzano istruzione e cura della salute mentale. Lo sviluppo soggettivo è considerato come un processo non universale, non-deterministico e sensibile al contesto, e considera la configurazione del soggetto come unità. Noi sosteniamo che tale discussione abbia un valore euristico per considerare la salute mentale come un processo attivo, al di là di entità diagnostiche e superando aspetti di oggettualizzazione e di gerarchia che spesso caratterizzano il rapporto tra gli utenti dei servizi e i lavoratori. Inoltre, si discute come le azioni professionali orientate allo sviluppo soggettivo potrebbero migliorare le relazioni dialogiche in grado di supportare gli individui e i gruppi nell'assumere posizioni attive nei loro percorsi di vita. Da questo punto di vista gli individui non sono considerati come un epifenomeno di forze sociali, ad esempio conseguenza di traiettorie di potere, ma come momento cruciale dell'esperienza sociale.

Soin en santé mentale et actions éducatives: de l'exclusion institutionnelle au développement subjectif

Cet article se fonde sur une étude qualitative menée au sein d'une communauté de service de santé mentale au Brésil. Il traite des actions professionnelles au sein du service de santé mentale en tant que sphère sensible au sein de laquelle peuvent se discuter les impasses et stratégies critiques pour favoriser les pratiques vers une la désinstitutionalisation. L'idée de développement subjectif considéré d'un point de vue culturel et historique est discutée de manière théorique afin de promouvoir des pratiques institutionnelles qui articulent éducation et soin en santé mentale. Le développement subjectif est considéré comme un processus non-universel, non-déterministe et sensible au contexte avec comme unité de mesure la configuration du sujet. Nous soutenons qu'une telle discussion a une valeur heuristique pour la compréhension de la santé mentale comme un processus en mouvement, transcendant les entités diagnostiques hermétiques, surmontant l'objectivisation et l'aspect hiérarchique qui caractérisent fréquemment la relation entre les utilisateurs et les travailleurs dans le champ de la santé mentale. De plus nous abordons en quoi les actions professionnelles orientées vers le développement subjectif pourraient améliorer les relations dialogiques capables d'aider les individus et les groupes à se positionner activement comme sujets de leur trajectoires de vie. À partir de ce point de vue les individus ne sont plus considérés comme épiphénomène des forces sociales comme par exemple un résultat d'effets de pouvoir mais comme moment crucial de l'expérience sociale.

Φροντίδα ψυχικής υγείας και εκπαιδευτικές δράσεις: από τον ιδρυματικό αποκλεισμό στην υποκειμενική ανάπτυξη

ΠΕΡΙΛΗΨΗ
Το άρθρο αυτό βασίζεται σε μια ποιοτική έρευνα που πραγματοποιήθηκε σε ένα Κοινοτικό Κέντρο Ψυχικής Υγείας στην Βραζιλία. Προσεγγίζει την επαγγελματική δράση στο πλαίσιο των υπηρεσιών ψυχικής υγείας ως ένα ευαίσθητο πεδίο, με βάση το οποίο συζητούνται τα αδιέξοδα και οι κρίσιμες στρατηγικές για την ανάπτυξη των πρακτικών με στόχο την αποϊδρυματοποίηση. Η ιδέα της υποκειμενικής ανάπτυξης από μια κοινωνικοϊστορική άποψη προσεγγίζεται ως μια μη καθολική, μη ντετερμινιστική και εξαρτώμενη από το πλαίσιο διαδικασία, που αναγνωρίζει τη διαμόρφωση του υποκειμένου ως βασική της μονάδα. Υποστηρίζουμε ότι η συζήτηση αυτή έχει ευρετική αξία για την κατανόηση της ψυχικής υγείας ως μιας ζωντανής διαδικασίας, πέρα από ερμηνευτικές διαγνωστικές κατηγορίες, που ξεπερνά την αντικειμενοποίηση και την ιεραρχική όψη που χαρακτηρίζουν συχνά τη σχέση μεταξύ των χρηστών των υπηρεσιών και των επαγγελματιών. Επιπλέον, συζητάμε πώς οι επαγγελματικές δράσεις που στοχεύουν στην υποκειμενική ανάπτυξη θα μπορούσαν να ενδυναμώσουν τις διαλογικές σχέσεις, ώστε να υποστηρίξουν τα άτομα και τις ομάδες να αποτελούν δρώντα υποκείμενα στη ζωή τους. Από αυτή την οπτική, τα άτομα δεν θεωρούνται επιφαινόμενο κοινωνικών δυνάμεων, όπως για παράδειγμα αποτέλεσμα της επίδρασης της εξουσίας, αλλά ως σημαντική στιγμή της κοινωνικής εμπειρίας.

Challenges within the Brazilian mental health care context

Historically, mental health care institutions have contributed to the pathologization of psychological processes (Amarante, 1995; Foucault, 1978; Mills, 2014). These processes have been largely criticized by psychiatric reform movements around the world during recent decades, leading to important transformations in mental health services (Arnkil & Seikkula, 2015; Moeller, 1999; Ramon, Healy, & Renouf, 2007).

In particular, Brazil was strongly influenced by Democratic Psychiatry in Italy, especially by authors like Basaglia (1980, 1985) and Rotelli (1994), who argue that 'mental disorders' should not be conceived of as illness, but as social, cultural productions and subjective production. According to them, mental health care should imply a process of deinstitutionalization which, from our point of view, demands not only social integration of these people, but also processes of subjective development[1] – a topic that has been radically excluded from mental health practices.

Such ideas about deinstitutionalization have begun to take shape in Brazil since the 1970s, making room for several transformations over the next decades. Mental health care has been gradually broadening its scope to include the constituent complexity of human processes, requiring interdisciplinary working beyond the traditional scope of areas of the health field (Amarante, 1995; Dimenstein, 2013).

In this context, Community Psychosocial Centres (*Centro de Atenção Psicossocial* – CAPS) are community-based mental health services which represent the main device of the Brazilian psychiatric reform process. They were designed as alternative services to the traditional asylums. Their services include searching for potential resources within the community in which they are established, so that all these resources are included in the assistance provided.

Nevertheless, even though the assistance is formally based on principles of democratic psychiatry, what happens in the daily routine of the services is quite different. In theory, the mental health service should work together with the community, taking into account the population's cultural productions. Therefore, the treatment should be a step in fostering social engagement and emancipation, as well as in promoting changes. However, in several situations, this articulation between service and community does not exist, and users have been assisted for many years only in activities inside the service, leading to several cases of institutionalized treatment.

Such difficulties, as argued elsewhere (Goulart, 2013, 2015, 2016), are the result of a process of new institutionalization, which represents the unilateral, hierarchical, and crystallized relationships between workers and users, who are treated as objects of technical procedures. In this sense, this situation is characterized by the maintenance of a 'mental hospital model' within the Community Psychosocial Centres (CAPS), not as walls and cages, but as social and individual subjective experiences. Through the process of new institutionalization, the institutional processes adopted in the treatment fail to combine subjective development together with assistance. As a consequence, the hypertrophied instrumental dimension of the institution's work seems to conceal the educational role played by the service (Goulart, 2013).

The case study of Sebatiao, which was part of a research project in a Community Mental Health Centre in the Federal District of Brazil (Goulart, 2013), is an example of such institutionalized process. The research was aimed at understanding social and individual subjective productions during the users' process of institutionalization and to find effective ways to help them emerge as subjects of their life. The field work for the research study was carried out uninterrupted over 36 months, which made it possible to create affective relationships with users and professionals of the service. This was an important condition for creating the social space within which the research could be realized (Goulart, 2013).

The research followed the principles of a constructive–interpretative methodology, based on the Qualitative Epistemology (González Rey, 1997, 2005), which conceptualizes the field work as a dialogical process that implies, from the very beginning, the construction of meanings by the researcher. Such meaning construction is based on the quality of the participants' expressions and not on their direct and intentional expression. The research is defined as a theoretical process oriented to produce theoretical models of intelligibility on the studied phenomenon. The researcher integrates a dynamic network of relationships and activities with the participants.

Sebastiao was 37 years old at the time the research began. He was diagnosed with schizophrenia and had been assisted by a Community Psychosocial Centre in Brazil for 7 years. His case study was chosen in order to make explicit this qualitative research standpoint and to demonstrate important theoretical issues arisen on the basis of this research experience.

The conversational sessions we had with Sebastiao were an important device in our dialogical approach. The researcher worked with Sebastiao in different contexts, within which different topics emerged and unpredictable situations occurred, allowing Sebastiao to generate different reflections and actions within his life, which were very relevant to the study. We will discuss some fragments, taken from our conversation with Sebastiao as well as from activities that the researcher shared with him during the research process. During an informal conversation we had, he said:

> Since I've started having those problems I have… of schizophrenia… I realized I needed treatment. So, I stopped everything I was doing to focus on my treatment, to get well soon. I think that's the way, isn't it? Firstly, one has to be well, to achieve good health conditions; only afterwards can one go out to do other things, such as work and leisure…

It is interesting how he convinced himself that he was not capable 'to do other things' before achieving 'good health conditions'. That is, at this moment, he felt that his treatment must be at the center of his life and that nothing else can be part of his daily routine. This position revealed indirectly the dominant institutional orientation addressed to the gap between treatment and social integration of service users, the gap between the so-called 'cure' and the subjective condition in which the users face the challenges of their lives within society. Besides this, during a conversation in a group session, Sebastiao said:

> The thing that bothers me most of all is when someone who does not know me looks at me and says, 'You're fine, you don't have anything'. How can they say that? I don't have this disease because I want it … No one knows how I am, just the psychiatrist…

In this second extract, the centrality of the psychiatrist to his own knowledge about himself is evident. In assuming this position, the 'mental illness' seemed to be understood as an object of the other's technical knowledge. That is, he did not acknowledge the relevance of his own actions in the course of his development.

The impact of the limitations of the mental health assistance given to Sebastiao also appears indirectly in Sebastiao's next statement: 'I get the job, I do the job properly. But suddenly, out of nowhere, man, I get discouraged, so I just walk away and leave. I resign! But that's because of these mental illness problems that I have'.

Sebastiao assumed his inability to work was due to his 'mental illness'. In this sense, he seems to be a prisoner of a situation in which he could do very little, centering his life on the 'illness' and not vice versa. We think that this expression indicates the existence of subjective productions that are beyond what was conscious to him, such as the production of subjective senses related to insecurity, devaluation of himself and fear, which can, in turn, be consequences of the lack of social bonds – a process which was intensified by the reification of his 'mental illness'. The ignorance of the complexity of the subjective configurations of Sebastiao's mental distress is one of the reasons that prevented the implementation of differentiated therapeutic actions which were addressed to his subjective development processes instead of to the elimination of symptoms.

In order to advance this hypothesis in process on how the institutionalization is subjectively organized in the mental health service, it would be necessary to expand on other theoretical constructions based on different case studies. Nevertheless, due to the intelligible articulation of singular processes, such as Sebastiao's, it becomes possible to address aspects of the social subjectivity of the institution that go beyond the individual dimension.

Clearly, the biomedical model that focuses on symptoms, as discussed by Canguilhem (2012), Foucault (1978), and Cooper (1967), prevails in the institutionalization framework discussed above. This logic conceives of 'mental disorder' as a deviation from an idealized general norm and treats it as an individual phenomenon, to the detriment of its subjective, social, and cultural dimensions. Consequently, together with the users' emotional fragility and lack of social bonds, an institutional configuration that associates mental disorder with social exclusion arises and crystallizes. Thereby, this situation generates an institutional vacuum that precludes the individual from developing a sense of citizenship, leaving him/her in a situation of marked vulnerability.

Hence, we have discussed that the challenges posed by this reality demand that mental health services (1) design institutional strategies that lie beyond the official discourse and the formality of public policy, and (2) have new theoretical perspectives to reflect on. In this sense, we have been advancing the theoretical articulation between education, mental health, and subjective development through a theoretical proposition of subjectivity from a cultural-historical approach (González Rey, 2002, 2012, 2015).

In order to briefly present these ideas, we would like, firstly, to introduce some general theoretical discussions related to the topic of subjectivity within the cultural-historical standpoint, which demands a brief discussion of Soviet psychology. Secondly, we will present ideas to construct these articulations between education, mental health and subjective development in the mental health care context in Brazil.

Subject and subjectivity from a cultural-historical standpoint: Deinstitutionalization beyond social ideals

Soviet psychology represents a broad heterogeneous movement, but its different trends had some principles in common, allowing it to be defined as a cultural-historical psychology (González Rey, 2011a, 2014a). Nevertheless, several deep contradictions among these trends also existed, but have not been studied in depth by Western and Russian psychologists until very recently (González Rey, 2014a). In general, Soviet psychology was largely influenced by the dramatic political and historical changes which characterized the Soviet era.

One of the most important theoretical contributions of Rubinstein's and Vygotsky's work was the transit from an element-based representation of psyche (such as traces and isolated psychological functions) to a representation based on principles in process and psychological units. For instance, Rubinstein (1964) elaborates the principle of the unity between consciousness and activity. For him, consciousness is already there in practice, and practice is an expression of consciousness. The problem is that neither of them clearly defined how consciousness is organized as a subjective system. Therefore, the presence of consciousness in activity within this theoretical standpoint has never been clarified.

Vygotsky discussed the notion of psychological units as living concepts, in a permanent process, making an important contribution to the topic of mental development, as Bozhovich (2009) argues. A very good example of that is the concept of *perezhivanie*, which expresses the unit that emerges as the dialectical expression of personality whenever facing a social influence. According to this concept, there is no external social influence apart from the person's personality (Vygotsky, 1994). Vygotsky highlights the generative character of the psyche, in which emotions play an essential role (González Rey, 2011a, 2014a, 2014b).

Nevertheless, Vygotsky's pioneering idea of units as part of a psychological system was never successfully developed by him. As Leontiev (1992, p. 43) explains, due to political and historical conditions, as well as to his premature death, the development of the idea of consciousness as a system of senses was never concretized. With the concept of *perezhivanie*, for example, Vygotsky did not make explicit how *perezhivanie* could be an expression of a subject's performance capable of integrating the current network of experiences, within which this performance takes place, with historical experiences that emerge during this performance.

Despite the advances of that psychology in recognizing the cultural genesis of human psychological processes, as a matter of fact, it did not advance toward a new ontological definition of the qualitative level of functioning of social and psychological processes in human beings under the conditions of culture. This challenge has returned the topic of subjectivity to relevance in terms of understanding a specific side of any human phenomenon, whether social or individual. The neglect of such topics, not only in the cultural-historical standpoint, but in psychology and social sciences in general, has led to a social reductionism, characterized by certain 'correct political positions' to be assumed.

Inspired by these overlooked theoretical contributions of Soviet psychology, González Rey advanced the conceptual construction of subjectivity from a cultural-historical standpoint, proposing a new ontological definition for the study of human processes (González Rey, 2002, 2007, 2009, 2011a, 2012, 2014a, 2014b, 2015). These works represent a step forward in the topic of motivation and subjectivity within this theoretical framework. González Rey's proposition integrates Vygotsky's idea to overcome the fragmentary approach to the study of psychological functions and, at the same time, it provides an opportunity to advance an ontological definition that was not clear in Vygotsky's concept of psychological unit. As González Rey stated: 'Subjectivity organizes itself as a complex configuration of subjective senses that is characterized by a chain of processes in which symbolical processes and emotions emerge together as a new quality that differs from all of the processes that participate in its genesis. These symbolic-emotional units specify the ontological character of human experience' (González Rey, 2016, p. 185).

Therefore, subjectivity is not a reflection of a given objective order, nor is it determined by external conditions, but by a symbolical–emotional production living these conditions. For this reason, it is very difficult to explain situations of mental distress traditionally associated with 'mental illness' based only on social conditions.

Within the history of the cultural-historical approach, another very inspiring concept for González Rey's theorization was Vygotsky's concept of *sense* which, according to Vygotsky, '(…) is the aggregate of all the psychological facts that arise in our consciousness as a result of the word. Sense is a dynamic, fluid, and complex formation which has several zones that vary in their stability' (Vygotsky, 1987, p. 276). Inspired by this definition, González Rey elaborated the concept of *subjective sense*, which represents the living system of actions as a subjective production, a 'unity embodied in dynamics and recursive relationships between emotions and symbolic processes within which one emerges as a result of the other without being its cause' (González Rey, 2002, p. 113).

Subjective senses are in every single action, in multiple ways, constituting *subjective configurations* of various types in different moments of the human performance. Therefore, *subjective configurations* represent a concept that expresses the integration of history and the present in a current experience, in such a way that these temporal dimensions appear as subjective senses at the present time. Also, *subjective configurations* integrate dimensions traditionally dichotomized, such as social/individual and external/internal. In this sense, as González Rey (2011a) argued, this concept embodies the metaphorical unity between consciousness and activity enunciated by Rubinstein.

A *subjective configuration* represents a relatively stable psychological formation that allows us to understand how the person's world and history are central elements of the ongoing experience. This stability should not be identified with a static organization, because it expresses itself by the congruence of a continuous flux of subjective senses generated by the configuration, but this congruence can be broken at any moment during the configured action; therefore, such stability expresses the resistance of the current dominant configuration to change.

Because of its flexibility, subjective configuration is a theoretical resource that helps us to articulate some dimensions of life that are artificially separated because of their formal differences, such as education, mental health, and subjective development. Therefore, the concept of subjective configuration allows the promotion of different levels of understanding to institutional processes around mental health care, which might be useful in overcoming some difficulties regarding the deinstitutionalization process.

The theoretical position of considering individual subjectivity as an inseparable part of the process of deinstitutionalization in mental health care allows greater understanding of how these social processes are articulated at the level of the subject. Consequently, it allows further theorization about how the individual subject's position can create disruptions in the imposed social norms which, by the force of the pathway they open, can creatively reconfigure new possibilities for social subjectivity. Therefore, individuals are not considered as epiphenomena of social forces, such as the results of the effects of power, but as crucial moments of social experience.

In this sense, socially developed processes only perform a transformative role when they are subjectively singularized and are able to change the individuals who constitute this social space. Also, this is what allows us to understand the study of a specific mental health service as a constituent unit of a complex social organization that transcends it. Such is the cross-disciplinary and flexible character that is expressed by the heuristic value of the category subjectivity within this theoretical framework.

Hegemonic notions of mental health, education and human development

In the scope of our research studies related to the articulation of mental health, education and human development (González Rey, Mitjáns Martinez, Rossato, & Goulart, in press; Goulart, 2015), we noticed that these dimensions are usually designed as fragmented because of their dominant and narrow representations, rather than their unity being considered as part of a subjective system. Specifically from the cultural-historical standpoint, we could say that mental health care was not even an object of research for historical reasons. Among the few works in psychotherapy from a cultural-historical standpoint (González Rey, 2007, 2012; Holzman & Mendez, 2003; Portes & Salas, 2011), there is a lack of publications addressing the educative and developmental processes, which overcome clinical semiology.

Education, in turn, has been thought of mainly from the perspective of assimilation of content and behavioral adjustments, rather than through the optic of the subjects who actively take part in their own educative processes. Therefore, education was directly linked with certain scholarly processes, and research in the educational field has not been contributing to some very problematic issues of social reality, such as mental health care. Education, in fact, has been confounded with instruction.

According to hegemonic standpoints, human development is not considered as a complex and systemic process. Burman (1994) says that the dominant Developmental Psychology has been studied through normative descriptions, which have slipped into naturalized prescriptions, as viewed through biological and evolutionary lenses.

However, if we conceive of both educational and mental health practices as processes that emphasize the quality of subjective development (González Rey, 2002, 2007, 2011b), it is fundamental to associate these practices in the various contexts where human development takes place. In this sense, considering the plasticity and mobility of the symbolic in relation to the emotional processes seems a powerful theoretical step in articulating different social contexts, not through the lenses of their formal functions, but through the quality of experiences of the people involved in these contexts. Subjectivity represents one attempt oriented to this goal. This could help mental health services to overcome the fragmentary and individualized perspective that is still dominant in mental health care.

Education, mental health, and subjective development: New pathways in the cultural-historical standpoint

Through the theoretical proposition of subjectivity within a cultural-historical approach, mental health care cannot be conceived of as a process having an inherent value, occurring outside the network of cultural-historical experience, because it cannot be disconnected from its consequences for the concrete life of the user. In fact, mental health care can only be considered to have achieved a therapeutic condition when it promotes changes that will help the user to develop alternatives to suffering and subjective paralysis.

Discussing the articulation between health, psychotherapy, and subjectivity, González Rey (2007, 2011b, 2012, 2015) argues that therapeutic actions within this theoretical framework do not emphasize the representation of conflict, but the creation of dialogical relationships which can foster the production of new subjective senses related to overcoming the subjective conflict. The psychotherapist's knowledge does not provide any direct answers according to the categorization of the service user's mental disorder. It is only a therapeutic tool when it is able to provide strategies that could promote educational processes that aim to build collective practices that will enhance subjective development, thereby providing different possibilities for social change.

Education is defined here as a system of actions addressed toward the subjective development of individuals and social groups. The ground on which these actions take place is the dialogical communications between the educator and the individual/group, as well as between the participants in the process (González Rey et al., in press). In this scenario, the field of education would contribute by promoting institutional changes and fostering reflections on possible institutional practices geared to the subject's social engagement and its creative character. Therefore, an experience is considered educative only when it triggers new reflections, emotions, and reactions among the participants in the process (González Rey, 2009). Education as such is very absent in social institutions, such as schools, hospitals, health care services, and prisons (González Rey et al., in press).

Subjective development, in turn, represents a way to overcome unilateral and absolute criteria of standardized children/people within universal stages without overlooking the uniqueness of this process, the dialectics between individual and social and the active role of the subject. As we argued elsewhere (González Rey et al., in press), subjective development results from different subjective configurations interwoven within different social networks from which actions emerge:

> One subjective configuration is a driving force of subjective development when it includes the development of new subjective resources that allows the individual to make relevant changes in the course of a performance, relations or other significant lived experiences leading to changes that define new subjective resources. (González Rey et al., in press, p. 30)

The subjective configurations on which the development of subjectivity takes place include changes in individual performances and positions that also lead to changes in different social spheres. Through this process, individuals or social groups becomes subjects of their actions by being capable of assuming positions, and of taking decisions and actions that open new pathways within the normative social system (González Rey, 2002, 2012, 2014a). In this sense, the subject emerges as a living agency, either social or individual, that actively generates new subjective senses during the action – a process that renders it possible to overcome any type of subjective or social determinism. Based on this perspective, the idea that there are positive and negative conditions of development which are independent of individuals and their relationships should be discarded once and for all (González Rey et al., in press).

Again, Sebastiao's process is useful in order to discuss a subjective development process. One of the greatest difficulties he had was to overcome his isolated routine. He used to keep himself in his bedroom the whole day, except when he was at the Community Psychosocial Centre. In order to address this situation, as a first approximation, he was invited by one of the service workers to participate in the 'Football Group' once a week. Although Sebastiao had never played football before, he accepted the challenge. After roughly a month, he said in a group conversation:

> The football match is good because nobody is better than anybody else. We go there, we run, we win, we lose (laughs) and it's okay. Our problems seem to disappear. I like people there so much.

From this statement, it is possible to appreciate the relevance of the individual's insertion into new social spaces, within which he/she can develop relationships and actions on his or her own within a complete different atmosphere from the dominant one in the mental health service. Probably for the first time, he was taking part in a group activity without feeling worse than or inferior to the others. This physical activity unfolded into new subjective senses related to self-worth through the feeling of being welcomed by a group. Evidence of this is that he spontaneously began to take occasional walks in his neighborhood. Then he started to do it more regularly and to walk longer distances, in places where before he had felt uncomfortable or even terrified. After a couple of weeks, he said:

> Now I'm not walking only three times a week, but every day! By the way, there are some days when I walk twice: in the morning and at the end of the afternoon.

And sometimes I go very far from home! I go out, I feel the sun, I see people on the streets. I get more excited! (…) And another thing that has changed my life is that I'm taking a shower every day. I used to take a shower twice a week. There were weeks when I didn't shower… and now I do it every day. If I walk twice a day, I take two showers! I'm getting better… I didn't use to shave myself, or brush my teeth. Today, I do it every day (laughs)!

Sebastiao's situation illustrates the first moment in a process of subjective development, not due to the type of activity he was practicing, let alone its frequency, but because the process represented a rupture within his social isolation and his feelings of fear, sadness, and lack of confidence. These feelings, along with the lack of social bounds, constituted the basis for his situation of distress. Through the process, Sebastiao was able to begin a chain of different actions related to social engagement, which were not restricted to the specific and isolated sphere of his life, such as hearing voices, doing physical exercises, or finding a job. Those actions were grounded in the emergence of a new subjective configuration involved in his active position as a subject, in such a way that he became able, at least partially, to overcome his psychiatric institutionalization.

The constructive-interpretative research, based on the Qualitative Epistemology, was the result of the demands raised by the definition of subjectivity assumed in this paper. The research, as briefly demonstrated previously, is a way to produce knowledge, but, at the same time, is a process within which the participants become active agents of new life pathways, in such a way that the research becomes also an important psychological and educational set of relationships and activities.

The creation of new social spaces within which the person can be integrated is an important condition for the transit from a patient identity to a citizen identity. Moreover, the dialogical condition of mental health care is a crucial aspect in overcoming the objectualization and hierarchical aspect which frequently characterize the relationship between service users and workers. Based on this perspective, the challenge is not only to overcome a specific institutionalized structure, such as the asylum, but to promote institutional conditions and social devices so that individuals and social groups are invited to cultivate critical and creative skills from their own subjective resources. To foster this, contradictory process demands educational actions based on an ethics of the subject, which implies a complex approach to the endless and dynamic movement between institutionalization and deinstitutionalization.

Final remarks

This paper has addressed, based on a qualitative research study within a Community Mental Health Centre in Brazil, the professional actions of community-based mental health services in Brazil, which are seen not as the only possibility for constructing a mental health network, but as a sensitive sphere in which to discuss deadlocks and critical strategies in order to expand the practices around deinstitutionalization.

In such an endeavor, the theoretical and practical challenge of advancing educational actions toward subjective development have heuristic value for understanding mental health as a living process, beyond hermetic diagnostic entities. Moreover, such theoretical articulation could enhance professional actions which emphasize the creation of dialogical relations capable of supporting individuals and groups to actively position themselves as subjects in their life pathways.

Therefore, the aim was to question the social and theoretical resources currently available and to reflect upon alternatives yet to be created. We think that such creative effort could help the overcoming of practices focused on solving specific problems, as well as the fragmentation of knowledge and practices around mental health care, enhancing practices which do not detach mental health, culture, and society.

Note

1. Later in this paper, we discuss in depth how subjective development is considered as a non-deterministic, non-universal, as well as a context-sensitive process, which has subjective configuration as its unit. In this way, subjective development represents a way in which to overcome absolute criteria as the basis to label people within standardized and universal stages.

Disclosure statement

No potential conflict of interest was reported by the authors.

Funding

This work was supported by the Brazilian Federal Agency for Support and Evaluation of Graduate Education – CAPES – under [grant number BEX 10348/14-0].

References

Amarante, P. (1995). *Loucos pela vida: a trajetória da reforma psiquiátrica no Brasil* [Mad at life: The trajectory of psychiatric reform in Brazil]. Rio de Janeiro: Panorama ENSP.

Arnkil, T. E., & Seikkula, J. (2015). Developing dialogicity in relational practices: Reflecting on experiences from open dialogues. *Australian and New Zealand Journal of Family Therapy, 36*, 142–154. doi:10.1002/anzf.1009

Basaglia, F. (1980). *A psiquiatria alternativa: Contra o pessimismo da razão, o otimismo da prática* [The alternative psychiatry: Against the pessimism of reason, the optimism of practice]. São Paulo: Brasil Debates.

Basaglia, F. (1985). As instituições da violência [Institutions of violence]. In F. Basaglia (Ed.), *A Instituição Negada: relato de um hospital psiquiátrico* [The denied institution: Report of a psychiatric hospital] (3rd ed., H. Jahn, Trad., pp. 34–72). Rio de Janeiro: Edições Graal.

Bozhovich, L. I. (2009). The social situation of child development. *Journal of Russian and East European Psychology, 47*, 59–86. doi:10.2753/RPO1061-0405470403

Burman, E. (1994). *Deconstructing developmental psychology*. London: Routledge.

Canguilhem, G. (2012). *Writings on medicine*. New York, NY: Fordham University Press.

Cooper, D. (1967). *Psychiatry and anti-psychiatry*. London: Tavistock Publications Limited.

Dimenstein, M. (2013). La reforma psiquiátrica y el modelo de atención psicosocial em Brasil: en busca de cuidados continuados e integrados em salud mental [Psychiatric reform and the psychosocial care model in Brazil: Looking for long-term and integrated care in mental health]. *CS (Cali), 11*, 43–71. doi:10.18046/recs.i11.1566

Foucault, M. (1978). *História da loucura* [History of madness] (J. T. Coelho Netto, Trad.). São Paulo: Perspectiva.

González Rey, F. (1997). *Epistemología Cualitativa y Subjetividad* [Qualitative epistemology and subjectivity]. São Paulo: Educ.

González Rey, F. (2002). *Sujeto y Subjetividad: Una aproximación histórico-cultural* [Subject and subjectivity: A cultural-historical approach]. México: Thomson.

González Rey, F. (2005). *Pesquisa qualitativa e subjetividade: os processos de construção da informação* [Qualitative research and subjectivity: The processes of construction of information] (2nd ed.). São Paulo: Cengage Learning.

González Rey, F. (2007). *Psicoterapia, subjetividade e pós-modernidade: uma aproximação histórico-cultural* [Psychotherapy, subjectivity and post modernity: A cultural-historical approach]. São Paulo: Pioneira Thomson Learning.

González Rey, F. (2009). Historical relevance of Vygotsky's work: Its significance for a new approach to the problem of subjectivity in psychology. *Outlines: Critical Practice Studies, 11*, 59–73. Retrieved from http://ojs.statsbiblioteket.dk/index.php/outlines/article/view/2589/2248

González Rey, F. (2011a). A re-examination of defining moments in Vygotsky's work and their implications for his continuing legacy. *Mind, culture and activity, 18*, 257–275. doi:10.1080/10749030903338517

González Rey, F. (2011b). *Subjetividade e saúde: superando a clínica da patologia* [Subjectivity and health: Overcoming the clinic of pathology]. São Paulo: Cortez.

González Rey, F. (2012). Sentidos subjetivos, lenguaje y sujeto: avanzando en una perspectiva postracionalista en psicoterapia [Subjective senses, language and subject: Advances in a post-rationalist perspective on psychotherapy]. *Rivista di psichiatria* [Journal of Psychiatry], *46*, 310–314. Retrieved from http://www.rivistadipsichiatria.it/r. php?v=1009&a=10978&l=14979&f=allegati/01009_2011_05/fulltext/8-Gonzalez%20 Rey(310-314).pdf

González Rey, F. (2014a). Advancing further the history of soviet psychology: Moving forward from dominant representations in western and soviet psychology. *History of Psychology, 17*, 60–78. doi:10.1037/a0035565

González Rey, F. (2014b). Human motivation in question: Discussing emotions, motives and subjectivity from a cultural-historical standpoint. *Journal for the Theory of Social Behavior, 45*, 1–18. doi:10.1111/jtsb.12073

González Rey, F. (2015). A new path for the discussion of social representations: Advancing the topic of subjectivity from a cultural-historical standpoint. *Theory and Psychology, 25*, 494–512. doi:10.1177/0959354315587783

González Rey, F. (2016). Advancing on the topics of the social and subjectivity from a cultural-historical approach: Moments, paths and contradictions. *Journal of the Theoretical and Philosophical Psychology, 36*, 175–189. doi:10.1017/CCOL0521831040

González Rey, F., Mitjáns Martinez, A., Rossato, M., & Goulart, D. M. (in press). The relevance of subjective configurations for discussing human development. In M. Fleer, F. González Rey, & A. Mitjáns Martinez (Eds.), *Cultural-historical perspectives on emotions: Advancing the concepts of perezhivanie and subjectivity*. Cambridge: Springer.

Goulart, D. M. (2013). *Institucionalização, subjetividade e desenvolvimento humano: abrindo caminhos entre educação e saúde mental* [Institutionalization, subjectivity and human development: Opening new paths between education and mental health] (Masters dissertation). University of Brasília. Retrieved from http://repositorio.unb. br/handle/10482/14958

Goulart, D. M. (2015). Clínica, subjetividade e educação: uma integração teórica alternativa para forjar uma ética do sujeito no campo da saúde mental [Clinic, subjectivity and education: An alternative theoretical integration to fostar na ethics of the subject]. In F. González Rey & J. Bizerril (Eds.), *Saúde, cultura e subjetividade: uma referência interdisciplinar* [Health, culture and subjectivity: An interdisciplinar standpoin] (pp. 34–57). Brasília: UniCEUB.

Goulart, D. M. (2016). The psychiatrization of human practices worldwide: Discussing new chains and cages. *Pedagogy, Culture & Society*. Advance online publication. doi:10.1080/14681366.2016.1160673

Holzman, L., & Mendez, R. (Eds.). (2003). *Psychological investigations: A clinician's guide to social therapy*. New York, NY: Brunner-Routledge.

Leontiev, A. A. (1992). Ecce homo. Methodological problems of the activity theoretical approach. *Multidisciplinary Newsletter for Activity Theory, 11/12*, 41–44.

Mills, C. (2014). *Decolonizing global mental health: The psychiatrization of the majority world*. London: Routledge.

Moeller, M. L. (1999). History, concept and position of self-help groups in Germany. *Group Analysis, 32*, 181–194. doi:10.1177/05333169922076653

Portes, P., & Salas, S. (2011). *Vygotsky in 21st century society: Advances in cultural historical theory and praxis with non-dominant communities*. New York, NY: Peter Lang.

Ramon, S., Healy, B., & Renouf, N. (2007). Recovery from mental illness as an emergent concept and practice in Australia and the UK. *International Journal of Social Psychiatry, 53*, 108–122. doi:10.1177/0020764006075018

Rotelli, F. (1994). Superando o manicômio: o circuito psiquiátrico de Trieste [Overcoming the hospice: The psychiatric circuit of Trieste]. In P. Amarante (Ed.), *Psiquiatria Social e Reforma* Psiquiátrica [Social psychiatry and psychiatric reform] (pp. 149–170). Rio de Janeiro: Editora FIOCRUZ.

Rubinstein, S. L. (1964). *El desarrollo de la psicología. Principios y métodos* [The development of psychology: Principles and methods]. Havana: Editora del Consejo Nacional de Universidades.

Vygotsky, L. S. (1987). Thinking and speech. In R. Rieber & A. Carton (Eds.), *The collected works of L. S. Vygotsky* (Vol. 1, pp. 43–287). New York, NY: Plenum.

Vygotsky, L. S. (1994). The problem of the environment. In R. Van Der Veer & J. Valsiner (Eds.), *The Vygotsky reader* (pp. 338–354). Oxford: Blackwell.

Displaying agency problems at the outset of psychotherapy

Jarl Wahlström and Minna-Leena Seilonen

ABSTRACT

In order to present him- or herself at the outset of psychotherapy as a credible client, the person needs to, on one hand, formulate a sense of lost agency in accounts of his/her life situation, and on the other, to present him- or herself as willing and able to take part in conversational self-exploration. In this study, we looked in detail at how one person, seeking psychotherapy, constructed accounts that served this double function. We sought to develop the usefulness of the concept of agency as an integrative theoretical construct of core processes in therapy and introduced a model of five aspects of agentic vs. non-agentic presentation, developed and applied in an earlier study on clients in semi-mandatory counselling. The results show how those aspects – relationality, causal attribution, intentionality, historicity and reflexivity – were present in, or lacking from, accounts given by this one client entering voluntary psychotherapy. We conclude that qualitative process research could benefit from considering loss of agency as one crucial object of psychotherapy and the ongoing discursive formulations and re-formulations of the client's more or less agentic positions as central to the process of therapy.

LAS DIFICULTADES DE LOS PACIENTES PARA DEMOSTRAR SU " SENTIDO DE SI MISMO" AL SOLICITAR PSICOTERAPIA

Para ser considerado como un cliente creíble, la persona que solicita psicoterapia debe demostrar desde el comienzo, por una parte,que ha perdido el 'sentido de sí mismo' como individuo en relación con el mundo y por la otra, debe mostrar interés en participar en conversaciones auto-exploratorias. En este sentido examinamos detalladamente, cómo una persona que solicita psicoterapia expresa su predicamento en relación con estos dos aspectos. Hemos buscado desarrollar la utilidad del concepto 'sentido de sí mismo' como un constructo teórico-integrativo de procesos centrales en terapia y hemos introducido un modelo de cinco aspectos para estudiar este proceso en su manifestación positiva o negativa en el cliente. Este modelo ha sido aplicado en un estudio anterior con clientes en orientación psicológica semi-obligatoria. Los resultados muestran cómo esos aspectos – relacionalidad, atribución causal,intencionalidad, historicidad y reflexibidad- estuvieron presentes o no en los contenidos narrados por este cliente al comenzar psicoterapia voluntaria. Concluimos que la investigación de procesos cualitativos podría beneficiarse si se considerase la pérdida del 'sentido de sí mismo' como un objeto crucial de la psicoterapia, así como también la consideración de todas las formulaciones y re-formulaciones del cliente en relación con su concepto de su 'sentido de sí mismo'.

L'attiva presentazione dei problemi all'inizio della Psicoterapia

Al fine di presentare se stessi come "clienti accettabili" all'inizio di una psicoterapia si deve, da un lato, enunciare un senso di smarrimento nei confronti della situazione di vita, e dall'altro, presentarsi come persona disponibile e capace di prender parte ad un dialogo di auto-esplorazione. In questo studio abbiamo esaminato in dettaglio il modo in cui una persona, in cerca di una psicoterapia, presenti spiegazioni che svolgano questa doppia funzione. Abbiamo cercato di presentare l'utilità del concetto "attivo" come un costrutto teorico integrativo dei principali processi in terapia e introdotto un modello composto da cinque aspetti della presentazione "attiva" vs. presentazione "non attiva", modello sviluppato e applicato in un precedente studio condotto su clienti in consulenza semi-obbligatoria. I risultati mostrano come questi aspetti - relazionalità, attribuzione causale, intenzionalità, storicità, e riflessività – possano essere presenti o assenti nelle presentazioni di un cliente che inizia volontariamente una psicoterapia. Concludiamo sottolineando come i processi di ricerca qualitativa potrebbero trarre vantaggio dal considerare come elemento cruciale della psicoterapia la mancanza di una presenza attiva così come la ricorrente formulazione discorsiva e ri-formulazione delle posizioni del cliente, più o meno attivo, come elemento centrale nel processo terapeutico.

Problèmes d'agencéité en début de thérapie

Pour se présenter comme un client crédible au début d'une thérapie, une personne doit à la fois formuler une certaine perte de contrôle lorsqu'elle fait le récit de sa situation et à la fois se montrer volontaire et capable de s'engager dans une auto-exploration conversationnelle. Cette étude examine en détail comment ayant fait une demande de psychothérapie, une personne construit ses récits ayant cette double fonction. Nous avons cherché à développer l'utilité du concept d'agencéité (agency) comme construction théorique intégrative du processus central en thérapie et avons introduit un modèle comprenant cinq aspects de présentation agentique et non-agentique que nous avions développé et appliqué lors d'une précédente étude portant sur des clients faisant une psychothérapie partiellement imposée. Les résultats montrent que ces aspects - relationalité, attribution causale, intentionnalité, historicité et réflexivité - étaient présents, ou absents, des récits fournis par ce client qui avait choisi d'entrer en psychothérapie. Nous concluons que le processus de recherche qualitative aurait avantage à considérer la perte de pouvoir décisionnaire comme élément crucial de la psychothérapie et les formulations et reformulations discursives des positions plus ou moins agentiques du client en tant que centrales au processus thérapeutique.

Η εμφάνιση προβλημάτων κυριότητας κατά την έναρξη της ψυχοθεραπείας

ΠΕΡΙΛΗΨΗ
Προκειμένου να παρουσιαστεί ως αξιόπιστος πελάτης κατά την έναρξη της ψυχοθεραπείας, το άτομο χρειάζεται, αφενός, να εκφράσει μια αίσθηση απώλειας της κυριότητας του στον τρόπο που περιγράφει τη συνθήκη της ζωής του, και από την άλλη, να παρουσιαστεί ως πρόθυμο και ικανό να συμμετέχει σε μια μέσω συνομιλίας αυτοδιερεύνηση. Στην παρούσα μελέτη εξετάσαμε λεπτομερώς πώς ένα άτομο, που αναζήτησε ψυχοθεραπεία, κατασκεύασε περιγραφές που εξυπηρετούν αυτή τη διπλή λειτουργία. Επιδιώξαμε να αναπτύξουμε τη χρησιμότητα της έννοιας της κυριότητας ως μια συνθετική θεωρητική έννοια των βασικών διεργασιών στη θεραπεία και εισαγάγαμε ένα μοντέλο αποτελούμενο από πέντε όψεις της παρουσίας με ή χωρίς κυριότητα, το οποίο αναπτύχθηκε και εφαρμόστηκε σε μια προηγούμενη μελέτη με πελάτες σε ημι-υποχρεωτική συμβουλευτική. Τα αποτελέσματα δείχνουν τον τρόπο με τον οποίο αυτές οι διαστάσεις -σχεσιακότητα, αιτιώδης απόδοση, προθετικότητα, ιστορικότητα, και αναστοχαστικότητα- υπήρχαν ή απουσίαζαν από το λόγο του συγκεκριμένου πελάτη που αναζήτησε ψυχοθεραπεία εθελοντικά. Καταλήγουμε στο συμπέρασμα ότι η ποιοτική έρευνα της ψυχοθεραπευτικής διεργασίας) θα επωφελούνταν από την αναγνώριση της απώλειας της κυριότητας ως κρίσιμο αντικείμενο στην ψυχοθεραπεία και από την αναγνώριση της συνεχιζόμενης δια του λόγου κατασκευής και ανακατασκευής θέσεων, με περισσότερη ή λιγότερη κυριότητα, του πελάτη ως κεντρικής σημασίας για τη θεραπευτική διαδικασία.

Introduction

Agency as a construct has different uses in psychotherapy research (Mackrill, 2009). The client's experience of loss of agency in his/her life has been conceptualized as a prime reason for seeking help from conversational therapy (Wahlström, 2006) and the participation of the client as an active agent is seen as prerequisite for the change process (Levitt, Pomerville, & Surace, 2016).

In this study, taking a constructionist and discursive stance, we look upon the process of therapy as an ongoing opening of new discursive formulations of the client's positions in regards to his/her problems (Avdi, 2012). Some of these positionings will be more, and some less agentic. From an institutional point of view, in order to act as an active participant in such a process, the person seeking treatment needs to present him- or herself as a credible client. This involves two interdependent discursive tasks: (1) to formulate a sense of lost agency in accounts of his/her life situation, and (2) to display him- or herself as willing and able to take part in conversational self-exploration. 'Credibility' here refers to the institutional role and position of a client, i.e. adopting a social discourse to which both the client and the therapist subscribe.

In the present single case study, we look upon how one prospective client presented her problems in her first psychotherapy session. Our interest is in how the client's problem formulations display and construct for her various agentic or non-agentic positions. With a background both in psychotherapy practice and in qualitative process research, we seek to develop the usefulness of the concept of agency as a theoretical construct which could further an integrative understanding of some core processes in therapy. To do this we see the need to acknowledge the complexity of the concept and the several aspects to it.

Agency refers to 'the power to do' or 'the force that causes effects' (Pope, 1998, pp. 242, 243), and the notion of an agent to someone capable of doing things and making things happen, implying some activity and independence. An essential feature of agency is being able to intentionally cause change in the world and to differentiate between actions and events caused by oneself and conditions attributable to external causes (Kögler, 2010, 2012). Thus, two salient aspects of agency are *intentionality* and *causal attribution*.

An agent is seen as capable of making intentional and constructive choices, changing the course of his or her actions, potentially reaching self-nominated goals, and thus of genuinely creating his or her life (Avdi, 2005; Jenkins, 2001). Reaching such an agentic stance calls for some distance to the self and critical self-observing, i.e. a reflexive position in relation to one`s thinking, acting and different aspects of the self (Dimaggio, 2011; Georgaca, 2001; Rennie, 2010). Such a reflexive posture affords also the possibility to view certain impulses or desires as problematic, unwanted or inauthentic (Kögler, 2012). Thus, a salient aspect of agency is *reflexivity*.

From a narrative perspective, agency is engaging oneself in narrative self-constructions (Bruner, 1990). In such construction, assuming a reflective perspective affords present experiences and actions to be presented as related to past, as well as future, events, experiences or actions, thus producing continuity in personal life stories (Georgaca, 2001). This conception outlines agency as a temporal process where the narrated past is reconstructed within the present and carried on into alternative forthcoming possibilities (Kupferberg & Green, 2005; Ogden, 1986). Thus a salient aspect of agency is *historicity*.

According to Harré (1995), the notion of agency has to be related to the position of the person within a social and moral order. Such a standpoint, emphasizing intersubjectivity as a fundamental constituent of agency, has been endorsed also by Gillespie (2012), Kögler (2012), Ogden (1986) and Markova (2003). Agentic actors, while embedded in one situation, transcend this and take more general perspectives, including those of other actors. Thus a salient aspect of agency is *relationality*.

Loss of agency, then, can be conceptualized in terms of the person constructing him- or herself as being in the position of an object or victim of some 'alien' entity, e.g. an experience, a circumstance or an illness, which is initiating some action, or is controlling or unduly influencing him or her (Avdi, Lerou, & Seikkula, 2015; Karatza & Avdi, 2011; Kupferberg & Green, 2005; Ogden, 1986). Non-agentic positions have been defined as not having a place in conversations where meanings pertinent to one's life are produced (Drewery, 2005), not having access to a self-authored autobiography (Bamberg, 2009), nor to have the option to take a reflexive, critical or evaluative standpoint in respect to the self and its actions (Avdi, 2012).

We look upon such loss of agency as being on one hand an actual state of affairs in a person's life – bringing about a genuine *sense* of lost agency – and on the other hand a discursive *presentation* or *display* of oneself as being in a non-agentic position. Paraphrasing Harré's (1995, p. 123) notion that 'being an agent and displaying oneself as an agent is one and the same', we argue that 'being a *non*-agent and displaying oneself as a *non*-agent is one and the same'. Thus problem formulations in psychotherapy, i.e. accounts of the sensation of lost mastery in some life situation(s), have a double function. Such accounts are simultaneously 'genuine' expressions of an experience *and* means of seeking a position in the actual situational context of the therapy session.

The aim of this study was to look in detail at how a person seeking voluntary psychotherapy constructed accounts that served the aforementioned double function of expressing the experiential loss of sense of agency and of taking the position as a potential client. When doing this, our second – and actually more definitive – aim was to introduce and try out the transferability (Lincoln & Guba, 1985) of a model of five aspects of agentic vs. non-agentic display, originally created by us in a study of disclaims of agency presented by repeated drunk driving clients entering semi-mandatory counselling (Seilonen & Wahlström,

2016). In that study it was found that the model could differentiate between the cases in a meaningful way, and contribute to an understanding of the clients' ways of positioning themselves in semi-mandatory counselling, as well as of their uses of the counselling context. In the present study, we ask how this model can show how the different aspects of agency constructions are present in, or lacking from, accounts given by the client entering voluntary psychotherapy.

Method

With the aim to review varieties of agentic vs. non-agentic self-presentations in psychotherapy, we performed a theory-guided qualitative content analysis (Mayring, 2014) of the speech turns of one client during her first visit to a university-based psychotherapy training clinic in Finland. The theoretical model that guided the analysis has been developed by us in an earlier study (Seilonen & Wahlström, 2016).

Participants and data

The client-participant was a female, married high school teacher, in her 30's, who had been on maternity leave for four and a half years, and returned to her work a couple of months before seeking therapy. Like all clients to the clinic she also was self-referred, but actually her father was the one who had first contacted the clinic. In her own initial telephone call and at the beginning of the first session, the client presented as her problem her social anxiety which caused her to be over conscientious in her work and fearful of her pupils' reactions. The work health service, which she had contacted a few weeks earlier, had diagnosed her as being burned out and moderately depressed. Later in the first session she talked a lot about the problems in her relationship with her husband, due partly to his drinking behaviour.

The therapist-participant was a female qualified psychologist in her early 30's who was at the time of the treatment specializing in integrative psychotherapy at the training clinic. The input of the therapist to the conversation in this session was remarkably small. After having asked the client to tell about her situation 'in her own words' she mainly used small continuers to signal her stance of empathic listening. There were a few important turns, though, in which she showed her responsiveness to the client's accounts. These had, without doubt, an important influence on the development of the client's telling but are not the object of analysis in this study.

The primary data of the study consisted of a video-recording of the first session, and the verbatim transcript thereof. The transcript amounted to 26 pages and 779 lines. The session was conducted in Finnish, and the analysis was performed on the original Finnish transcript. Short excerpts from the transcript have been translated into English for the purpose of this article. The participants gave their informed consent to the use of the data according to a protocol reviewed by the university's Ethical Committee.

Analysis

As a first step of analysis both authors read independently the data and coded the client's turns according to the model of aspects of agency display, determining what aspect the passage in question expressed, and whether it was agentic or non-agentic. In consensus meetings, the coding of the passages was reviewed. Then as a second step, the displays of agency vs. non-agency in the evolving problem formulations and life accounts according to each aspect were subjected to consensual qualitative content analysis.

The Five Aspect Model

The model that informed the content analysis (Seilonen & Wahlström, 2016) argues that five interrelated aspects of agency – relationality, causal attribution, intentionality, historicity and reflexivity – can be identified as present in, or missing from, life-accounts given by clients in counselling or therapy contexts. The presence or absence of an active formulation of the aspect contributes to rendering the presentation of the client as agentic or non-agentic.

Relationality is defined as presentations of others in relation to self, intersubjective perspective-takings, boundaries between self and others and connections between the self and others.

Causal attributions are defined as presentations of varied phenomena and the doings of actors (self and others) as caused either externally or by the actors, including the speaker him- or herself.

Intentions are defined as presentations of the actors' aims and purposes in varied life situations (including the presenting problems) and in the situation of giving the account (the therapy session).

Historicity is defined (1) as the temporal sequencing of events within the account into an understandable story, and (2) as the dialectics between temporal, experienced positions in the life situation accounted for and their interpretation in the present moment of telling.

Reflexivity is defined as evaluative and reflective talk in regard to the life situation or problem accounted for. When present in an account, reflexivity is usually connected to some other aspect of agency.

Results

In the course of analysis, passages relevant to each aspect of agency were identified. Reading the passages assigned to different aspects, it became evident that the client's presentation of agency or non-agency changed and evolved as her accounting of her difficulties and her different life-situations carried on. It also became obvious that the different aspects diverged in relation to how they contained agentic vs. non-agentic display. In the following we present condensed expositions of each aspect. The presentation includes short illustrative excerpts from the data. Their locations in the transcript are indicated with line-numbers.

Relationality

Within the relational field that emerged through her accounts, the client mainly displayed herself as non-agentic. There was, though, variations both in respect to topics and to how the telling progressed as the session went on. The relational field included her husband and children (mentioned for the first time in line 11), her pupils and their parents (line 42), her sisters and friends (line 82), her parents (line 107), the headmaster of her school (line 108), the physician and the psychologist from her work health services (lines 122 and 132), and some women in an Al Anon group (line 427).

In relation to her sisters and parents she presented herself at the beginning of the session as emotionally reactive and helpless – she 'bursts into tears' (line 61) when talking to them, and they are the ones who urge her to seek help. In that respect she pictured herself as utterly non-agentic: 'then again this my other sister said that now one has to seek some help' (line 102). Later in the session she says that her parents described her as always having been 'so nice' (line 686) and that she was the good girl in the family who, unlike her sisters, did not cause any trouble.

In relation to her pupils and their parents she presented herself as fearful and on her guard – she has to beware that they do not 'catch her' (line 96) for not knowing enough about her subject. She feels tense and anxious before entering the class room, and the parents' meetings are 'of course an entirely different case' (line 44), meaning that they are even worse.

In relation to the headmaster she pictured herself as expecting him to be surprised at her announcement of staying out of work: 'because in school I haven't said anything [about my problems]' (line 118). Then she herself appears to be astonished by how he showed an understanding attitude towards her, evidently not being as astounded by the news as she had expected.

In relation to the health professionals she described herself as opposing, but at the same time accepting, their assessment of her situation. She felt intimidated by the diagnoses: 'depression that sounds as such a terrible strong word' (line 141). However, she did not contest the assessments of her condition, and she followed the prescriptions of taking medicine and to seek therapy but in her telling these are pictured as strange and alarming.

In relation to her husband she presented herself in various positions. She mostly referred to him as 'the husband', instead of using his first name. He can be called upon when she needs help but his attitude is not told as helpful. He says that she does not need to reveal the real reason for staying out of work but she cannot 'pretend anymore' (line 110). Later in the session she tells about her husband's drinking problem and untoward behaviour: 'there is this kind of psychological abuse' (line 317). She says that 'they are there somewhere as a lump all those things' (line 362). Her relation to him appears as blurred – his words and doings affect her in a way which she has difficulties to articulate: 'so this is what this man is like (…) can this man act like this' (lines 323–324). The relationship is presented as alienated and her attitude as increasingly critical.

This questioning of her relationship with the husband, and of the position she has assumed within it, is also expressed in her telling of her experience of participating in an Al Anon group. She has found it difficult to accept the other women's attitude: 'they are married to an alcoholic and still they can somehow live their own lives' (lines 436–437). For her it had felt odd that 'somehow you don't let it [the drinking] bother you but still you have there the alcoholic by your side' (lines 449–450).

In relation to the therapy the client, by strongly taking the initiative to talk and give meticulous descriptions of her situation and problems, gave the impression of seeking the position of a compliant client. Then, on the other hand, her mode of telling was that of reporting and full of details, creating an image of an outsider perspective, and of her as participating only due to the circumstances. This changed when she started to talk about the marital problems and her relations to her parents and sisters. Interestingly, after having dwelled on these issues for some time, she says: 'are these issues relevant here but if I still [say something] about myself …' (lines 663–664); as if asking whether she is permitted to take ownership of her own experience and perspective.

Causal attributions

In the initial problem formulation the client's causal attributions were mostly external and situational: 'all the spring I was anxious about returning to work' (lines 35); 'even just being in front of others, before the class only [is difficult] for me' (line 42); 'I start to have also these kind of physical symptoms' (line 69); 'There was not a single day that I wouldn't have thought about returning to work' (lines 70–71). Attributions were also given to essentialized characteristics of herself: 'I am too conscientious' (line 76); 'I am sensitive, I observe myself' (line 155).

In later accounts of her life situations the attributions became more internal and personal: 'such a terrible kind of checking, I know' (lines 94–95); 'I started to have this feeling am I now really crazy' (line 197); 'I have somehow noticed [this] am I that kind of nice girl all the time' (lines 665–666). Thus, in such attributions, the reasons for her troubles were not placed in outer or inner circumstances but in her own ways of taking stances ('checking', 'having a feeling', 'having noticed'), thus rendering her a more agentic position in relation to the problems.

Intentionality

The client mainly presented her intentions as non-agentic, in the sense that they were mostly adapted to her perceived expectations of others towards her. In work, her intention had been to prepare her classes conscientiously and make sure that the pupils do not 'catch' her for not knowing something. She struggled not to show her insecurity to her colleagues and this changed only when the anxiety and the feeling of burn out got too strong: 'I thought that I can't pretend anymore' (lines 110–111). Still, she pictured herself as overtly responsible: 'The doctor suggested a longer sick leave but I said I cannot be away even two weeks' (lines 123–124). In her account the main intention presented is one of enduring difficulties and avoiding causing troubles to others.

Also in close relationships she presented her intentions as have been, throughout her history, to comply with others' wishes, to endure misbehaviours, and take responsibility for conflicts. In relation to her parents her intention was told as having been to be 'a good girl' who does not make troubles: 'I would never have dared to do like that [as her sister did] … I still think about what mum and dad would say about this or that' (lines 682–684). She told how she 'apologized' for taking this kind of husband who is not well educated and is ill-behaved when drunk: 'I used to have these feelings of guilt … that I know that he is not the ideal son-in-law' (lines 707–711).

When accounting for her relation to her husband and his abusive behaviour the client presented her intentions with some self-reflection. Her aim, which she now started to question, had been to tolerate and endure all: 'I take in everything and sometimes it feels that I am even guilty for his drinking' (line 260). She had been trying to control her husband's drinking, and even keeping records of it, but now she doubtfully asked 'if there is anything that I can do about it' (line 422).

In the client's account intentions were closely connected to relations. Her main intention in regards to others appeared as having been to hide herself, as showing herself as not having intentions, i.e. demands or requests, of her own. That intention then placed her outside mutual intersubjective connections in her relational field and positioned her as less agentic.

Historicity

In the earlier part of the session, when the client was describing her symptoms and problems, history was present in the form of detailed descriptions of events just following each other. History-telling in the form of such temporal sequencing of events – creating a chronology – pictured her as an external observer of what happened to her: 'already last year I started to terribly [worry] somehow that how am I going to cope' (lines 38–39). Thus, her problem accounts were mostly ahistorical in the sense that they were mainly reports of her affective and bodily reactions, the doings of herself and others, and other events; not including her own subjective point of view. She does not give any interpretations to her reactions, nor does she evaluate their possible reasons or consequences.

Later in the session she articulated detailed biographical stories of her relationships in her family of origin and in her present family. She repeatedly presented her own position as a 'good girl' (conscientious, forgiving, asking forgiveness, obeying) in her important relationships, and as a reactive – not active – person being influenced by circumstances and the decisions of others.

Historicity in the sense of temporal dialectics between the experienced past and the present moment of telling was scarce in her accounts. She adopted an interpreting subject position very cautiously. Talking about her family of origin she stated: 'I have the sense that I have always somehow been told that I am so, that I don't demand anything, I am so nice ...' (lines 685–686). After having told many stories about her subjugated position in the couple relationship she, responding to a question by the therapist, pondered: 'Somehow it often feels like is he using to his advantage this that I am so terribly forgiving ...' (lines 691–692). Thus, she did make an effort to relate patterns and positionings to each other, but her interpretations of the meaning of the past for her present situation were uncertain and tentative and without her own subjective point of view.

Reflexivity

In the client's accounts the presence of evaluative and reflective talk was scarce. When occurring, reflexivity contributed in various degrees to the display of agency in the other aspects. Connected to relationality reflexivity increased during the session. Talking about her husband she elaborated her reflections starting with a question ('Is he like this?'); then an evaluative statement of facts ('He did things against my will.'); then questions implying related positionings ('Am I so unimportant for him?', 'Is he using my forgiveness?'). This last question related her forgiving attitude to his abuse, thus displaying a mutual, intersubjective positioning and a more agentic stance. Still, her intersubjective position remains that of a passive object.

Talking about her family of origin she reflected on her position as a 'good girl' by pondering on the expectations put on her: 'There were not necessarily any kind of direct messages that were given me [but] a little bit like that that I somehow felt that something is expected of me' (lines 673–675); and by comparing her position to that of her two sisters who did things that 'she would never have dared to do' (lines 681–682).

In the client's attributions of reasons for her work-related problems, reflexivity was hardly present. She, on one hand, described her anxiety and physical reactions, loss of appetite and her constant crying and thinking about her work, as self-evident things just happening to her. On the other hand, she blamed her own attitudes (e.g. 'I'm too conscientious') for her troubles. This did not appear as a reflection, though, rather as still another way of naming causes outside her power of impact.

Reflexivity was missing from the client's presentations of intentionality. Her intentions were hardly outspoken and her main intention appeared to be to hide herself from others, and even from herself. That intention could not afford a reflective stance towards the purposes of her actions. In her narratives of the past, however, increasing reflexivity was present and contributed to the tentative construction of a historical, agentive position were the past started to be related to the present experience.

Discussion

We performed a theory-guided qualitative content analysis on accounts of problems and life-situations given by a female client in her first psychotherapy session. The aim was to try out how a model of discursive agency construction – The Five Aspect Model – could embrace the different ways in which the client adopted the double position of presenting herself as having a lost sense of agency, and a willingness to address her problems in conversational therapy. This model of agentic vs. non-agentic display had been developed in an earlier study on (non)agency constructions of clients in semi-mandatory counselling for repeated drunk driving offenders (Seilonen & Wahlström, 2016). The present study can be seen as an attempt to assess the transferability (Lincoln & Guba, 1985) of that model to a different kind of case, i.e. one in which the client enters psychotherapy voluntarily.

The analysis showed that the model was able to specify how the client's account constructed her positions in regard to her problems, her relations to others, herself and the therapy in various ways as more or less agentic. The quality of non-agentic positioning varied between the different aspects suggested by the model, and with respect to topics and/or contexts:

Relationality

When talking about her presenting problem (social anxiety) and action to be taken in respect to it, she pictured herself as depending on others. In regard to her close relationships she presented herself as a person who accommodates to the image she has of what others expect from her. This non-agentic self-positioning lessened, when in her account she started to adopt a budding reflective stance, and hence a potential differentiation within self/other related agency ascriptions.

Causal attribution

She moved from external and situational attributions to self-related ones. The latter took, though, mainly the form of giving essentialized characteristics as causes, and hence did not contribute to the construction of agentic formulations.

Intentionality

She presented herself as non-intentional, i.e. as not wanting to impact her social surroundings. Her ultimate intention appeared to be to endure her troubles and hide her 'true self' from others, and even from herself.

Historicity

She started by giving very detailed, but not reflected, accounts of events in her life but adopted gradually, although with caution, a more reflecting and interpreting stance in her narration of past events in her life. However, her own subjective point of view was mostly lacking.

Reflexivity

Reflection, as a quality of accounting, increased in the presentations of relationality and historicity, as she took more of a subjective position in her account. In the presentations of causal attributions or intentionality reflexivity was not present.

In our earlier case study on three clients in semi-mandatory counselling for repeated drunk driving (Seilonen & Wahlström, 2016), we could, using the Five Aspects Model, distinguish between different discursive strategies used by the clients for constructing non-agency, and for actually evading a position as a credible client. In the present study, we could notice how the client, over the course of the first session, moved from a pointedly non-agentic self-positioning towards an emerging reflexivity in the account. In this respect, she clearly presented herself as a credible psychotherapy client.

The comparison between the 'non-willing' clients of the former study and the 'willing' one in the present study is multi-faceted, though. A reactive and adoptive positioning to others was observed also in one of the earlier cases, whose agency display was labelled as 'unconcerned'. Still, the functions of such a positioning appeared to be different – in the drunk-driving case that of getting over and managing troubles, in the social anxiety case that of avoiding causing any trouble. The positioning of herself as helpless could be understood as an attempt to influence her social surroundings by assuming a non-agentic position. In the drunk-driving case the adoptive position to others seemed to be situationally useful for the client.

In respect to causal attributions, two of the drunk-driving cases exhibited only situational, external causes for their actions, whereas one, labelled as 'akratic' (i.e. acting against his own will) in his agency display, referred to his inner states as causes for action. The present case seems to obtain a place in between. Her account moved a step towards internal attribution, without actually including such presentations.

The three cases of drunk-driving clients differed clearly from each other in respect to how intentionality was presented in their accounts. Intentions were actively warded off (the so called 'disowned' agency display), ambivalent or irrelevant ('unconcerned' agency), or reflected ('akratic' agency). In the social anxiety case, interestingly, intentionality appeared as the aspect least in use in the constructing of an agentic display. Non-intentionality was not, though, presented bluntly as in the case of 'disowned' agency, but rather as something self-evident not even in need of consideration.

It appears that reflexivity was the one aspect of agency display in which the client seeking voluntary psychotherapy differed the most from those signed up for semi-voluntary counselling. The clients representing 'disowned' and 'unconcerned' agency display exhibited no reflexive stance in respect to their actions, while the one representing 'akratic' agency did so otherwise, but not so when a moral evaluative position of the self would have been called upon. The present case, again, clearly moved during the course of the session from a non-reflective stance towards evaluative and pondering statements on her relational positions.

Of the three cases in semi-mandatory counselling, only one – the 'akratic' one – took up an actual client-position by presenting himself as a person with subjectively experienced problems. The self-positioning within the therapy-context of the self-referred and voluntary client of the present study clearly changed during the session. In the earlier parts of the session she presented herself as being more or less forced by circumstances to seek help (a stance underlined by the fact that her father was the original caller). Later she, in a rather inconspicuous way, assumed the position of a client with an active interest in exploring her troubles within the contexts of her present relationships and personal history.

We conclude that the Five Aspects Model of agency display – integrating viewpoints from epistemology, cognitive psychology, psychoanalysis, constructionism and contemporary conceptualizations of relationality – contributed to a detailed description of how the client-participant in this case study successfully fulfilled the institutional task of a prospective psychotherapy client. It should be noted that the analysis in this study was 'closed' in the sense that we did not look for possible new categories that might have emerged from an open analysis. It is also obvious that due to the very limited number of cases analysed so far, the Five Aspects Model is only tentative. We need further case studies to determine to what degree the model saturates the variety of agentic vs. non-agentic display in problem formulations.

We also want to underline that this discursive work was mainly performed by the client, and to suggest the importance of further studies on how clients contribute to the construction of psychotherapeutic encounters as curative contexts. We conclude that qualitative process research could benefit from considering loss of agency as one crucial object of psychotherapy and the ongoing discursive formulations and re-formulations of the client's more or less agentic positions as central to the process of therapy. This view on restoring agency as a prime objective of psychotherapy allows for an integration of other aspects of the therapeutic change process, which have been studied in qualitative process research.

Disclosure statement

No potential conflict of interest was reported by the authors.

References

Avdi, E. (2005). Negotiating a pathological identity in the clinical dialogue: Discourse analysis of a family therapy. *Psychology and Psychotherapy: Theory, Research and Practice, 78*, 493–511.

Avdi, E. (2012). Exploring the contribution of subject positioning to studying therapy as a dialogical enterprise. *International Journal for Dialogical Science, 6*, 61–79.

Avdi, E., Lerou, V., & Seikkula, J. (2015). Dialogical features, therapist responsiveness, and agency in a therapy for psychosis. *Journal of Constructivist Psychology, 28*, 329–341.

Bamberg, M. (2009). Identity and narration. In P. Huehn, J. Pier, W. Schmid, & J. Schoenert (Eds.), *Handbook of narratology* (pp. 132–143). Berlin: Walter de Gruyter.

Bruner, J. (1990). *Acts of meaning*. Cambridge, MA: Harvard UP.

Dimaggio, G. (2011). Impoverished self-narrative and impaired self-reflection as targets for the psychotherapy of personality disorders. *Journal of Contemporary Psychotherapy, 41*, 165–174.

Drewery, W. (2005). Why we should watch what we say: Position calls, everyday speech and the production of relational subjectivity. *Theory & Psychology, 15*, 305–324.

Georgaca, E. (2001). Voices of the self in psychotherapy: A qualitative analysis. *British Journal of Medical Psychology, 74*, 223–236.

Gillespie, A. (2012). Position exchange: The social development of agency. *New Ideas in Psychology, 30*, 32–46.

Harré, R. (1995). Agentive discourse. In R. Harré & P. Stearns (Eds.), *Discursive psychology in practice* (pp. 120–136). London: Sage Publications.

Jenkins, A. H. (2001). Individuality in cultural context: The case for psychological agency. *Theory & Psychology, 11*, 347–362.

Karatza, H., & Avdi, E. (2011). Shifts in subjectivity during the therapy for psychosis. *Psychology and Psychotherapy: Theory, Research, and Practice, 84,* 214–229.

Kögler, H.-H. (2010). Recognition and the resurgence of intentional agency. *Inquiry, 53,* 450–469.

Kögler, H.-H. (2012). Agency and the other: On the intersubjective roots of self-identity. *New Ideas in Psychology, 30,* 47–64.

Kupferberg, I., & Green, D. (2005). *Troubled talk: Metaphorical negotiation in problem discourse.* New York, NY: Mouton de Gruyter.

Levitt, H., Pomerville, A., & Surace, F. (2016). A qualitative meta-analysis examining clients' experiences of psychotherapy: A new agenda. *Psychological Bulletin, 142,* 801–830.

Lincoln, Y. S., & Guba, E. G. (1985). *Naturalistic inquiry.* Beverly Hills, CA: Sage.

Mackrill, T. (2009). Constructing client agency in psychotherapy research. *Journal of Humanistic Psychology, 49,* 193–206.

Markova, I. (2003). Constitution of the self: Intersubjectivity and dialogicality. *Culture and Psychology, 9,* 249–259.

Mayring, Ph. (2014). *Qualitative content analysis: Theoretical foundation, basic procedures and software solution.* Klagenfurt. Retrieved from http://nbn-resolving. de/urn:nbn:de:0168-ssoar-395173

Ogden, T. H. (1986). *The matrix of the mind. Object relations and the psychoanalytic dialogue.* Northvale, NJ: Jason Aronson Inc.

Pope, R. (1998). *The English studies book.* London: Routledge.

Rennie, D. L. (2010). Humanistic psychology at York University: Retrospective: focus on clients' experiencing in psychotherapy: Emphasis of radical reflexivity. *The Humanistic Psychologist, 38,* 40–56.

Seilonen, M.-L., & Wahlström, J. (2016). Constructions of agency in accounts of drunk driving at the outset of semi-mandatory counseling. *Journal of Constructivist Psychology, 29,* 248–268.

Wahlström, J. (2006). The narrative metaphor and the quest for integration in psychotherapy. In E. O`Leary & M. Murphy (Eds.), *New approaches to integration in psychotherapy* (pp. 38–49). London: Routledge.

How do people cope with post traumatic distress after an accident? The role of psychological, social and spiritual coping in Malaysian Muslim patients

Rafidah Bahari⬛, Muhammad Najib Mohamad Alwi⬛, Nasrin Jahan, Muhammad Radhi Ahmad and Ismail Mohd Saiboon⬛

ABSTRACT

Introduction: Post traumatic distress, acute stress disorder and even post traumatic stress disorder may occur following traumatic events such as a motor vehicle accident (MVA). Instead of presenting to mental health service, many turn to psychosocial and spiritual strategies to cope with symptoms. The objective of this study is to explore the psychosocial and spiritual coping strategies utilised by MVA victims to deal with the distressing post traumatic symptoms.

Methods: An exploratory qualitative study using individual in-depth interview was conducted from May to September 2015. Purposive sampling was done to optimise wide exploration. Only Muslim participants were included. The interviews were recorded, transcribed verbatim and analysed using thematic approach.

Results: All participants interviewed employed psychological, social and spiritual coping strategies to help manage their post traumatic stress symptoms. Positive thinking and rationalisation are examples of psychological coping mechanisms used. Many have supportive families. Common spiritual coping strategies practised include the use of different Quranic verses and prayers.

Conclusion: Psychosocial and spiritual coping strategies are popular, highly tolerable and useful for post traumatic distress. Psycho-socio-spiritual therapy may be an effective treatment for post traumatic stress in Muslim Malaysian patients. Further research is needed in this area.

COMO LAS PERSONAS SOBRELLEVAN LA ANGUSTIA POST-TRAU-MATICA CAUSADA POR UN ACCIDENTE: el papel de la asistencia psicológica, social y espiritual en pacientes malasios musulmanes.

Introducción: Angustia post-traumática, angustia estresante aguda e inclusive estrés post-traumático pueden ocurrir después de un evento traumatizante tal como un accidente automovilístico (AA). En lugar de ir a un servicio de salud mental, muchas personas tornan hacia estrategias psico-sociales o espirituales para sobrellevar los síntomas causados por el accidente. El objetivo de este estudio es explorar las estrategias psico-sociales y espirituales utilizadas por las víctimas de AA para sobrellevar los síntomas de angustia después del accidente.

Métodos: se realizó un estudio cualitativo exploratorio empleando entrevistas exhaustivas individuaes desde Mayo hasta Septiembre 2015. Se estableció una muestra intencional para optimizar una exploración amplia. Se incluyeron participantes musulmaes sólamente. Las entrevistas fueron grabadas, transcritas verbatum y analizadas por temas.

Resultados: todos los participantes emplearon estrategias psicológicas, sociales y espirituales para sobrellevar y ayudarse a controlar los síntomas de la angustia post-traumática. Ejemplos de los mecanismos psicológicos fueron: racionalización y pensamiento positivo. Algunos pacientes recibieron apoyo familiar. Una estrategia espiritual común fue la utilización de versos y oraciones del Koran.

Conclusión: Las estrategias psicosociales y espirituales son populares, altamente tolerables y útiles para sobrellevar la angustia post-traumática. La terapia psico-socio-espiritual puede ser un tratamiento efectivo para esta angustia con pacientes malasios musulmanes. Se necesita mayor investigación en esta área.

Come le persone affrontano il disagio post-traumatico dopo un incidente? Il ruolo del coping psicologico, sociale e spirituale nei pazienti musulmani malesi.

Introduzione: Il distress post traumatico, il disturbo acuto da stress e il disturbo da stress post traumatico possono verificarsi a seguito di eventi traumatici, come un incidente automobilistico (MVA). Invece di presentarsi ai servizi di salute mentale, molte persone utilizzano strategie psicosociali e spirituali per gestire i sintomi. L'obiettivo di questo studio è quello di esplorare le strategie di coping psicosociali e spirituali utilizzati dalle vittime MVA per affrontare gli angoscianti sintomi post-traumatici.

Metodo: uno studio esplorativo che ha utilizzato l'intervista individuale approfondita è stato condotto da maggio a settembre 2015. È stato utilizzato un campionamento intenzionale, così da ottimizzare l'ampiezza dell'indagine. I partecipanti sono tutti musulmani. Le interviste sono state registrate, trascritte parola per parola e analizzati utilizzando l'approccio tematico.

Risultati: Tutti gli intervistati hanno utilizzato strategie di coping psicologico, sociale e spirituale per gestire i sintomi dello stress post-traumatico. Il pensiero positivo e la razionalizzazione costituiscono un esempio dei meccanismi di coping psicologico utilizzati. Molti hanno il supporto delle famiglie. Le comuni strategie di coping spirituale utilizzate includono l'uso di versetti coranici e di preghiere.

Conclusioni: le strategie di coping psicosociali e spirituali risultano comuni, altamente accettate e utili per la gestione dell'angoscia post traumatica. La terapia psico-socio-spirituale può dunque essere un trattamento efficace per lo stress post-traumatico nei pazienti malesi musulmani, sebbene siano necessarie ulteriori ricerche in questo settore.

Gestion de la détresse post traumatique après un accident? Le rôle de l'aide psychologique, sociale et spirituelle chez les patients malais musulmans.

Introduction: la détresse post traumatique, le syndrome de stress aigu et même le syndrome de stress post traumatique peuvent survenir à la suite d'un événement traumatique tel qu'un accident de la circulation. Au lieu de s'adresser aux services de santé mentale, beaucoup se tournent vers des stratégies psychologiques et spirituelles pour faire face aux symptômes. L'objectif de cette étude était d'explorer les stratégies psychologiques et spirituelles utilisées par les victimes d'accidents de la circulation pour gérer les symptômes post traumatiques problématiques.

Méthode: une étude qualitative a permis cette exploration à partir d'entretiens individuels approfondis ayant eu lieu de mai à septembre 2015. Un échantillonnage ciblé a été préféré afin d'optimiser cette exploration. Seuls les participants musulmans ont été inclus. Les entretiens ont été enregistrés, retranscris mot à mot et analysés selon une approche thématique.

Résultats: tous les participants interviewés avaient eu recours à des stratégies psychologiques, sociales et spirituelles pour les aider à gérer leurs symptômes de stress post traumatique. La pensée positive et la rationalisation sont des exemples de stratégies psychologiques utilisées. Beaucoup ont bénéficié du soutien de leur famille. Les stratégies spirituelles pratiquées les plus répandues incluent l'utilisation de versets Coraniques et des prières.

Conclusion: les mécanismes psychosociaux et spirituels de gestion de ces symptômes sont populaires, bien tolérés et utiles pour gérer la détresse post traumatique. La thérapie psychosociale spirituelle peut être un traitement contre le stress post traumatique auprès de la population malaise d'obédience musulmane. Ce domaine mérite d'être recherché plus avant.

Πώς διαχειρίζονται οι άνθρωποι τη μετατραυματική δυσφορία μετά από ένα ατύχημα; Ο ρόλος που παίζουν ψυχολογικοί, κοινωνικοί και πνευματικοί τρόποι διαχείρισης από μουσουλμάνους Μαλαισιανούς ασθενείς

ΠΕΡΙΛΗΨΗ

Εισαγωγή: Η μετατραυματική δυσφορία, η διαταραχή από οξύ στρες, ακόμη και η διαταραχή μετά από μετατραυματικό στρες μπορεί να εμφανιστούν μετά από τραυματικά γεγονότα, όπως ένα τροχαίο ατύχημα. Αντί να απευθυνθούν σε μια υπηρεσία ψυχικής υγείας, πολλοί στρέφονται σε ψυχοκοινωνικές και πνευματικές στρατηγικές προκειμένου να διαχειριστούν τα συμπτώματα. Ο στόχος της παρούσας έρευνας είναι η διερεύνηση των ψυχοκοινωνικών και πνευματικών στρατηγικών που υιοθετούν τα θύματα τροχαίων ατυχημάτων στη διαχείριση των μετατραυματικών συμπτωμάτων.

Μεθοδολογία: Πραγματοποιήθηκε μια διερευνητική ποιοτική μελέτη με τη χρήση εις βάθος ατομικών συνεντεύξεων από το Μάιο έως τον Σεπτέμβριο του 2015. Χρησιμοποιήθηκε η σκόπιμη δειγματοληψία με στόχο να διερευνηθεί το ζήτημα ευρέως. Συμμετείχαν μόνο μουσουλμάνοι συμμετέχοντες. Οι συνεντεύξεις μαγνητοφωνήθηκαν, απομαγνητοφωνήθηκαν αυτολεξεί και αναλύθηκαν με τη χρήση της θεματικής προσέγγισης.

Αποτελέσματα: Όλοι οι συμμετέχοντες φάνηκε να χρησιμοποιούσαν ψυχολογικές, κοινωνικές και πνευματικές στρατηγικές αντιμετώπισης στη διαχείριση των συμπτωμάτων του μετατραυματικού στρες. Η θετική σκέψη και η εκλογίκευση αποτελούν παραδείγματα των ψυχολογικών στρατηγικών διαχείρισης που χρησιμοποιούνται. Πολλοί δέχονται την υποστήριξη της οικογένειας τους. Κοινή πνευματική στρατηγική διαχείρισης αποτελεί η χρήση διαφορετικών στίχων και προσευχών του Κορανίου.

Συμπεράσματα: Οι ψυχοκοινωνικές και πνευματικές στρατηγικές αντιμετώπισης είναι δημοφιλείς, ιδιαίτερα αποτελεσματικές και χρήσιμες στην αντιμετώπιση του μετατραυματικού στρες. Οι ψυχοκοινωνικοπνευματικές παρεμβάσεις μπορεί να είναι αποτελεσματικές στη θεραπεία του μετατραυματικού στρες στους μουσουλμάνους Μαλαισιανούς ασθενείς. Σε αυτόν τον τομέα απαιτείται περαιτέρω έρευνα.

Introduction

In many countries worldwide, injuries due to motor vehicle accidents (MVA) are common and are a frequent cause of presentation to hospitals. About 20–50 million injuries including 1.24 million road deaths occur annually making it one of the major cause of morbidity globally (World Health Organization, 2013).

Following such a traumatic event, psychological distress regularly occurs (Kupchik et al., 2007).

Most research in the past 30 years on the subject of post traumatic stress and post traumatic stress disorder (PTSD) has been done among military personnel and civilians exposed to war (Jones, 2010; Rae, 2007). Recently, studies on this topic have broadened to include non-combative situations such as natural disasters, violence and MVA. Incidence of PTSD after MVA varies from 7.4% in Malaysia to 24–33% in the United States of America (Bahari, Alwi, Ahmad, & Saiboon, 2015). Symptoms of PTSD are highly correlated with time; being worst at two weeks and then reducing significantly after one month and continue to reduce (Hepp et al., 2008). Hence, for most people, time heals and they required no formal intervention from mental health services.

Nevertheless, even when the symptoms are self-limiting, they can be distressing when they are present. Given that there is a discrepancy between the number of MVAs happening daily and the rate of PTSD after one month of the event, Malaysian MVA victims must be doing something right in handling their own symptoms. The objective of this study is to explore the coping strategies used, in particular the psychological, social and spiritual approached employed by MVA victims in Malaysia to cope with their symptoms of post traumatic stress.

Methods

Design

This study required an in-depth exploration of thoughts, beliefs, values, experiences and emotions of participants who had been through MVA in Malaysia. An exploratory qualitative design was chosen since it was deemed the best method to achieve the study's objective (Creswell, 2014). The main vehicle of exploration was in-depth interviews guided by semi-structured interview schedules. Participants were interviewed in great detail, either individually or in pairs and usually more than once.

Participants

A list of eligible participants was drawn from a previous quantitative cross-sectional study which aimed to estimate the incidence of PTSD occurring in Malaysia following MVA. These people were presented to the Emergency Department of University Kebangsaan Malaysia Medical Centre (UKMMC) from August 2014 to October 2014. However, for the qualitative study, only those who were Malaysian, aged 18 or above and fluent in Malay or English were included and offered to be interviewed one year after the accident. Since Malaysia is a Muslim country and published research on Muslims with PTSD is virtually non-existent, we decided to focus the qualitative study on Muslim participants only. Lastly, those who suffered head injury during the accident and had severe communication difficulty were excluded.

Purposive sampling was done to ensure maximum variation among the participants and different age groups, gender, marital status, education, socio-economic status and transport during accident were represented. Recruitment went on until we reached the point of saturation. In other words, when no new information was obtained from the last person, we stopped recruiting and interviewing. However, we did have a rough idea of the number of participants we wanted to recruit prior to commencing the study. In accordance with recommendations from current literature, we aimed to include 3 to 10 participants in the study (Mason, 2010; Miles, Huberman, & Saldana, 2014).

Setting

The UKMMC is a large public hospital situated in Kuala Lumpur which serves not only the city, but also suburban and rural areas surrounding the city. It is a government hospital which charges patrons minimal fees for consultations and treatments. Hence, patients attending the hospital come from all walks of life, but those of higher income are underrepresented.

Interviews were done in venues chosen by participants themselves. Most preferred to have the interviews in their own homes but some chose to have them in their place of work, and some in other venues. Our only instructions for the venue were that participants feel comfortable there, privacy was maintained and disruptions were minimal.

Materials

A semi-structured interview schedule was developed based on the objective of the study. The draft of the interview schedule was pretested on three participants who satisfied the inclusion and exclusion criteria but were not involved in the main study. Their feedback was obtained and then used to modify the semi-structured interview schedule.

Procedures

The study obtained ethical approval from the UKMMC Ethics Committee prior to its commencement. One hundred and twelve patients presented to the UKMMC Emergency department in that period, but only 68 consented to be part of the cross-sectional study. A further 39 were then excluded from the qualitative study because they either did not fulfil the criteria or were not contactable or deceased. The final list was 29 participants who agreed to take part in interviews conducted 1 year after they first presented to the department.

All of the interviews were led by the main researcher (RB) and were done with at least another team member present. At every interview, observations were documented and participants' responses were noted down in the interview schedule. The interviews were also recorded as audio and video if the participant consented. Most of the time, we interviewed the participant again for a second time to obtain more information and fill in lapses and gaps of the previous interviews. For a few of the participants we even interviewed them further after the second interview informally through the phone. Especially in cases where the interview was done in pairs and we felt that one person dominated the interview, we sought out the less-dominating participant in the pair and interviewed them individually in another session to ensure independent views were obtained. Interviews lasted for at least 45 min and in cases of multiple interviews, for at least 3 h in total. Visual tools such as emotion recognition stickers and Venn diagrams were used to complement findings and aid participants in elaborating their answers.

A total of four key informants were also interviewed based on need to validate findings from participants. They consisted of a senior consultant psychiatrist, a Malay culture expert with special interest in Malay traditional medicine, an Islamic Medicine practitioner and an academician in Islamic Studies who is a part-time Islamic Medicine practitioner.

Data analysis

Prior to analysis, audio recordings of the interview were transcribed verbatim and then converted into analysable text. Data analyses were done based on themes and sub-themes according to the study objective and aided by Atlas. ti software.

Data collection and analysis were done continuously and parallel to each other. This allowed in-depth understanding of descriptions given by participants, helped to overcome unmet needs and decisions on subsequent steps. Also, this process helped to find the saturation point of which participant recruitment can cease.

Trustworthiness of the findings was determined by triangulating information obtained from participants, key informants and other tangible products. By tangible product we meant any phrases from books, quotes from websites, verses from the Quran and captions from magazines and newspapers that were referred to by participants were looked up and used to verify participants' information. Similarly, materials obtained from key informants were not included in the analysis, but were only used to check our findings. Debriefing immediately following interviews and meetings to share information between team members were regularly held which also strengthened the validity of findings.

Table 1. Participants' characteristics.

ID	Age	Sex	Marital status	Ethnicity	Highest education	Occupation
IDI 1	41	Female	Married	Malay	SPM	Housewife
IDI 2	50	Male	Married	Malay	SPM	Police officer (Special Force)
IDI 3	64	Male	Married	Malay	SPM equivalent	Retired (army)
IDI 4	20	Male	Single	Malay	Foundation studies	Undergraduate student
IDI 5	21	Male	Single	Malay	Foundation studies	Undergraduate student
IDI 6	23	Female	Married	Rohingya	Certificate	Translator
IDI 7	35	Female	Married	Malay	Diploma	Nurse
IDI 8	24	Male	Single	Malay	Degree	Bank executive
IDI 9	29	Female	Single	Malay	Degree	Engineer

Results

Participants' characteristics

At point of saturation, nine participants were interviewed and their character-istics are presented in the following table (Table 1).

Post traumatic stress symptoms

All participants reported having post traumatic stress symptoms immediately following the event. For most participants, the symptoms resolved after about two weeks. Two of the female participants continued to have symptoms one year on, one having mild symptoms but the other slightly worse.

The most common symptoms reported were intrusion symptoms usually in the form of intrusive memories and sometimes dreams (Figure 1). Many partic-ipants reported alteration in mood, commonly anger and irritability following the event and some continued to have alteration in cognition in which they continue to feel unsafe on the road. Despite that, very few avoided the area or getting on motorcycles due to the fact that those options were not open to them.

Coping

When faced with a stressful situation, a person may develop psychological dis-tress depending on how they appraise the situation (primary appraisal) and their evaluation of their ability to control their situation or their own reactions (secondary appraisal). Strategies employed to reduce these distress either by mediating primary or secondary appraisal are called coping (Glanz, Rimer, & Viswanath, 2008). There are different ways to classify coping, one popular way is to divide them into problem-focused and emotion-focused coping (Folkman & Lazarus, 1980). We have taken elements of that, but for this paper, we decided on a pragmatic approach of classifying coping into psychological, social and spiritual.

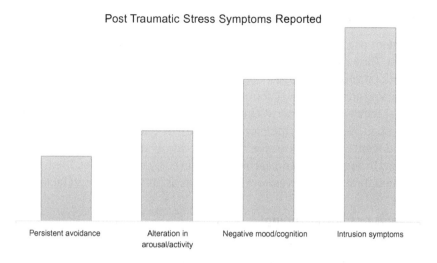

Figure 1. Post traumatic stress symptoms experienced by subjects.

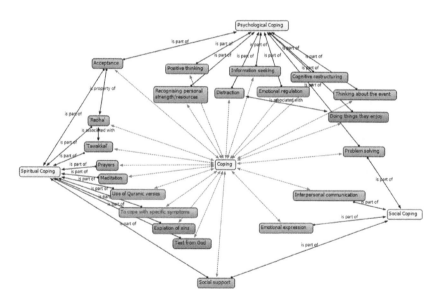

Figure 2. Coping strategies employed by subjects to deal with their post traumatic stress symptoms.

A MVA is regarded as a stressful situation by most people and having post traumatic stress symptoms following it is not uncommon (Beck & Coffey, 2007). In this study, all participants admitted to having some symptoms immediately after the event. However, none of the participants actually presented to mental health services, but rather coped with post traumatic symptoms themselves using a variety of strategies (Figure 2).

Psychological coping

The use of psychological coping is common to all participants in one form or another. They can be subdivided further into two sub-themes: cognitive and behavioural coping strategies. Cognition refers to the mental activity engaged in obtaining and processing information while behaviour applies to the action or physical activity of the person (Colman, 2015). Hence in cognitive coping, participants coped by processing the information and eventually came up with beliefs so that the event no longer distresses them. A person who used behavioural coping preferred to keep busy or engage him/herself in enjoyable activities. This is better illustrated through narratives from participants as presented below (Table 2).

Religious or spiritual coping

Participants were also familiar with the use of religious or spiritual coping. In Islam, spirituality and religiosity point towards the same construct, namely Muslims' relation to Allah (God) (Bonab, Miner, & Proctor, 2013). Hence for most

Table 2. Some narratives illustrating psychological coping strategies used.

Cognitive type	Examples
Acceptance	'I think when I got back from hospital, it was then I started to accept what happened. My friend was okay, safe. So I can accept what happened.' (20-year-old male Malay student)
Positive thinking	'Positive. Whatever it is, just be positive. When something happens, try to become positive and then we can really think.' (24-year-old male Malay bank executive)
Recognising personal strength/resources	'It's how you handle yourself. How you gather your resources, for example if you want to cool down you can get and air-conditioner.' (48-year-old male Malay Special police officer)
Information seeking	'Then I went blank. I just knew that I was in pain and what I needed to do. I need to know what was happening (why I was in so much pain). I wanted to see the doctor, to know if anything was broken.' (41-year-old Malay housewife)
Emotional regulation	'I think if a person can regulate his/her emotions, they can think better, they will know what to do.' (20-year-old male Malay student).
Cognitive restructuring	'So I thought that it is not a big deal. Just a small matter. It (motor vehicle accident) always happen in our community. That's life. Like when I fell off my motorcycle (in the accident). It was slippery. (I just fell), even a banana peel could have made me slip. So no big deal.' (64-year-old male Malay army veteran)
Thinking about the event	'I think I kept thinking about the event to reflect on it, to learn from it. Next time I will not use car lanes (when I am riding a motorcycle), even if I am in a hurry (laughed).' (29-year-old female engineer)
Behavioural type	*Examples*
Distraction	'My mom and husband are very intelligent. They don't want me to think (about the accident). They buy all my favourite movies and put them at home. So when I got time, I just turn on my TV.' (23-year-old Rohingya female interpreter)
Doing things they enjoy	'For example, I do things that I enjoy, like playing futsal. Indulge in my hobbies so that I will forget (the accident).' (21-year-old Malay male student)
Problem solving	'Maybe that's just me. There is no use to keep thinking about something bad that has happened in the past. Just move on. Let say we lose something … no need to continue to be sad about it. Try to find a solution!' (24-year-old male Malay bank executive)

Muslims, the terms have similar meaning and often used interchangeably. Here, three sub-themes were identified: the use of religion or spirituality to make sense of post traumatic symptoms, to reduce general distress and to handle specific symptoms. The main strategy is to accept the symptoms as fated by God which is related to the Islamic concepts of 'redha' and 'tawakkal'. 'Redha' can be translated as acceptance that whatever happened had been fated by God. 'Tawakkal' on the other hand means to rely on God completely (Utz, 2011). Again, they are best demonstrated through quoting participants' own narratives (Table 3).

Social coping

Participants were unanimous in stating that strong social support was what kept them from falling apart following their MVA. However, while most relied on friends and family for support, a few had extremely extensive support network.

Table 3. Religious and spiritual coping sub-themes.

Making sense of symptoms	Examples
'Redha'	'There is no need to think about these things (the accident), because it is already written (fated by God). If it was going to happen, then it will happen.' (20-year-old Malay male student)
'Tawakkal'	'I wasn't well (had symptoms)…I think as Muslims we just return to God. We can pray. I accepted the situation and just "tawakkal" (relied on God completely). Like that.' (41-year-old housewife)
A test	'This is a test. To me, God will not test me beyond my limit of patience. That is what I believe.' (41-year-old Malay housewife)
Expiation of sins	'We wondered why it happened to us. What did we do (to deserve it)? Maybe this is what God wanted to show us. People say that pain can expiate sins. So we are given a second chance. For us to change (to be good).' (20-year-old Malay male student)
Reducing distress	*Examples*
Solat or Prayers	'When I felt stressed, I make solat (prayers). Then I feel calmer. No special solat, just a normal solat.' (24-year-old Malay male banker)
Quranic verses	'Nowdays, when I have the breathing problem, I feel so restless like being in a tent. I could not talk to anyone. I want to talk, I want to tell my feelings, but I could not express. Something is going on my mind. Even sometimes I tell my mom; (23-year-old Rohingya female interpreter)
Meditation	'When I am stressed, I say *Innalillahi wainna ilaihi rojiun* three times, then I inhale and exhale while saying 'I accept whatever is happening to me'. I practice that when I feel stress. Just once each time, and I feel okay afterwards." (41-year-old Malay housewife)
Support	'My classmates from my (informal) Islamic Studies class and even the "ustazah" (female Islamic Studies teacher) came to visit. So I was comforted. People cared.' (41-year-old housewife)
Handling specific symptoms	*Examples*
Intrusive memory	'No, I did not want to think of the accident, but the memories came suddenly. I heard of that happening to other people. And they did say that the memories came in flashes. So I do the zikir (chants). I say *subhanallah wal hamdulillah, allahuakhbar* and *astaghfirullah*.' (41-year-old housewife)
Avoidance	'So after the accident everytime I am about to mount a motorcycle, I felt I should read some prayers. Especially the prayer that you read before mounting your vehicle. Then I feel more confident (not afraid) to ride my motorcycle.' (21-year-old male student)

This is perhaps better demonstrated with the Venn diagram (Figure 3) and narrative below (Table 4).

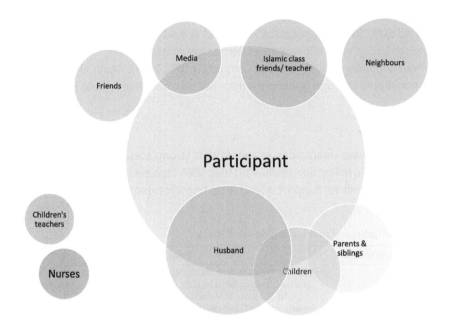

Figure 3. Venn diagram representing a subject's extensive social network.
Note: The size represents the importance and the distance represents how beneficial they are.

Table 4. The participant's narrative expanding on the above Venn diagram.

Support according to importance – size	'First, husband. Then children and parents and siblings (equally). Then friends, my classmates from my Islamic Studies class and the teacher, social media, neighbours, my children's school teachers and nurses'
	'Nurses, (they supported me) only during my (physical) illness. Smaller size for friends because I now have fewer friends. The usual story, friends forsake you sometimes when you are in difficulty. Fortunately, I have good neighbours. Who understand me, and helped me during difficult times'
Support according to benefit – distance	'Husband, children and my parents and siblings should be very close to me. In fact, the children, my husband and family should overlap because my children also need my husband and they also need my family. Friends a bit further, because now I am reacquainted with my school friends and they are very helpful. Neighbours slightly further. Social media needs to be very close to me because I find them extremely beneficial, every single day. The same for my Islamic Studies class (classmates and teacher). Nurses and school teachers further away from everybody because they are only beneficial for specific things. Same goes to friends and neighbours, you have to be selective on what you want to share with them'
	'The Islamic Studies class is beneficial all the time because every time I go there I feel happy. Like a release. I can ask so many questions, not just related to Islamic Studies. I also ask their opinion on personal problems I might have. I relied on them heavily, I can't go to counsellors (or mental health service providers), I don't know any. And sometimes your family can't motivate you either'

Discussion

All participants admitted to having post traumatic stress symptoms, but a few fulfilled diagnoses of acute stress disorder and even fewer PTSD. The most frequently reported symptoms were intrusion symptoms, mainly in the form of intrusive memories. Despite that, only one of the participant ever reported to their doctor that they had symptoms. Most interviewees implied that they were not aware that what they had experienced were symptoms of mental disorder. Even if they were aware, there was palpable reluctance to present to mental health services due to stigma. Nevertheless, reasons for not presenting to mental health services were beyond the scope of this study and hence were not pursued further.

Coping as a participant has been extensively studied. Common strategies such as cognitive restructuring, social support, acceptance and religious coping kept cropping up again, regardless whether the study had been done the United States of America, Gaza or anywhere else in the world (Bisson, 2007; Spence, Nelson, & Lachlan, 2010; Thabet, El-Buhaisi, & Vostanis, 2014). This demonstrates that some responses are part of human nature and can be applied across different religions, races and cultures.

Many of the participants used psychological approaches to deal with their post traumatic distress. This is interesting since psychological awareness is still lacking in the community and stigma is rife. Its environment then makes compliance to recommended psychotherapeutic approaches like trauma-focused cognitive behaviour therapy (TF-CBT) and eye movement desensitisation and reprocessing problematic (Bisson & Andrew, 2009; Roberts, Kitchiner, Kenardy, & Bisson, 2012). On the other hand, processing the event by thinking about it, positive thinking, and the use of distraction to name a few are techniques integral to CBT and EMDR anyway. This may give researchers in Malaysia some grounds to develop a briefer intervention for ASD and PTSD which incorporates these familiar strategies.

There are currently growing interests in researches on mental illness and spirituality (D'Souza, 2007, 2012; Hook et al., 2010; Koenig, 2012). Some strategies have been described, such as the use of repeating a useful phrase or 'mantram' during stressful times (Bomyea & Lang, 2012). We found similar strategy in our participants and other approaches such as the use of specific prayers to counter intrusion and avoidance symptoms. Furthermore, our participants had no reservations about employing spiritual or religious approaches, a common finding in communities in the East (Chiu, 2005). It is hence beneficial to combine spiritual and religious themes in psychotherapy, an idea that is already being put into practice by some researchers (Pearce et al., 2015).

In general, it was apparent that our participants relied heavily on social support to tide them through their period of distress. In some participants, their social network was so extensive to even include their children's school teachers and friends. Many also implied that the helping spirit of the members of the community that sustained them and eventually prevented them from developing PTSD. This culture has been observed in many less affluent countries in which the more traditional values of community rather than individuality still prevails (Maercker & Hecker, 2016). Duckers et. al. while trying to explain the vulnerability paradox also referred to this idea that perhaps the less individualistic nature of the people in less affluent countries is an important factor protecting them from the condition (Duckers, Alisic, & Brewin, 2016).

Ultimately, in the end, participants agreed that due to that difficult period of time in their life, they have now become better people. This positive outcome is well described in literatures as post traumatic growth in which it also includes spiritual growth in the case of our participants (Fang et al., 2011; Maercker, Zöllner, Menning, Rabe, & Karl, 2006). Since post traumatic stress can be a catalyst for self-development, it is not necessarily a bad thing in itself. Our role as mental health professionals in the management of PTSD should probably be as facilitators for this positive growth while monitoring our clients carefully.

Strength

In keeping with current literatures, most participants employed not one, but a variety of coping strategies at the same time (Morris & Rao, 2013). While it was natural for people to do that, this made it difficult in research to truly establish which approaches were effective and which were more of a hindrance. This was where the strength of the qualitative design of this study lay. By employing an exploratory design, participants were given the free reign to expand on their answers and a better picture was obtained.

Limitations

The use of purposive sampling is common in qualitative research. Although employing a non-probability sampling method normally introduces bias, in order to study a certain phenomenon, it is the most effective method since responses from a variety of people were sought after and knowledgeable experts were also included. The method stays robust even when compared against random probability sampling, and its inherent bias contributes to the efficiency (Tongco, 2007).

Only one participant was a car passenger while the rest were riding motorcycles during the accident. While this seems contradictory to the purposive nature of sampling in this study, this reflected the true picture of MVAs in Malaysia where an overwhelmingly large number of those riding motorcycles are annually involved in accidents. This could be due to the attitudes of motorcyclists themselves who prefer this mode of transport so that they can easily, and most of the time dangerously weave through heavily congested traffic. Also, they are not as protected as car drivers and are often injured even in minor accidents, contributing to the higher number of presentations to emergency departments.

Finally, the setting of this study may favour those people from lower to middle socio-economic classes as indicated by their occupation, educational attainment and mode of transport. Malaysia has two health services, private and public. Those who are more affluent or those who possess good health insurance coverage due to their employment often opt to attend private hospitals due to their less crowded nature and short waiting times. The setting of this study is a public university hospital which may explain the difficulty in recruiting people of the higher social classes.

Conclusion

Psychosocial and spiritual coping strategies were widely used. They appear effective in reducing post traumatic stress since participants recovered from their symptoms without intervention from mental health services. Apart from reinforcing strategies such as use of social support, cognitive restructuring, acceptance and religious coping which had been established in other studies, specific techniques were identified to effectively manage intrusion and avoidance symptoms.

In managing post traumatic stress in the Malaysian population, incorporating social and spiritual approaches into current psychotherapeutic practices could be the way forward. Apart from integrating them into the treatment of ASD and PTSD, they may be advocated as strategies to reduce distress in the immediate aftermath of MVAs. Prevention of PTSD is especially important in Malaysia and other developing countries whose mental health services may not be so widely available as to avoid overwhelming the service.

Disclosure statement

No potential conflict of interest was reported by the authors.

Funding

This work was supported by grants from Cyberjaya University College of Medical Sciences Grants Scheme (CRGS); KolejUniversiti Sains PerubatanCyberjaya [CRG/01/02/2015].

ORCID

Rafidah Bahari ⓘ http://orcid.org/0000-0002-4991-8029
Muhammad Najib Mohamad Alwi ⓘ http://orcid.org/0000-0002-2397-4321
Ismail Mohd Saiboon ⓘ http://orcid.org/0000-0003-3972-9803

References

Bahari, R., Alwi, M. N. M., Ahmad, M. R., & Saiboon, I. M. (2015). PTSD after motor vehicle accidents in Malaysia. In *The 5th world congress of asian psychiatry*, Fukuoka, Japan.

Beck, J. G., & Coffey, S. F. (2007). Assessment and treatment of posttraumatic stress disorder after a motor vehicle collision: Empirical findings and clinical observations. *Professional Psychology: Research and Practice, 38,* 629–639.

Bisson, J., & Andrew, M. (2009). Psychological treatment of post-traumatic stress disorder (PTSD). *The Cochrane Collaboration, 1,* 1–115.

Bisson, J. I. (2007). Post-traumatic stress disorder. *Occupational Medicine, 57,* 399–403. doi:10.1093/occmed/kqm069

Bonab, B. G., Miner, M., & Proctor, M.-T. (2013). Attachment to God in Islamic spirituality. *Journal of Muslim Mental, 7,* 77–104. Retrieved from http://quod.lib.umich.edu/j/jmmh/10381607.0007.205/–attachment-to-god-in-islamic-spirituality?rgn=main;view=fulltext

Bomyea, J., & Lang, A. J. (2012). Emerging interventions for PTSD: Future directions for clinical care and research. *Neuropharmacology, 62,* 607–616. doi:10.1016/j.neuropharm.2011.05.028.

Chiu, L. (2005). Spirituality and treatment choices by South and East Asian women with serious mental illness. *Transcultural Psychiatry, 42,* 630–656. doi:10.1177/1363461505058920

Colman, A. M. (2015). *A Dictionary of Psychology. Oxford paperback reference* (Vol. 3). Oxford: Oxford University Press. doi:10.1093/acref/9780199534067.001.0001

Creswell, J. W. (2014). The selection of a research approach. In *Research design: Qualitative, quantitative and mixed methods approaches* (4th editio). London: Sage. ISBN 978-1-4522-2610-1.

D'Souza, R. (2007). The importance of spirituality in medicine and its application to clinical practice. *The Medical Journal of Australia, 186* (10 Suppl), S57–S59. Retrieved from http://www.ncbi.nlm.nih.gov/pubmed/17516886

D'Souza, R. (2012). Spirituality and psychiatry: Special series. *Asian Journal of Psychiatry*, *5*, 179 p. doi:10.1016/j.ajp.2012.05.008

Duckers, M. L. A., Alisic, E., & Brewin, C. R. (2016). A vulnerability paradox in the cross-national prevalence of post-traumatic stress disorder. *The British Journal of Psychiatry*, *209*, 300–305. doi:10.1192/bjp.bp.115.176628

Fang, C. K., Li, P. Y., Lai, M. L., Lin, M. H., Bridge, D. T., & Chen, H. W. (2011). Establishing a 'Physician's spiritual well-being scale' and testing its reliability and validity. *Journal of Medical Ethics, 37*, 6–12. doi:10.1136/jme.2010.037200

Folkman, S., & Lazarus, R. S. (1980). An analysis of coping in a middle-aged community sample. *Journal of Health and Social Behavior, 21*, 219–239.

Glanz, K., Rimer, B. K., & Viswanath, K. (2008). *Health behaviour and health education* (Vol. 63). San Francisco, CA: Jossey-Bass. doi:10.1016/S0033-3506(49)81524-1

Hepp, U., Moergeli, H., Buchi, S., Bruchhaus-Steinert, H., Kraemer, B., Sensky, T., & Schnyder, U. (2008). Post-traumatic stress disorder in serious accidental injury: 3-Year follow-up study. *The British Journal of Psychiatry, 192*, 376–383. doi:10.1192/bjp.bp.106.030569.

Hook, J. N., Worthington, E., Davis, D., Jennings, D., Gartner, A., & Hook, J. P. (2010). Empirically supported religious and spiritual therapies. *Journal of Clinical Psychology, 66*, 46–72. doi:10.1002/jclp

Jones, E. (2010). Shell shock at Maghull and the Maudsley: Models of psychological medicine in the UK. *Journal of the History of Medicine and Allied Sciences, 65*, 368–395. doi:10.1093/jhmas/jrq006

Koenig, H. G. (2012). Commentary: Why do research on spirituality and health, and what do the results mean? *Journal of Religion and Health, 51*, 460–467. doi:10.1007/s10943-012-9568-y

Kupchik, M., Strous, R. D., Erez, R., Gonen, N., Weizman, A., & Spivak, B. (2007). Demographic and clinical characteristics of motor vehicle accident victims in the community general health outpatient clinic: A comparison of PTSD and non-PTSD subjects. *Depression and Anxiety, 24*, 244–250. doi:10.1002/da.20189

Maercker, A., & Hecker, T. (2016). Broadening perspectives on trauma and recovery: A socio-interpersonal view of PTSD. *European Journal of Psychotraumatology, 7*, 29303. doi:10.3402/ejpt.v6.29303.

Maercker, A., Zöllner, T., Menning, H., Rabe, S., & Karl, A. (2006). Dresden PTSD treatment study: Randomized controlled trial of motor vehicle accident survivors. *BMC Psychiatry, 6*, 29. doi:10.1186/1471-244X-6-29

Mason, M. (2010). Sample size and saturation in PhD studies using qualitative interviews. *Forum Qualitative Sozialforschung/Forum, 11*, 1–19. Retrieved from http://www.qualitative-research.net/index.php/fqs/article/viewArticle/1428

Miles, M. B., Huberman, A. M., & Saldana, J. (2014). *Qualitative data analysis: A methods sourcebook* (3rd Editio). Sage. Retrieved from http://www.amazon.com/Qualitative-Data-Analysis-Methods-Sourcebook/dp/1452257876

Morris, M. C., & Rao, U. (2013). Psychobiology of PTSD in the acute aftermath of trauma: Integrating research on coping, HPA function and sympathetic nervous system activity. *Asian Journal of Psychiatry, 6*, 3–21. doi:10.1016/j.ajp.2012.07.012

Pearce, M. J., Koenig, H. G., Robins, C. J., Nelson, B., Shaw, S. F., Cohen, H. J., & King, M. B. (2015). Religiously integrated cognitive behavioral therapy: A new method of treatment for major depression in patients with chronic medical illness. *Psychotherapy, 52*, 56–66. doi:10.1037/a0036448

Rae, R. (2007). An historical account of shell shock during the First World War and reforms in mental health in Australia 1914–1939. *International Journal of Mental Health Nursing, 16*, 266–273.

Roberts, N., Kitchiner, N., Kenardy, J., & Bisson, J. I. (2012). Early psychological interventions to treat acute traumatic stress symptoms. *The Cochrane Collaboration,* (1), 1–82. Retrieved from http://onlinelibrary.wiley.com/doi/10.1002/14651858.CD007944.pub2/full

Spence, P. R., Nelson, L. D., Lachlan, K. A (2010). Psychological responses and coping strategies after an urban bridge collapse. *Traumatology, 16,* 7–15. doi:10.1177/15347 65609347544

Thabet, A., El-Buhaisi, O., & Vostanis, P. (2014). Trauma, PTSD, anxiety and coping strategies among Palestinians adolescents exposed to War on Gaza. *The Arab Journal of Psychiatry, 25,* 71–82.

Tongco, M. (2007). Purposive sampling as a tool for informant selection. *Ethnobotany Research & Applications, 5,* 147–158. Retrieved from http://scholarspace.manoa.hawaii.edu/handle/10125/227

Utz, A. (2011). *Psychology from the Islamic perspective.* Riyadh: International Islamic Publishing House.

World Health Organization. (2013). WHO global status report on road safety 2013: Supporting a decade of action, 304. Retrieved from http://apps.who.int/iris/handle/10665/78256

Communities, psychotherapeutic innovation and the diversity of international qualitative research in mental health

David Harper

ABSTRACT

The articles in this special issue are hugely varied in terms of their country of origin (Brazil, Finland, Italy, Malaysia and the UK); theoretical influences (e.g. Lacanian theory, cultural-historical approaches and relational theories) and method of qualitative analysis (e.g. content and thematic analyses, Lacanian discourse analysis, Grounded theory, ethnography and auto-ethnography). In this commentary, I will discuss each article in turn before moving on to address some common issues including: the relationship between therapeutic innovation and research; differing implicit models of subjectivity; the need for theoretically pluralistic approaches to interpretation; and the need to incorporate the views of service users.

LA DIVERSIDAD EN LA INVESTIGACION CUALITATIVA EN SALUD MENTAL A NIVEL INTERNACIONAL: Comentarios acerca de los articulos en esta edición

Los artículos en esta edición especial son muy variados en términos del país de origen (Brasil, Finlandia, Malasia y el Reino Unido), influencias teóricas (ej: teoría lacaniana, métodos historico-culturales y teorías relacionales) y métodos de análisis cualitativo (ej: análisis temático y de contenido, análisis lacaniano del discurso, "ground theory"), etnografía y auto-etnografía). El uso de métodos de investigación cualitativa en ciencias sociales como la Psicología, se ha incrementado mucho (Carrera-Fernández; Guardia-Olmos & Pero-Cebollero 2014) y en el campo de la salud mental (Harper -en imprenta-) y resulta inspirador ver semejante amplitud de trabajo internacional y de diversidad teóricay metodológica representados en el presente número de esta revista. En este comentario analizaré cada artículo antes de pasar a tratar algunos planteamientos communes.

La varietà della ricerca qualitativa internazionale nel campo della salute mentale: un commento agli articoli nello special issue

Gli articoli di questo numero sono estremamente variegati rispetto al paese di origine (Brasile, Finlandia, Italia, Malesia e Regno Unito), influssi teorici (ad esempio: la teoria lacaniana, approcci storico-culturali e le teorie relazionali) e metodo di analisi qualitativa (ad esempio: analisi dei contenuti e tematiche, analisi lacaniana del discorso, Grounded Theory, etnografia e auto-etnografia). I metodi di ricerca qualitativa sono sempre più utilizzati nelle scienze sociali quali la psicologia (Carrera-Fernandez, Guardia-Olmos & Peró-Cebollero, 2014) e in tutto il dominio della salute mentale in generale (Harper, in corso di stampa) ed è stimolante vedere un tale gamma di lavoro e tale diversità di teorie e metodi rappresentati in questo special issue. Nel presente commento vorrei discutere ciascun articolo prima di affrontare alcune questioni comuni.

Diversité de la recherche qualitative internationale en santé mentale : commentaire des articles formant l'édition spéciale

Les articles qui composent cette édition spéciale sont très divers quant à leur origine (Brésil, Finlande, Italie, Malaisie and Royaume-Uni), leurs influences théoriques (théorie lacanienne, approches historico-culturelles ou théories relationnelles par exemple) et les méthodes d'analyse des données (analyse thématique de contenu, analyse lacanienne du discours, théorie ancrée, ethnographie et auto-ethnographie par exemple). Les méthodes de recherche qualitatives sont de plus en plus utilisées dans les sciences sociales telles que la psychologie (Carrera-Fernández, Guàrdia-Olmos & Peró-Cebollero, 2014) et dans le domaine de la santé mentale de manière plus générale (Harper, sous presse). Il est donc stimulant de voir un tel éventail de travaux internationaux et une telle diversité dans les théories et méthodes représentées dans ce numéro spécial. Ce commentaire passe d'abord en revue chaque article puis aborde des questions fréquentes.

Η ποικιλομορφία στη διεθνή ποιοτική έρευνα στην ψυχική υγεία: Ένα σχόλιο για τα άρθρα στο ειδικό τεύχος

Τα άρθρα σε αυτό το ειδικό τεύχος διαφοροποιούνται σημαντικά ως προς τη χώρα προέλευσης (Βραζιλία, Φινλανδία, Ιταλία, Μαλαισία και Ηνωμένο Βασίλειο), ως προς τη θεωρητική κατεύθυνση (π.χ. Λακανική θεωρία, πολιτισμικο- ιστορικές προσεγγίσεις και σχεσιακές θεωρίες) και ως προς την μέθοδο της ποιοτικής ανάλυσης (π.χ. ανάλυση περιεχομένου και θεματική ανάλυση, Λακανική ανάλυση λόγου, Θεμελιωμένη Θεωρία, εθνογραφία και αυτοεθνογραφία). Οι ποιοτικές ερευνητικές μέθοδοι χρησιμοποιούνται ολοένα και περισσότερο στις κοινωνικές επιστήμες, όπως είναι η ψυχολογία (Carrera-Fernández, Guàrdia-Olmos &Peró-Cebollero, 2014) και γενικότερα στο πλαίσιο της ψυχικής υγείας (Harper, υπό δημοσίευση) και αποτελεί έμπνευση να βλέπει κανείς το ευρύ φάσμα της ερευνητικής εργασίας διεθνώς και την ποικιλομορφία όσον αφορά τη θεωρία και τη μέθοδο που εκπροσωπούνται σε αυτό το ειδικό τεύχος. Σε αυτό τα άρθρο, θα συζητήσω κάθε άρθρο ξεχωριστά και στη συνέχεια θα συζητήσω κάποια κοινά σημεία.

Therapeutic community for children with diagnosis of psychosis: What place for parents? The relation between subject and the institutional 'Other'

Qualitative research methods are increasingly being used in social sciences like psychology (Carrera-Fernández, Guàrdia-Olmos, & Peró-Cebollero, 2014) and across the domain of mental health more generally (Harper, in press; Harper & Thompson, 2012) and it is inspiring to see such a range of international work and such diversity of theory and method represented in the special issue. The structural location of journal commentaries tends to invite monological rather than dialogical communication and so where I have raised issues I hope the authors will take these comments in the constructive spirit in which they are offered. As a qualitative researcher myself I am all too aware that all studies are open to challenge on a variety of grounds. Indeed, there are several studies of my own which would be conducted differently with the benefit of hindsight.

In this study, conducted in Northern Italy at a therapeutic community for children and young people with diagnoses of psychosis or autistic spectrum disorders, the author/s present an analysis of two of the five patterns identified in transcripts of 'Parents' Place' meetings between staff at the therapeutic community and parents of children living in the community. The community and researchers are theoretically informed by a Lacanian approach in their understanding of psychosis and the researchers also use this approach in analysing the transcripts, drawing on Parker and Pavón-Cuéllar's Lacanian discourse analysis (2013), with a particular focus on blockages and deadlocks in discourse, using the notion of anchoring or 'quilting points'. A verbatim recording (i.e. including only what was said and no subsequent psychotherapeutic interpretation) of the Parents' Place meetings was provided to parents at the next meeting as a 'receipt' of their concerns. These transcripts were analysed both by the authors and staff at the therapeutic community. The two themes they focused on concerned the parents' talk about their relationship with the general institutional network (social services agencies, the courts, etc.) and their relationship with the therapeutic community.

For anyone who has been involved with families where social services agencies are concerned about risk to the child or where the child and family are struggling to manage psychological distress, there was much that rang true in the extracts from the meetings: the sadness of parents missing their child; their concern about the child's care; their helplessness in the face of action by the courts; their anger at professionals and the courts; and their fears about the future. The authors wrote sensitively about the parents' predicament and also identified patterns in the relationships that could be set up between parents and those involved in a psychotherapeutic intervention (idealization of therapists and criticism of other agencies, homogenization of professionals and agencies, etc.) and they drew on Lacanian theory, particularly the Hegelian concept of the master–slave relationship. As someone who has found some Lacanian work theoretically dense, I thought the authors' account of the relevance of his ideas here was clear.

One of the strengths of broadly humanistic approaches to psychotherapy and qualitative research has been their focus on the meaning of human interactions but often there is a desire to produce a final narrative which is coherent and makes sense. Yet, as the psychoanalyst, clinical psychologist and qualitative researcher Stephen Frosh warns us, this is impossible:

> The human subject is *never* a whole, is always riven with partial drives, social discourses that frame available modes of experience, ways of being that are contradictory and reflect shifting allegiances of power as they play across the body and the mind. (Frosh, 2007, p. 638, emphasis in original)

One of the strengths of discourse analytic approaches is their focus on the variable and contradictory nature of talk – something that conventional psychological approaches avoid through a methodological focus on the issue of reliability. There are different approaches to understanding this variability. Discursive approaches might focus on the movement between different discursive repertoires or the serving of different social functions, whereas a Bakhtinian dialogical approach (Bakhtin, 1981, 1984) might draw on notions of polyphony – that talk is comprised of multiple voices – and unfinalizability – that meaning is never finally fixed because something new can often be said. Of course, the area of affect and emotion, so often neglected by psychologists preferring to focus on more rationalist constructs, is infused with contradiction and has been a key site where new approaches have been developed (e.g. Ellis & Tucker, 2015; Wetherell, 2012), particularly in the field of psychosocial studies. Psychoanalytic approaches to this variability also have much to contribute and Parker and Pavón-Cuéllar's (2013) Lacanian approach to textual indeterminacy is a useful intervention and the authors here show what value such an approach can have in understanding relational and affective ambivalence.

As someone whose psychotherapeutic theoretical preferences lie elsewhere (e.g. critical community psychology and narrative and systemic approaches), I found myself considering alternative formulations of the community's therapeutic practices and the researchers' interpretations. It seemed to me that the practice of giving parents a record of their concerns, free from psychotherapeutic interpretation – what the authors termed a 'receipt' – was, at a basic human level, a valuable intervention in itself in that the parents could then see evidence that at least their voices had been heard. Written forms of communication with therapy clients have seen considerable growth in the last 20–30 years. This can be particularly valuable given research findings suggesting that patients attending GPs often have a very poor memory of the consultation (Ley, 1979) and particularly if emotionally intense material has been discussed. Indeed, in other settings, health professionals have experimented with giving people recordings of their consultations (Tsulukidze, Durand, Barr, Mead, & Elwyn, 2014).

I know family therapists who have given video recordings of sessions to clients and Depree (2016) has invited couples to watch videos of their sessions with some interesting results. Such communications between psychotherapists and clients are a topic worthy of future investigation. I can recall when therapeutic letters were really only found in approaches like cognitive analytic therapy and narrative therapy, whereas written formulations and therapeutic letters to clients are now common across all areas of therapeutic practice in the UK's National Health Service.

These kinds of communications include not only what the clients said but questions or interpretations from the therapist and one of the interesting aspects of the therapeutic community's approach to this here was that such interpretation was omitted. Given that parents can often feel positioned as helpless victims of the legal, health and social service systems, such acknowledgement is likely to be therapeutic in itself, regardless of the theoretical basis of the record. Similarly, positioning parents as experts on their own child would, from a range of therapeutic perspectives, be seen as a valuable way of engaging parents in therapeutic work and of restoring confidence in their parenting ability. A final aspect likely to appeal to a range of theoretical perspectives is the way in which the community seeks to put a range of possibilities before clients rather than an overly prescriptive approach.

Displaying agency problems at the outset of psychotherapy

In this Finnish study, the researcher/s attempted to assess the transferability of a system for categorizing elements of talk into one of five categories of agency. These categories had been developed in a previous study of semi-mandatory counselling for drink-driving (Seilonen & Wahlström, 2016). A transcript of a first psychotherapy session with a female teacher was analysed using a theory-guided content analysis. No new examples of agency were looked for.

Agency is a key issue in psychotherapy and the approach to it here reminded me of social cognition studies of attributions in therapy – for example, in family therapy sessions (e.g. Munton, Silvester, & Stratton, 1999). The use of such categorical approaches can be useful in that raters can calculate interrater reliabilities of coding judgements and can report on the frequency with which certain kinds of attributions are used.

An alternative, more discursive approach to agency might emphasize fluidity, flux and the multiple meanings of discourse rather than a categorical system where necessarily global judgements need to be made. Positioning theory (Davies & Harré, 1990) might offer an alternative approach. A discursive approach might also note the influence of the therapist's turns on the interaction as these set the context for the client's response. This is a first therapy session and clients are faced, as noted in the article's introduction, with a series of interactional demands – how to account for why they are there, how to ask for help without appearing too helpless and so on. One implication of a focus on agency as produced within an interaction rather than as an inherent property of an individual is that therapists could learn about what kinds of interaction tend to lead to more agentic talk and this might have implications for training. Of course, one would need to be careful that a descriptive account is not transformed by others into a normative account. For example, historically, descriptive accounts of narratives as consistent have been used to cast doubt on the narratives of those who have been traumatized and so have fragmented narratives (Hyvärinen, Hydén, Saarenheimo, & Tamboukou, 2010).

How do people cope with post traumatic distress after an accident? The role of psychological, social and spiritual coping in Malaysian Muslim patients

This Malaysian study focused on the coping strategies drawn on by Muslim participants who had received hospital treatment following their involvement in motor vehicle accidents and experiencing post-traumatic stress responses like intrusive thoughts, images, low mood and so on. Interviews with 29 participants were analysed using a broadly thematic approach (no specific theoretical model was stated). Three aspects of coping responses were presented: psychological (i.e. cognitive and behavioural strategies); religious and spiritual; and social coping which included discussion of the network of support around a person (family, friends, neighbours and members of religious groups and classes). The religious and spiritual strategies were differentiated further by whether they were oriented to making sense of the experience (e.g. promoting acceptance of one's situation), reducing distress (e.g. through praying, reciting Quranic verses, practicing meditation or gaining social support from religious groups) or focusing on specific experiences like intrusive memories or avoidance of similar situations.

Religion and spirituality are important aspects of many mental health service users' lives though, often, mental health professionals are much more secular than the general population (Delaney, Miller, & Bisonó, 2013). Vieten et al. (2013) have suggested some religious and spiritual competencies for therapists and Griffith and Griffith (2002) offer some suggestions of how therapists might talk about these issues with clients. Studies like this can be very useful in helping professionals understand more about these important resources in people's lives.

This article was helpfully contextualized in relation to key Malaysian Islamic concepts – for example, the notions of Redha (which emphasized how events were fated) and Tawakkal (which emphasized acceptance and reliance on God). A key finding of the study was the importance of support from a variety of interlocking communities: family; friends; neighbours; and religious groups and classes. Although the wider study from which these findings were gathered utilized mixed methods, it was unclear whether these participants were experiencing a level of post-traumatic stress responses which would have warranted psychotherapeutic intervention.

It was interesting to see how different kinds of spiritual practices might be useful with different kinds of stress responses. Thus, reciting Quranic verses seemed to be useful when dealing with intrusion responses. A brief reference was made to a participant's use of social media and I wondered whether this might be an aspect of further study. For example, how might social media be used to facilitate community support if, for example, members of different communities cannot be physically present at the hospital bedside?

The authors conclude by discussing the possibility of developing therapies adapted for use with participants from different backgrounds. This would, no doubt, be useful, but I also found myself wondering whether there might be broader public health implications of the study. Given the existence of discrimination and stigma about mental health problems, one possibility might be to develop a preventative intervention like a leaflet given out to those who have experienced such accidents, normalizing what are regarded as mental health 'symptoms' as, rather, understandable human responses to situations of threat. For example, in such accidents, some participants may have feared they would lose their life or suffer catastrophic injury. Such a leaflet might outline useful psychological and spiritual coping strategies and encourage the seeking out of support from a range of sources of support in the community.

Mental health care and educational actions: From institutional exclusion to subjective development

The relationship between the individual and social structures was also a theme of this Brazilian study. Here, the researcher/s developed a cultural-historical approach to an analysis of a case study informed by three years of fieldwork at a Community Psychosocial Centre. The case study was used as an illustration of more theoretical points the author/s wished to make. They argued that de-institutionalization could be viewed as simply about closing asylums but that this was insufficient because, if I have understood them correctly, there were still institutionalizing attitudes shared within the mental health system and by society at large, including many of those experiencing psychological distress. Their theoretical approach was informed by Soviet psychology, especially the ideas of Sergei Rubinstein and Lev Vygotsky – the latter more well known internationally than the former. In addition, the researchers drew on educational ideas, emphasizing dialogical and transformative approaches rather than normative ones. They argued that interventions should aim to promote the development of the subject. As an illustration, they discussed Sebatiao, who was hearing voices and was in receipt of mental health services. He had given up his job and was becoming more socially isolated and beginning to neglect his self-care. Subsequently, he was invited to participate in a football group, after which he began to go out walking on his own and, feeling much more positive and energetic, reported he was engaging in more regular self-care.

As Rose (1986) has noted, psychiatry is now conducted across a range of sites following international policies of de-institutionalization. The article was a useful reminder that a de-institutionalization of buildings must be accompanied by a de-institutionalization of the mind and of society. A key issue in such social change is how psychological distress is conceptualized in society – Read, Haslam, Sayce, and Davies (2006), for example, suggest that a biomedical 'illness' explanation of distress is more associated with continuing discrimination and stigma and that a more thoroughgoing social account is associated with better outcomes. Developing public campaigns to promote a more psychosocial approach to mental health, involving people with direct personal experience, is required as well as a de-institutionalization of buildings.

Transformative models of education provide a powerful alternative metaphor for psychological change than models rooted in the history of more pathologizing approaches to psychotherapy, and one is reminded of the work of the Brazilian pedagogical theorist Paula Freire and his linking of education with the development of a critical consciousness through reflection and action – conscientization (Freire, 1970). Vygotsky's ideas also have huge potential – one could see therapeutic work as about collaborating to create zones of proximal development, for example.

The innovation of the football group seemed a useful one regardless of theoretical rationale. For example, Spandler, Roy, and Mckeown (2014) have utilized the football metaphor and football venues to promote therapeutic work, though they note that its use is filled with complexity, particularly with regard to gender relations (Spandler & McKeown, 2012).

Hurting and healing in therapeutic environments: How can we understand the role of the relational context?

This article also focused on the relational context of therapeutic communities. It presented findings from three British studies: a narrative ethnography based on a large amount of data collected over 8–12 months of fieldwork (participant observation, interviews, etc.) from two therapeutic communities (a residential and a day programme) for people with diagnoses of personality disorder; a grounded theory of interviews of an open therapeutic faith community by a researcher occupying different positions at different times (e.g. as client, as a health professional and as a member of the community's management team); and an auto-ethnography of vignettes based on the researcher's experiences in hospital and staying in a family home, part of a therapeutic community. This pluralistic approach to the topic was interesting, though perhaps a little ambitious in that it was a challenge to do justice to the complexity of each study in the space available.

J.M. Clarke's study (study 1) included a beautiful quote from one of the community members who noted 'it is people that hurt us and people that heal us', and this neatly summarized the key theme of the whole article. This study provided a useful illustration of the ways in which communities can both provide solidarity (e.g. in the narrative about Julie) which might facilitate emotional expression and can also be experienced as excluding (e.g. in the narrative about Robert).

As someone influenced by systemic therapy ideas and who has worked with couples and families, I know it can be difficult to understand what is going on in a relationship when one only hears a fragment of one person's experience at one particular point in time. I found myself wondering about what the perspectives of others in the community might be about Robert's relationship with them. What were Robert's previous experiences of relationships? For example, might he have experienced victimizing relationships which might have made him wary of others? If so, how might this be perceived by other community members? I also thought about the problematic interactional cycles in which human relationships can become trapped. One would hope that therapeutic communities might usefully focus on the psychological meaning of such patterns for all those involved.

The community was focused on care for those with diagnoses of personality disorder – a hugely contentious diagnosis (Cromby, Harper, & Reavey, 2013) – and one received by service users in different ways, some feeling it is profoundly insulting, others feeling it explains their difficulties. It would have been interesting to hear more about what role, if any, the diagnosis and the heterogeneous experiences often associated with it played in the relationships in the community.

The second study, by Brown, focused on an open therapeutic faith community. It drew on a wider mixed methods study which had utilized standardized outcome measures as well as qualitative methods. Brown's reflection on how the community clients talked about how they had been fearful about completing the evaluation forms was salutary and a useful reminder that such measures are not unproblematic and transparent windows to a person's emotional state. Instead, when we complete these measures, we do so within a biographical and social context. Since many of the clients had experienced compulsory psychiatric treatment, it is, perhaps, not surprising that they might be wary of services and Brown's dual relationship (e.g. as, at different times, peer and professional) added a further layer of complexity. However, it seemed that, subsequently, Brown had been able to develop a relationship whereby clients were able to talk in more detail about their experiences. The description of the clients' survival strategies and the ways in which they had been both hurt by and healed by relationships was useful. It would have been interesting to hear further reflection on how Brown thought their multiple roles might have influenced the analysis.

I wondered whether the processes discussed here as examples of 'dissembling', 'withholding information' and 'performing' could have been seen within an interactional context. The danger is that such terms could be heard, particularly by the clients, as pathologizing. However, when we dissemble or withhold information, this is usually in a context where someone is asking information of us that we are wary of giving for a variety of reasons. We may feel the questions are overly intrusive, we may not trust the person who is asking the questions or we may fear who else they may tell or what will be done with the information. Given the focus on the link between negative life experiences and survival strategies, an alternative interpretation of such actions is to see them as part of a cautious or guarded repertoire and means of engaging the world developed as a strategy in response to adverse events in one's life.

S.P. Clarke's study (study 3) was an auto-ethnography drawing on vignettes of two very different experiences – one in a hospital experienced as anxiety-provoking and unwelcoming, the other in the context of a supportive family home. Clarke helpfully delineated the effects of a relational climate of permissiveness.

Three key themes were drawn out in the discussion: the role of emotion and emotional climate; the utility of expertise from experience in identifying the importance of belonging and hope; and the way in which fluid rather than rigid hierarchies might be more therapeutically beneficial. The authors drew primarily on dyadic conceptualizations of relationships, primarily from a Rogerian perspective, and I wondered whether further layers of meaning could be drawn out by examining relationships within therapeutic communities from a critical community psychology (e.g. Kagan, Burton, Duckett, Lawthom, & Siddiquee, 2011) and systemic perspective (e.g. Tomm, George, Wulff, & Strong, 2014). Covering three studies in a short space imposes constraints on what can be said and a lot was, necessarily, left unsaid.

Some common themes

Considering the articles as a whole, there seemed to be a number of cross-cutting themes. For example, relationships and communities were key topics and I've already suggested that systemic and interactional perspectives might be of value here. In addition, the kinds of participatory research strategies found within the critical community psychology tradition (e.g. Kagan et al., 2011) might also be of use.

It was good to see a range of data being used as well as interviews (which have become dominant in qualitative research – Harper, in press). Thus, we saw the use of ethnography and auto-ethnography as well as therapy transcripts and participant observation fieldwork. However, where researchers are summarizing large amounts of data from long-term fieldwork, it might be helpful to give some indication of the criteria used in selecting themes or extracts and whether strategies like negative case analysis were used.

One of the issues which occurred to me in the articles discussing particular psychotherapeutic innovations was the link between theory and practice. Part of the task of socialization into a psychotherapeutic tradition through professional training is to ensure that the two are closely linked but, often, textbook descriptions of this process view practice as emerging from theory, with the latter always primary. However, social scientists suggest that, often, theory seems to follow developments in practice (Gabbay, 1982). Potter, for example, has noted that 'it is not hard to conceive of theories being used as a gloss on application which has been undertaken for quite different reasons' (1982, p. 46). A case could be made for therapeutic practice innovations occurring in an unpredictable and serendipitous manner with the therapist then seeking to develop, in a *post hoc* manner, a theoretical rationale for it. This should not be viewed negatively, though, and recent years have seen models of reflective practice develop, drawing on active philosophies of learning and emphasizing an iterative and mutually influential relationship between action and reflection.

Sometimes, therapeutic innovations emerge because of ideas circulating in the broader culture – for example, we often see similar developments occurring in different traditions. For example, in a tongue-in-cheek chapter, Epstein, Wiesner, and Epstein (2007) suggest that the Reflecting Team approach (where families hear the reflections of a team who have listened to the therapy session) pioneered by the systemic family therapist Tom Andersen might have owed a lot to Woody Allen's 1971 film *Play it Again, Sam* where internal dialogues were made audible and visible through the scenes between the Woody Allen and the Humphrey Bogart characters!

There were some differences between the articles in relation to the implicit assumptions made about subjectivity. Parker (1994) delineates three models of subjectivity found in qualitative research: an 'uncomplicated subjectivity' found in much humanistic work where the assumption is that the data 'speaks for itself'; the 'blank subjectivity' found in much discursive research where the discourse user is seen as the product of clashing cultural discourses where human agency is untheorized; and a 'complex subjectivity' which sees individual agency as tangled up in the social structures and discursive forms found in culture. In addition, the narrative therapist White (2004) reminds us of the danger of essentialist and naturalistic accounts which may offer somewhat 'thin' readings of therapeutic change by drawing on notions like inner 'insight' or 'resilience'. With further exploration, it often becomes clear that people use such terms as shorthand descriptions of much more complex processes (Harper, 2014). Moreover, when people have experienced significant emotional trauma, it is important to understand their sometimes complex relationships with others in a biographical and interactional context.

More theoretically pluralistic approaches offer one way of appreciating such complexity. The Wertz et al. (2011) collection offers an example of how this might be done by drawing on phenomenological psychology, grounded theory, discourse analysis, narrative research and intuitive inquiry to analyse a text and the transcript of an interview with a young woman who also offered her reflection on the analyses of the researchers. Of course, such an ambitious approach is a challenge in the context of articles for scholarly journals, but it offers a way of addressing the challenge of a pluralistic approach and the need to incorporate the views of participants.

It is important in qualitative research for there to be a good balance between data and theory, lest the research participant's voice is lost (Waddingham, 2015). An issue less discussed in the articles was whether the views of research participants had been sought on the analyses (though this obviously does not apply to the auto-ethnography in Hurting and healing in therapeutic environments: How can we understand the role of the relational context?). Respondent validation is an important criterion for evaluating qualitative research (Elliott, Fischer, & Rennie, 1999), though this is complicated as qualitative methods differ in the kinds of their epistemological claims they make (Reicher, 2000). Certainly, service user researchers could be more involved in qualitative research (Faulkner, 2012) and Sweeney, Greenwood, Williams, Wykes, and Rose (2013) have suggested a novel approach where several researchers, including service users, are involved in the process of analysis, creating an opportunity for discussion of different interpretative perspectives.

Reading the articles, it is clear that there is theoretically and rich research being conducted internationally, on a range of important social topics in mental health and psychotherapy. The editors of the issue are to be commended for collating such an interesting, thought-provoking and diverse range of articles.

Disclosure statement

No potential conflict of interest was reported by the author.

References

Bakhtin, M. M. (1981). *The dialogic imagination: Four essays.* (M. Holquist, Ed., C. Emerson & M. Holquist, Trans.). Austin: University of Texas Press.
Bakhtin, M. M. (1984). *Problems of Dostoevsky's poetics.* (C. Emerson Ed., Trans.). Minneapolis: University of Minnesota Press.

Carrera-Fernández, M. J., Guàrdia-Olmos, J., & Peró-Cebollero, M. (2014). Qualitative methods of data analysis in psychology: An analysis of the literature. *Qualitative Research, 14*, 20–36.

Cromby, J., Harper, D., & Reavey, P. (2013). *Psychology, mental health & distress*. Basingstoke: Palgrave Macmillan.

Davies, B., & Harré, R. (1990). Positioning: The discursive production of selves. *Journal for the Theory of Social Behaviour, 20*, 43–63.

Delaney, H. D., Miller, W. R., & Bisonó, A. M. (2013). Religiosity and spirituality among psychologists: A survey of clinician members of the American Psychological Association. *Spirituality in Clinical Practice, 1(S)*, 95–106.

Depree, J. (2016). *Video-recording for therapeutic purposes in couple counselling* (Thesis, doctor of philosophy (PhD)). University of Waikato, Hamilton.

Elliott, R., Fischer, C. T., & Rennie, D. L. (1999). Evolving guidelines for publication of qualitative research studies in psychology and related fields. *British Journal of Clinical Psychology, 38*, 215–229.

Ellis, D., & Tucker, I. (2015). *Social psychology of emotion*. London: Sage.

Epstein, E., Wiesner, M., & Epstein, M. (2007). True stories: Acts of informing and forming. In H. Anderson & P. Jensen (Eds., 2007), *Innovations in the reflecting process: The inspirations of Tom Andersen* (pp. 137–148). London: Karnac.

Faulkner, A. (2012). Participation and service user involvement. In D. Harper, & A. R. Thompson (Eds.), *Qualitative research methods in mental health and psychotherapy: An introduction for students and practitioners* (pp. 39–54). Chichester: Wiley.

Freire, P. (1970). *Pedagogy of the oppressed*. (M. B. Ramos, Trans.). New York, NY: Continuum.

Frosh, S. (2007). Disintegrating qualitative research. *Theory & Psychology, 17*, 635–653.

Gabbay, J. (1982). Asthma attacked? Tactics for the reconstruction of a disease concept. In P. Wright & A. Treacher (Eds.), *The problem of medical knowledge: Examining the social construction of medicine* (pp. 23–48). Edinburgh: Edinburgh University Press.

Griffith, J. L., & Griffith, M. E. (2002). *Encountering the sacred in psychotherapy: How to talk with people about their spiritual lives*. New York, NY: Guilford Press.

Harper, D. (2014, April). Continuing the conversation: A response to Anne and friends. *Clinical Psychology Forum, 256*, 26–29.

Harper, D. (in press). Chapter 23: Clinical psychology. In C. Willig & W. Stainton Rogers (Eds.), *Handbook of qualitative research in psychology* (2nd ed.). London: Sage.

Harper, D., & Thompson, A. (Eds.). (2012). *Qualitative research methods in mental health and psychotherapy: An introduction for students and practitioners*. Chichester: Wiley.

Hyvärinen, M., Hydén, L. C., Saarenheimo, M., & Tamboukou, M. (Eds.). (2010). Introduction. In *Beyond narrative coherence: An introduction* (pp. 1–15). Amsterdam: John Benjamins.

Kagan, C. M., Burton, M., Duckett, P. S., Lawthom, R., & Siddiquee, A. (2011). *Critical community psychology*. Oxford: Wiley-Blackwell.

Ley, P. (1979). Memory for medical information. *British Journal of Social and Clinical Psychology, 18*, 245–255.

Munton, A. G., Silvester, J., & Stratton, P. (1999). *Attributions in action: A practical approach to coding qualitative data*. Chichester: Wiley.

Parker, I. (1994). Reflexive research and the grounding of analysis: Social psychology and the psy-complex. *Journal of Community & Applied Social Psychology, 4*, 239–252.

Parker, I., & Pavón-Cuéllar, D. (2013). *Lacan, discourse, event: New psychoanalytic approaches to textual indeterminacy*. London: Routledge.

Potter, J. (1982). "... Nothing so practical as a good theory": The problematic application of social psychology. In P. Stringer (Ed.), *Confronting social issues* (pp. 23–49). London: Academic Press.

Read, J., Haslam, N., Sayce, L., & Davies, E. (2006). Prejudice and schizophrenia: A review of the 'mental illness is an illness like any other' approach. *Acta Psychiatrica Scandinavica, 114*, 303–318.

Reicher, S. (2000). Against methodolatry: Some comments on Elliott, Fischer, and Rennie. *British Journal of Clinical Psychology, 39*(1), 1–6.

Rose, N. (1986). Psychiatry: The discipline of mental health: The power of psychiatry. In P. Miller & N. Rose (Eds.), *The power of psychiatry* (pp. 43–84). Cambridge: Polity Press.

Seilonen, M. L., & Wahlström, J. (2016). Constructions of agency in accounts of drunk driving at the outset of semi-mandatory counseling. *Journal of Constructivist Psychology, 29*, 248–268.

Spandler, H., & McKeown, M. (2012). A critical exploration of using football in health and welfare programs: Gender, masculinities, and social relations. *Journal of Sport & Social Issues, 36*, 387–409.

Spandler, H., Roy, A., & Mckeown, M. (2014). Using football metaphor to engage men in therapeutic support. *Journal of Social Work Practice, 28*, 229–245.

Sweeney, A., Greenwood, K. E., Williams, S., Wykes, T., & Rose, D. S. (2013). Hearing the voices of service user researchers in collaborative qualitative data analysis: The case for multiple coding. *Health Expectations, 16*, e89–e99.

Tomm, K., George, S. S., Wulff, D., & Strong, T. (Eds.). (2014). *Patterns in interpersonal interactions: Inviting relational understandings for therapeutic change.* London: Routledge.

Tsulukidze, M., Durand, M. A., Barr, P. J., Mead, T., & Elwyn, G. (2014). Providing recording of clinical consultation to patients – A highly valued but underutilized intervention: A scoping review. *Patient Education and Counseling, 95*, 297–304.

Vieten, C., Scammell, S., Pilato, R., Ammondson, I., Pargament, K. I., & Lukoff, D. (2013). Spiritual and religious competencies for psychologists. *Psychology of Religion and Spirituality, 5*, 129–144.

Waddingham, R. (2015). Whose voice are we hearing, really? *European Journal of Psychotherapy & Counselling, 17*, 206–215.

Wertz, F. J., Charmaz, K., McMullen, L. M., Josselson, R., Anderson, R., & McSpadden, E. (2011). *Five ways of doing qualitative analysis: Phenomenological psychology, grounded theory, discourse analysis, narrative research, and intuitive inquiry.* New York, NY: Guilford Publications.

Wetherell, M. (2012). *Affect and emotion: A new social science understanding.* London: Sage.

White, M. (2004). Narrative practice and the unpacking of identity conclusions. In M. White (Ed.), *Narrative practice and exotic lives: Resurrecting diversity in everyday life.* Adelaide: Dulwich Centre.

Everyday life, manifesto-writing and the texture of human agency

John McLeod

ABSTRACT

Qualitative research provides a flexible array of methodologies that can be applied to the understanding of different aspects of psychotherapy practice. This paper offers commentary and reflection around the contribution of a set of qualitative studies included in the current issue of this journal. Conceptual and methodological issues are discussed in relation to the aims, methods and findings of these studies. Key themes that are highlighted across these studies include the relevance for psychotherapy of a focus on everyday life, the tension between description and theorising in qualitative inquiry, and the nature of human agency. Suggestions are made regarding possible strategies for enhancing the relevance and impact of qualitative research within the field of counselling and psychotherapy.

LA VIDA COTIDIANA, LA ESCRITURA DE MANIFIESTOS Y LA TEXTURA DEL SENTIDO DEL SI MISMO

La investigación cualitativa ofrece un conjunto flexible de métodologías que pueden aplicarse a diferentes aspectos en la práctica de la psicoterapia. Este articulo ofrece comentarios y reflexiones acerca de la contribución de los estudios cualitativos incluidos en el presente número de esta revista. Se discuten aspectos conceptuales y metodológicos en relación con las metas, métodos y resultados de estos estudios.Los temas claves que se destacan a través de ellos incluyen la relevancia para la psicoterapia, de tener un foco en la vida cotidiana, la tensión entre la teoría y la descripción en la investigación cualitativa y la naturaleza del sentido del sí mismo. Se hacen sugerencias en relación con la posibilidad de usar estrategias para aumentar la relevancia y el impacto de la investigación cualitativa en el campo de la psicoterapia y la orientación psicológica.

La vita quotidiana, il manifesto-scrittura e lo spessore dell'azione umana

La ricerca qualitativa fornisce un range flessibile di metodologie che può essere applicato alla comprensione dei diversi aspetti della pratica psicoterapeutica. Questo contributo offre commenti e riflessioni relativi a una serie di studi qualitativi inclusi in questo numero della rivista. Aspetti concettuali e metodologici sono discussi in relazione a obiettivi, metodi e risultati degli studi presentati. I temi chiave evidenziati in questi studi includono la rilevanza della vita di ogni giorno per la psicoterapia, la contrapposizione tra descrizione e teorizzazione nella ricerca qualitativa e la natura dell'umano. Le proposte sono orientate a suggerire possibili strategie per migliorare la rilevanza e l'impatto della ricerca qualitativa nel campo della consulenza e della psicoterapia.

Vie quotidienne, écriture de manifeste et texture de l'agenceité humaine

La recherche qualitative fournit un éventail de méthodologies pouvant entre utilisées pour comprendre les différents aspects de la pratique psychothérapeutique. Cet article offre un commentaire et une réflection quant à la contribution d'une série de d'études qualitatives publiées dans ce numéro spécial. Des questions conceptuelles et méthodologiques sont évoquées en relation avec les objectifs, les méthodes et les résultats de ces études. L'accent est mis sur des thèmes-clés dont ceux de la pertinence pour la psychothérapie de se centrer sur la vie quotidienne, la tension entre description et théorisation en recherche qualitative et la nature de l'agencéité humaine.

Καθημερινή ζωή, συγγραφή διακήρυξης και η υφή της ανθρώπινης κυριότητας

Η ποιοτική έρευνα προσφέρει ένα ευέλικτο εύρος από μεθοδολογίες, οι οποίες μπορούν να εφαρμοστούν στην κατανόηση διαφορετικών όψεων της ψυχοθεραπευτικής πράξης. Αυτό το άρθρο προσφέρει σχολιασμό και στοχασμό αναφορικά με τη συμβολή μιας σειράς ποιοτικών μελετών που φιλοξενούνται στο συγκεκριμένο τεύχος του περιοδικού. Συζητούνται εννοιολογικά και μεθοδολογικά ζητήματα σε συνάρτηση με τους στόχους, τις μεθόδους και τα αποτελέσματα αυτών των ερευνών. Τα σημεία- κλειδιά που τονίζονται σε αυτές τις έρευνες περιλαμβάνουν τη σημασία που έχει για την ψυχοθεραπεία η εστίαση στην καθημερινή ζωή, την ένταση ανάμεσα στην περιγραφή και στη θεωρητικοποίηση στην ποιοτική έρευνα, και τη φύση της ανθρώπινης κυριότητας. Παρέχονται προτάσεις αναφορικά με πιθανές στρατηγικές για την προώθηση της σύνδεσης και της επίδρασης της ποιοτικής έρευνας στο πεδίο της συμβουλευτικής και της ψυχοθεραπείας.

The links between art and psychotherapy are widely recognised, but perhaps not fully examined. At the heart of both enterprises is the act of 'making', and in particular the making of something special (Dissanayake, 2000). There is also the display of what has been made. Art is disseminated in many ways – in homes, in unexpected places in the countryside and city streets, through performance, on the web. Mainly, though, we tend to think about art as being displayed at an exhibition or in a room in a gallery. What is made through psychotherapy is primarily displayed through performance. In some instances, however, a researcher documents the making process of psychotherapy, and creates a text that can be displayed on a wall (conference poster), performed as a lecture or published in a research journal.

If the yellow covers of the *European Journal of Psychotherapy and Counselling* can be regarded, for a moment, as an exhibition space, this brief introductory paper can be viewed as similar to a review of an exhibition written by an art critic. Clearly, what is of primary importance when reading the articles in this special issue is to listen to your own response, and reflect on how these studies connect with your own interests. What a critic has to say is secondary. Hopefully, it may motivate you to visit the exhibition, or enable you to see the work in a different light.

The studies in this issue of the journal reflect a range of different qualitative methodologies, applied to a variety of therapeutic settings. Apart from being interesting and valuable examples of qualitative inquiry, there was no pre-determined rationale for including them in this particular exhibition space. Nevertheless, I suggest that they can be viewed as representing two vitally significant emergent themes within contemporary psychotherapy theory and practice: the implications of adopting more of a focus on everyday life, and the concept of human agency as a means of opening up new understandings of the life difficulties experienced by clients. In addition, these articles exemplify a central polarity within the methodology of qualitative inquiry, at one end characterised by a grounded and descriptive approach, and at the other by a theory-driven perspective.

Psychotherapy and everyday life

One of the common factors across both art and psychotherapy resides in their relationship to everyday life. Art and psychotherapy, in their different ways, allow a person to step outside everyday life. In this respect, they offer a 'special' experience, which is memorable and which has the potential to highlight some of the underlying significance of what it means to be human. While the notion of the therapeutic space as a 'cultural island' (Back, 1972) has been around for a long time within the psychotherapy literature, it could be argued that its potency has not been sufficiently acknowledged. The commitment to attend therapy, in itself, involves making an adjustment to the personal scheduling of everyday life activities. Combined with travel time to and from therapy sessions, participation in therapy calls for a two-hour block of time (at least) each week, that is a departure from the usual routine of everyday life.

A series of studies by Dreier (1998, 2000, 2008, 2015) and his colleagues has shown how therapy clients use the movement from everyday life into therapy sessions, and then back out again, as a means of re-positioning themselves in relation to elements of their everyday life, and, in time, rearranging these elements. Göstas, Wiberg, and Kjellin (2012) showed how clients in successful therapy shifted from a state at the start of therapy of being absorbed by personal issues and as a consequence unable to participate fully in everyday life, to a state of re-engagement in everyday matters. However, these are somewhat isolated studies. For the most part, psychotherapy research has concentrated on an examination of what happens in the therapy room, and has largely defined the outcomes of therapy in terms of symptom changes. These are important research topics, but have been pursued at the expense of developing a comprehensive understanding of the everyday context of psychotherapy.

Some of the papers in this issue of the journal make important contributions to the task of mapping out the links between therapy and everyday life. In the study by Bahari, Mohamad Alwi, Jahan, Ahmad and Mohd Saiboon (2016), people who had experienced a motor vehicle accident were interviewed about whether they had symptoms of psychological trauma, and how they had coped. Most of them indicated at least some trauma symptoms. None of those who were interviewed had made use of any formal counselling or psychotherapy interventions. All of them described a range of everyday resources that they exercised in the process of coming to terms with what had happened to them. The most important of these resources were their social network, and spiritual beliefs/practices. Technically, this was a nice study, conducted with a high level of ethical sensitivity and care. The findings of the study draw our attention to the coping resources that are available to most people. It is not unusual for a therapy client to mention that he or she has been involved in a motor vehicle accident or similar incident. Typically, such reports trigger therapist formulations in terms of post-traumatic stress disorder (PTSD). What the study by Bahari et al. (2016) tells us is that it may be just as relevant to explore why and how the everyday resources of the client were not sufficient, or to examine how they can be utilised more effectively.

The format of the paper by Clarke, Clarke, Brown and Middleton (2016) comprises a synthesis of findings from three studies of relational healing processes in therapeutic communities, rather than a report of a single study. In some respects this structure is frustrating for the reader, in so far as there is not enough space to explain the details of data collection and analysis in each of the studies. On the other hand, the different methodologies employed in the studies add credibility to the conclusions that are offered. This paper offers some extremely helpful insights into the healing characteristics of everyday contexts. People who are given the opportunity to spend time in a therapeutic community have usually been exposed to toxic and abusive interpersonal environments in their past.

Clarke et al. (2016) describe some of the ways in which therapeutic communities can be enormously helpful in enabling participation in curative and supportive micro-interaction sequences. They also illustrate forms of interaction in therapeutic communities that have harmful effects, and hinder recovery.

Although the other papers in this issue of the journal less directly address the question of everyday life aspects of therapy, it may still be instructive to view them from an everyday perspective. Wahlström and Seilonen (2016) analyse the way that a client talked about herself in a first session of therapy. What is particularly striking about this client is the extent to which her narrative lacks agency – things happen to her, rather than her making them happen. This analysis is discussed more fully below. However, when reading the paper by Wahlström and Seilonen (2016), it can be instructive to attempt to imaginatively recreate a sense of what the everyday life of this person could be like. The studies by Romelli and Pozzi (2016) and Goulart, and González Rey (2016), also discussed more fully below, also refer to important aspects of the relationship between everyday life and the process of therapy, in two contexts: a therapeutic community for children (Romelli & Pozzi, 2016), and a community mental health project (Goulart, and González Rey, 2016). The latter study develops an analysis of a useful way of thinking about everyday life: the idea that it is structured, at least in part, around a network of socially defined 'pathways' that the person can follow.

Description and interpretation in qualitative research

The field of qualitative research is characterised by a complex mesh of methodological traditions, each of which draws on a slightly different set of epistemological influences. In practical terms, one way of organising this complexity is to view all qualitative research as seeking to accomplish three tasks: description, analysis and interpretation. From this perspective, competing qualitative methodologies can be understood as providing different blends of these features. In this respect, the articles in this issue of the journal represent radically different approaches. The study of coping strategies following a road traffic accident (Bahari, et al., 2016) is mainly descriptive of the experiences of those who were interviewed, with analysis of categories of coping strategy but minimal theoretical interpretation. By contrast, in the papers by Romelli and Pozzi (2016) and Goulart, and González Rey (2016), much of the text consists of presentation of theory, with vivid but brief descriptive evidence used to illustrate theoretical points. The other two papers fall between these extremes.

My own initial response to the papers by Romelli and Pozzi (2016) and Goulart, and González Rey (2016) was to experience some degree of frustration and confusion. Frustration, because I wanted to know more about the lived experience and cultural context of the people being studied (i.e. more description). Confusion, because the limits of a journal article did not allow sufficient space to offer an adequate account of the underlying theory. Further reflection on parallels between psychotherapy (and psychotherapy research) and art brought me to a realisation that I am willing to accept, or even embrace frustration and confusion when confronted by a piece of art. So why do I require psychotherapy research to conform to my expectations and fit into my comfort zone? Surely, there is a value to being challenged by a therapy research report, and to be required to invest work and effort to make sense of it.

An intriguing area of common ground between psychotherapy and art is the tendency to make pronouncements about the way the world is, or how it should be. In psychotherapy, this takes the form of theories and approaches. In art, it takes the form of artists' manifestos (Danchev, 2011). For a psychotherapist, it is interesting to read artists' manifestos. They tend to come across as self-contained definitions of reality that are not in fact particularly interested in persuading anyone else, but instead serve the function of defining a set of ideas that are significant to a particular group of people at a particular point in time. Within the community of adherents to the manifesto, brilliant work is carried out, because the freshness of the new vision enables members to see and do things in a different way. In some respects, the papers by Romelli and Pozzi (2016) and Goulart, and González Rey (2016) can be regarded as examples of manifesto-writing as much as examples of social science.

One of the key differences between manifesto-writing and science is that the latter allows for the possibility that the theory is open to change in the face of observation and evidence. Most of the time, the principle that scientific theories is open to refutation functions as an underlying value statement rather than as a procedural reality. After all, it is not often that theories are refuted. But it does promote a respect for curiosity and willingness to report observations that do not quite fit. An example of the latter can be found in the study by Clarke et al. (2016), who found that patients in the therapeutic community faked their responses to symptom questionnaires in order to control their length of stay. In the context of the overall aims of the Clarke et al. (2016) study, this observation had minimal relevance. As a contribution to broadening our understanding of the validity of symptom measures in psychotherapy research, it is potentially highly significant.

The tension between description and interpretation in qualitative research can never be resolved, and can be regarded as a source of creative possibility. One strategy that can be helpful, which is used to great effect in Interpretative Phenomenological Analysis (IPA: Smith, Flowers, & Larkin, 2009) is to do the descriptive work first, and allow the reader to see what you (the investigator) saw, and only then offer an interpretative account. The other way round (starting with the interpretative scheme, and then selecting observations that are of interest to that perspective) has the effect of placing the reader in a take-it-or-leave-it position. When there is sufficient description, the reader can, to some degree, make up their own mind. If qualitative research is to be true to its roots in hermeneutics (McLeod, 2011), it needs to keep in mind that traditions of interpretative inquiry in fields such as theology, law and literary criticism are based in the practice of all interlocutors having access to the same text.

The texture of human agency

In an art exhibition, there is often one piece that stands out. Within this issue of the journal, I suggest that the paper by Wahlström and Seilonen (2016) will function in that way. This is an analysis of a first session of psychotherapy, with the aim of analysing how the client described herself as agentic (i.e. having intentions and purposes, as opposed to being at the mercy of events). The session was recorded, and transcribed. Part of the impact of this paper lies in the selection of the case. The therapist said little in the session, which meant the researchers did not need to take account of any possibility that the way that the client was describing her life was significantly influenced by the therapist's responses to her. Another distinctive feature of this session was that the client was relentlessly non-agentic. It is then not a typical case but an extreme case, selected because it highlights certain themes.

The analysis carried out by Wahlström and Seilonen (2016) possesses the depth and authority of being informed by a long line of inquiry, including philosophical perspectives on human agency (Macmurray, 1961) and previous studies of client agency by many investigators, including Hoener, Stiles, Luka, and Gordon (2012), Mackrill (2009), and the authors themselves. What they have accomplished is the construction of a model of five key aspects of client agency: relationality, causal attribution, intentionality, historicity and reflexivity. For many therapists, client agency is an important factor but one that is hard to pin down: 'he does not seem to be willing to accept responsibility for his actions, but I can't figure out how to get him to look at it'. The framework developed by Wahlström and Seilonen (2016) offers therapists a way of making sense of agency as not merely a general attribute of the client's way of being and talking, but as a set of specific constituent processes, each of which can serve as the focus for therapeutic conversation, reflection and change. This development has the potential to make a highly significant contribution to the gradual shift away from self-contained schools of psychotherapy, in the direction of a structure of practical psychotherapeutic knowledge that draws on all traditions. The concept of 'agency' is part of a common language of therapy. Different approaches to therapy have evolved their own distinctive methods for promoting client agency. The five-process model of agency allows us to see how these methods fit together, and to make distinctions between scenarios in which each of them may be more or less helpful.

Conclusions

The articles in this issue of the journal confirm the vigour and relevance of qualitative research in counselling, psychotherapy and related disciplines. This commentary has offered some perspectives that invite further critical reflection on the part of readers of these contributions. Other perspectives are available, and the reader's own response always needs to be the primary starting point for evaluating the meaningfulness and practical utility of a research study. As with art, there is a difference between casually looking at an exhibit, and making the commitment to imaginatively enter its world. The latter involves a willingness to look more than once, and to engage in dialogue in which the horizon of one's own assumptions and beliefs may begin to shift. It is to the credit of the authors of the papers in this collection, and the reviewers and editors who have assisted them in their work, that their efforts have had the capacity to make an impact of this kind.

Disclosure statement

No potential conflict of interest was reported by the author.

References

Back, K. W. (1972). *Beyond words. The story of sensitivity training and the encounter movement.* New York, NY: Russell Sage Foundation.

Bahari, R., Mohamad Alwi, M. N., Jahan, N., Ahmad, M. R., & Mohd Saiboon, I. (2016). How do people cope with post traumatic distress after an accident? The role of psychological, social and spiritual coping in Malaysian Muslim patients. *European Journal of Psychotherapy and Counselling, 18* (4), forthcoming.

Clarke, S., Clarke, J., Brown, R., & Middleton, H. (2016). Hurting and healing in therapeutic environments: How can we understand the role of the relational context? *European Journal of Psychotherapy and Counselling, 18* (4), forthcoming.

Danchev, A. (2011). *100 artists' manifestos: From the futurists to the stuckists.* London: Penguin.

Dissanayake, E. (2000). *Art and intimacy: How the arts began.* Seattle: University of Washington Press.

Dreier, O. (1998). Client perspectives and uses of psychotherapy. *European Journal of Psychotherapy & Counselling, 1,* 295–310. doi:10.1080/13642539808402315

Dreier, O. (2000). Psychotherapy in clients' trajectories across contexts. In C. Mattingly & L. Garro (Eds.), *Narratives and the cultural construction of illness and healing* (pp. 237–258). Berkeley: University of California Press.

Dreier, O. (2008). *Psychotherapy in everyday life.* New York, NY: Cambridge University Press.

Dreier, O. (2015). Interventions in everyday lives: How clients use psychotherapy outside their sessions. *European Journal of Psychotherapy & Counselling, 17,* 114–128. doi: 10.1080/13642537.2015.1027781

Göstas, M. W., Wiberg, B., & Kjellin, L. (2012). Increased participation in the life context: A qualitative study of clients' experiences of problems and changes after psychotherapy. *European Journal of Psychotherapy & Counselling, 14,* 365–380. doi:10.1080/1364253 7.2012.734498

Goulart, D., & González Rey, F. (2016). Mental health care and educational actions: From institutional exclusion to subjective development. *European Journal of Psychotherapy and Counselling,18* (4), forthcoming.

Hoener, C., Stiles, W. B., Luka, B. J., & Gordon, R. A. (2012). Client experiences of agency in therapy. *Person-Centered & Experiential Psychotherapies, 11*, 64–82. doi:10.1080/14 779757.2011.639460

Mackrill, T. (2009). Constructing client agency in psychotherapy research. *Journal of Humanistic Psychology, 49*, 193–206. doi:10.1177/0022167808319726

Macmurray, J. (1961). *Persons in relation*. London: Faber.

McLeod, J. (2011). *Qualitative research in counselling and psychotherapy* (2nd ed.). London: Sage.

Romelli, K., & Pozzi, G. (2016). Therapeutic community for children with diagnosis of psychosis: What place for parents? The relation between subject and the institutional 'Other'. *European Journal of Psychotherapy and Counselling, 18* (4), forthcoming.

Smith, J. A., Flowers, P., & Larkin, M. (2009). *Interpretative phenomenological analysis: Theory, method and research*. London: Sage.

Wahlström, J., & Seilonen, M.-L. (2016). Displaying agency problems at the outset of psychotherapy. *European Journal of Psychotherapy and Counselling, 18* (4), forthcoming.

'Not dead … abandoned' – a clinical case study of childhood and combat-related trauma

Julianna Challenor

ABSTRACT

This clinical case study examines inter-subjective processes with a counselling client who presented with symptoms of complex trauma including severe anxiety, low mood, dissociation and suicidality. Therapy lasted 12 months and was ended abruptly by the client. Psychoanalytic and phenomenological hermeneutic frameworks are drawn on in theorizing the work. From this perspective, loss associated with trauma is conceptualized as relational, as traumatic states threaten psychological organization and the continuing experience of relational ties that are needed for survival. Dissociation is understood as a defensive state that changes the way that temporality is experienced. The client's capacity for dissociation appeared to have developed in early childhood in response to physical abuse, predisposing him to further ongoing and severe trauma as an adult soldier. There will be a focus on the way that dissociation and enactment in the therapeutic relationship limited the therapist's capacity to provide the client with inter-subjective regulation of disavowed affect. The client's unconscious experience of unbearable affect led to a breakdown of the therapeutic relationship and termination of therapy. Using detailed session and supervision notes and correspondence received from the client, theory and practice links will be evaluated, as well as some methodological aspects of case study research.

"NO MUERTO ... ABANDONADO" Estudio clínico del caso de un niño y el trauma de lucha por la sobrevivencia

El estudio clinico de este caso examina procesos inter-subjetivos con un cliente en orientación psicológica que presentaba complejos síntomas de trauma incluyendo severa ansiedad, bajos estados de ánimo, disociación y tendencias suicidas. La terapia duró doce meses y fue abruptamente terminada por el cliente. Se utilizan el marco teórico psicoanalítico y hermenéutico fenomenológico como apoyo teórico para el trabajo. Desde este punto de vista se conceptualiza el trauma relacionado con la pérdida como relacional, ya que los estadios traumáticos amenazan la organización psicológica y la experiencia de continuidad en los contactos relacionales ncesarias para la supervivencia. Se ve la disociación como un estado defensivo que contribuye a cambiar la manera en la cual se experimenta la temporalidad. La capacidad del cliente para la disociación parece haber sido puesta en marcha en su niñez temprana como respuesta al abuso físico, predisponiéndolo a un continuo y fuerte trauma en su vida adulta como soldado. Enfocamos cómo la capacidad del terapeuta para proporcionarle al cliente una regulación inter-subjetiva de sus afectos no reconocidos, se vió limitada por la disociación del cliente and su tendencia al "acting-out"en la relación terapéutica. La experiancia inconsciente de afecto insoportable por parte del cliente llevó a la ruptura de la relación terapéutica y a la terminación de la terapia.Se evalúan las conexiones entre la teoría y la práctica utilizando notas detalladas de la sesiones con el cliente y de la supervisión y correspondencia recibida del cliente, así como también aspectos metodológicos de la investigación en el estudio de casos.

'Non morto ... abbandonato' – Uno studio clinico su un caso di infanzia con traumi

Questo studio clinico esamina i processi inter-soggettivi in un caso di consulenza con un cliente che presenta sintomi riferibili a traumi complessi, ad esempio forte ansia, tono dell'umore depresso, dissociazione e rischio suicidario. La terapia, durata 12 mesi, è stata conclusa bruscamente dal cliente. Quadri ermeneutici a orientamento psicoanalitico e fenomenologico sono descritti in base alla teorizzazione del lavoro. Da questo punto di vista, la perdita associata ad un trauma viene concettualizzata in termini relazionali, poiché le condizioni indotte da eventi traumatici costituiscono una minaccia per l'organizzazione psicologica e l'esercizio di legami relazionali necessari per la sopravvivenza.

La dissociazione è intesa come uno condizione difensiva che cambia il modo di vivere la temporalità. La propensione verso la dissociazione, che sembra essersi sviluppata nella prima infanzia in risposta ad abusi fisici, predispone il cliente all'esposizione ad ulteriori e severi traumi, in qualità di militare. Ci si focalizza sul modo in cui la dissociazione nella relazione terapeutica limiti la capacità del terapeuta di offrire al cliente una regolazione inter-personale di impatto emozionale negato. L'esperianza inconscia del cliente di sentimenti intollerabili ha determinato la rottura della relazione terapeutica e l'interruzione della terapia. Utilizzando particolari delle sessioni, note di supervisione e la corrispondenza ricevuta dal cliente, si valuteranno le connessioni tra teoria e pratica, così come alcuni aspetti metodologici della ricerca sul caso in oggetto.

'Pas mort ... abandonné': un cas clinique de trauma infantile et lié au combat

Ce cas clinique examine les processus intersubjectifs client-thérapeute pour un client en situation thérapeutique présentant des symptômes signes d'un traumatisme complexe en particulier: angoisse sévère, état dépressif, dissociation et suicidalité. La thérapie a duré douze mois et fut interrompue abruptement par le client lui-même. Un cadre de référence psychanalytique et phénoménologique-herméneutique ont aidé à la théorisation du travail. Grâce à cette perspective, la perte associée au trauma a été conceptualisée comme étant relationnelle, puisque les états traumatiques menaçaient à la fois l'organisation psychologique et l'expérience du maintien des liens relationnels, nécessaires à la survie.La dissociation est considérée comme un état défensif ayant la capacité d'altérer la manière dont est vécue la temporalité. La capacité du client à dissocier semble s'être développée dans sa prime enfance en réaction à des violences physiques, le prédisposant ainsi à un traumatisme sévère et persistant dans sa vie de soldat adulte. Nous nous concentrerons ici sur la façon dont la dissociation et le passage à l'acte au sein de la relation thérapeutique ont limité la capacité du thérapeute à fournir au client une régulation intersubjective de l'affect dénié. L'expérience inconsciente du client d'un affect insupportable a conduit à une rupture de la relation thérapeutique et une fin du travail.

A l'aide de notes détaillées des séances et des supervisions ainsi que de la correspondance émanant du client, les liens théorie/pratique seront évalués ainsi que certains aspects méthodologiques de la recherche basée sur les études de cas.

«Όχι νεκρός ... εγκαταλελειμμένος» – Μια μελέτη κλινικής περίπτωσης της παιδικής ηλικίας και τραυμάτων που συνδέονται με πόλεμο

Η παρούσα μελέτη κλινικής περίπτωσης εξετάζει τις διυποκειμενικές διεργασίες με έναν πελάτη συμβουλευτικής, με συμπτώματα σύνθετου τραύματος, στα οποία συμπεριλαμβάνονταν έντονο άγχος, χαμηλή διάθεση, διάσχιση και αυτοκτονικότητα. Η θεραπεία διήρκεσε 12 μήνες και τερματίστηκε αιφνίδια από τον πελάτη. Για τη θεωρητική κατανόηση της ψυχοθεραπευτικής δουλειάς χρησιμοποιούνται ψυχαναλυτικά και φαινομενολογικά ερμηνευτικά πλαίσια. Από αυτή την οπτική, η απώλεια που σχετίζεται με το τραύμα προσεγγίζεται ως σχεσιακό φαινόμενο, καθώς οι τραυματικές καταστάσεις απειλούν τη ψυχολογική οργάνωση και τη συνέχιση της εμπειρίας των σχεσιακών δεσμών που απαιτούνται για την επιβίωση.

Η διάσχιση κατανοείται ως ένας αμυντικός μηχανισμός που μεταβάλει τον τρόπο με τον οποίο βιώνεται ο χρόνος. Φάνηκε ότι η τάση του πελάτη για διάσχιση είχε εμφανιστεί στην πρώιμη παιδική ηλικία, ως απάντηση σε σωματική κακοποίηση, προδιαθέτοντας τον για συνεχιζόμενο και σοβαρό τραύμα ως ενήλικο στρατιώτη. Θα εστιάσουμε στον τρόπο με τον οποίο η διάσχιση ή αποσύνδεση και η εκδραμάτιση στη θεραπευτική σχέση περιόρισε τη δυνατότητα της θεραπεύτριας να προσφέρει στον πελάτη τη δυνατότητα διυποκειμενικής ρύθμισης των συναισθημάτων που είχε απαρνηθεί. Η ασυνείδητη εμπειρία αβάσταχτων συναισθημάτων του πελάτη οδήγησε στη διάλυση της θεραπευτικής σχέσης και στον τερματισμό της θεραπείας.

Χρησιμοποιούνται λεπτομερείς σημειώσεις από τις συνεδρίες και από την εποπτεία, και αλληλογραφία από τον πελάτη, για να αξιολογηθεί η σύνδεση ανάμεσα στη θεωρία και στην πράξη, όπως και κάποιες μεθοδολογικές όψεις της έρευνας στις μελέτες περίπτωσης.

Introduction

In this article, I present a single clinical case study that aims to explore some key relational processes from an inter-subjective, relational psychoanalytic approach to working with complex and chronic trauma. There will be a particular focus on my understanding of the client's dissociative experience and the abrupt ending of the therapy as an enactment of this.

Almost one year after beginning work with the client, 'Peter',[1] I received the following email:

> ... I feel that our sessions have become more dangerous for me as it is raising my consciousness of suicide. I find myself thinking and obsessing about dying and what it would mean for others (in my more inclusive thoughts). I feel, maybe incorrectly that I do not at the moment have the energy to deal with the pain that comes with looking inward ... I would like to stop coming to our sessions and just delve back into numbness and do the best I can with the tools and space you have created for me, with me.

The abrupt, unplanned ending came as a shock, yet it was not entirely a surprise. There had been many times during the previous 12 months of therapy in which Peter and I had tried to make sense of why the therapy was increasingly being experienced by him as dangerous and persecutory. With hindsight and a close reading of the case, I am going to argue that this is something that I should have foreseen. Whether it could have been prevented, however, I am not certain. My aim in this report is to suggest one possible way of understanding what happened.

The complexity of Peter's presentation can be understood through his experience of extensive physical abuse and domestic violence from early childhood until his teens. This experience created in him the dissociative capacity necessary for a highly successful military career in which further multiple traumas were experienced. Cumulatively, this was psychologically devastating, but the trauma did not fully manifest itself in symptoms until some years after the end of his military service, when he was in a civilian job and a stable relationship with a supportive partner.

Discussion of methodological validity

The current case study draws on process notes that were completed immediately after every session, together with ongoing self-reflection and regular supervision with an experienced psychoanalytically trained clinical supervisor. Process notes focused on the main themes of the session, the dominant affect and the transference/countertransference relationship and were drawn on in clinical supervision. Supervision offered the opportunity to develop the formulation over the course of the therapy, discuss the use of interpretations and as a place for containing countertransferential responses to Peter and the work.

The use of the case study as a research method can be argued to possess value through its power to inform theory and practice and '… provide the groundwork for hypotheses that can be tested empirically' (Kudler, Krupnick, Blank, Herman, & Horowitz, 2009; p. 355). The selection can be justified as an example of an extreme case, which reveals information not available in representative cases (Flyvbjerg, 2006). Integrating qualitative research methodology with experiential clinical material, particularly that from a psychoanalytically informed perspective, is wrought with tensions however. Throughout, attention was paid to minimizing these tensions by staying as close as possible to qualitative methodology. The research questions can be summarized as: What is my (subjective, theoretically informed) understanding of the process of the therapy with this client? How useful and effective is the particular case formulation and to what extent have I been able to implement the formulation in practice?

Drawing on the structure of the pragmatic case study research method of Fishman (2005), and an analytic strategy that can be described as a deductive, or theoretical, thematic analysis (Braun & Clarke, 2006), coding of the text was for the clinical concepts of dissociation and enactments (Bromberg, 2011) and temporality and trauma (Stolorow, 2007) that had been identified through the theoretical understanding of the case. The final stage of the analytic process was to shape the interpreted themes into a meaningful narrative.

A particular strength of this research is that it covers 12 months of therapy and is able to take into account contextual factors and a sufficient number of incidents of the phenomenon being examined (McLeod, 2010) and therefore constitutes a phase analysis that makes sense of complex material (Yin, 2009).

An important limitation is that empirical validity is difficult to argue for in clinical case study research when transcripts of sessions are unavailable. There is an inevitable subjectivity at work when the therapist and researcher are same person, with the risk of '… selective remembering and reporting' (McLeod, 2010; p. 15). Psychoanalytic epistemology can be argued to be a depth hermeneutic tool based in self-reflection (Habermas, 1971). Stolorow (1997) describes psychoanalysis as a phenomenological, intersubjective inquiry, and within that inquiry, subjective emotional experience is considered to be regulated in relational systems. The in-depth approach of the research method can be argued to be mirroring the therapeutic process with the analytic strategy of the current research essentially a continuation of the clinical relational process, in which the subjectivity of the therapist is employed in making meaning of the client's experience. The interpretation of my subjective experience of the client takes place at two points in time. First, in the session itself, and for a second time in the analysis of the process notes as text. There are two hermenuetics at work here; phenemonological inquiry meeting the psychoanlytic hermeneutic. Yet, the application of this method lacks the intersubjective, moment-to-moment responses of the client to the therapist's interpretations that take place in sessions, and is therefore limited and necessarily tentative in its findings. To try to ensure that I have represented the joint experience of the therapy as accurately as possible, I asked for consent to write it and invited a response to the material at draft stage. Peter chose his own pseudonym and did not ask for any changes to be made. The account remains, however, predominantly a subjective one of my experience, rather than Peter's, and in this respect, the research findings themselves can only be considered to be partially inter-subjectively produced. This inevitably moves the research away from the relational paradigm on which the clinical process was founded.

Many valuable alternative methods exist for evaluating clinical process. A conversation analysis approach to transcripts of sessions could provide a close reading of micro-processes and say something useful about what is happening inter-subjectively, yet would not provide answers to the research questions outlined above. Another qualitative research approach would be for (another researcher) to interview the client about his experience of the therapy and for this text to be subjected to a narrative analysis or a hermeneutic method such as Interpretative Phenomenological Analysis (Smith, Flowers, & Larkin, 2009). This too would generate useful findings, but would necessarily represent the lived experience of the client, not mine. I argue that this would create an ethical problem by imposing a specific theoretical understanding – a psychoanalytic discourse – on the client's experience, that he may not share.

Theoretical understanding of the case – Inter-subjectivity systems theory

I have drawn on the inter-subjectivity theories of Stolorow (2007) and Bromberg (2011), integrated with Schore and Schore's (2008) contemporary extension of attachment theory, to outline a developmental understanding of affective bodily based processes and regulation that is consistent with psychoanalytic thinking about unconscious and conscious experience of trauma and of therapeutic change.

In this approach, affect regulation is considered as a pragmatic framework to understand psychopathology and therapeutic change. The goal within the therapy is to empathically regulate the client's arousal state using the transference–countertransference relationship (Schore & Schore, 2008). These relational psychoanalytic theories have been drawn on in order to provide a framework for my understanding of the experience of dissociation in the client and in the therapeutic dyad, and the subsequent possible enactments that may arise. They provide an account of trauma that can incorporate both unconscious and conscious aspects of the experience of the particular therapeutic relationship currently under scrutiny.

The effectiveness of psychodynamic psychotherapy as a treatment for PTSD and trauma related to combat, childhood physical abuse, domestic violence and PTSD is supported in a review by the Task Force of the International Society for Traumatic Stress Studies in the US (Kudler et al., 2009). The PTSD Task Force provides treatment guidelines based on extensive reviews of the clinical and research literature and states that the aim of such an approach is to progressively understand the psychological meaning of traumatic events in the survivor's unique historical context, their individual personality structure and their goals (Kudler et al., 2009). Psychodynamic therapy for trauma aims to address '... wishes, fantasies, fears and defences ...' generated in the therapy and the therapeutic relationship should emphasize '... safety and honesty' (Kudler et al. p. 583).

The theoretical concept of attunement is privileged in relational psychoanalytic accounts of development and the therapeutic process. Founded in Kohut's (1971) self psychology, it can be defined in the parent–infant relationship as the parent's appropriate reactiveness to the child's experience, such as offering comfort when the child is distressed (Stern, 1985), a psychobiological (involving both autonomic and central nervous systems) regulation of affective states that has an integrating effect and forms the attachment bond (Schore, 2001). A lack of attunement in childhood, such as that which occurs in abuse or neglect, leads to the absence of integration of affect, and dissociation or disavowal of affective responses. The child who has developed in this way is unable to feel that their emotions are an integrated part of themselves, and throughout their life will be vulnerable to traumatic states which threaten their psychological organization and the continuing experience of relational ties that are needed for survival.

> Lacking a holding context in which painful affect can live and become integrated, the traumatised child ... must disassociate painful emotions from his or her ongoing experiencing, often resulting in psychosomatic states or in splits between the subjectively experienced mind and body. (Stolorow, 2007, p. 10)

In the therapeutic relationship, affect or emotion needs to be defended against and there will be a fear or anticipation of re-traumatization. Developmental trauma is thus understood as the experience of unbearable affect (Stolorow, 2007).

Developmentally, a child's recurring experience of mal-attunement leads them to become unconsciously convinced that their experience of yearning for their unmet needs and painful feeling states is due to some inherent inner badness or defect in themselves (Stolorow, 2007). The neurological effect of this mal-attunement is summarized in a strikingly appropriate military metaphor by Cozolino (2014):

> In the face of early interpersonal trauma, all the systems of the social brain become shaped for offensive and defensive purposes ... when the brain is shaped in this way, social life is converted from a source of nurturance into a minefield' (p279).

Cozolino (2014) describes an experience of 'core shame' that results from childhood abuse or neglect in which the self is felt to be 'fundamentally defective, worthless, and unlovable … . (p. 282).

Stolorow (2007) argues that the client in this situation will experience their emerging feeling states as intolerable to the therapist. Their inability to believe that they can or will ever be understood by another person will make itself felt in the transference. Additionally, when a child has experienced early trauma, the capacity to use affects as 'guiding signals' for understanding subjective experience has not developed.

Therapeutic impact will thus be determined by the extent to which the client experiences the therapist as attuned to their subjective affective experience, as well as the transference meaning of the experience. Stolorow (2007) draws on Heidegger's existential notion of 'resoluteness' to conceptualize the possibility for change: '… in resoluteness, one seizes upon or takes hold of possibilities into which one has been thrown, making these possibilities one's *own* (p. 43).

Within this relational model of trauma, the capacity for the therapist to provide an experience of attunement for the client is mediated by the capacity for dissociation. Dissociation in trauma is a defensive state and is experienced as a shattering of time and its unifying nature (Stolorow, 2007). Temporality, the experience of a past, present and future at any given moment, is relationally or inter-subjectively derived – our belief that we will continue to exist in a stable, ongoing and predictable way comes through our shared experience of time in relationships with others (Stolorow, 2007). By taking away the experience of the world as stable and predictable, emotional trauma destroys this structural experience of temporality, altering one's very sense of selfhood as a unitary being, and of being in time (Stolorow, 2007). The world and other people thus lose their significance and ability to anchor the person, leading to an experience of total aloneness, estrangement and detachment. This creates unendurable anxiety that must be disassociated from in order to survive it.

Bromberg's theory of multiple self-state, trauma and enactments

Bromberg (2011) draws on the notion of a unitary experience of self vs. multiple self-states to explain dissociation. The capacity to dissociate is a 'normal hypnoid capacity of the mind' that can become part of the structure of personality. It is used as a defence against trauma so as to allow the self to bear what is unbearable by disconnecting the mind (Bromberg, 2011, p. 178). 'Hypnoid capacity' in this context refers to the capacity to create an experience of the absence of consciousness. This dissociative structure becomes active to allow incompatible self-states to continue to function without awareness of other self-states. In situations with the potential for dangerous (shame-inducing) inter-subjectivity, dissociation is needed to prevent a potentially traumatizing encounter with the mind of the needed other. Dissociation protects from the storm of emotions meaning that in this state, inter-subjective regulation of affect such as that which is intended in the therapeutic relationship is impossible.

When the client experiences unprocessed trauma in the company of the therapist, there is '… almost always' a '… dissociated here-and-now shame experience' (Bromberg, 2011; p. 180). In bringing alive the trauma, the client's (developmentally unmet) hunger for relief, comfort and soothing is also brought back to life but cannot be communicated symbolically, leading to the experience of shame and triggering dissociation. As it cannot be symbolized, this experience can only be communicated through enactment. The therapeutic relationship itself then becomes dangerous to the traumatized client, arousing affect that cannot be contained as internal conflict within an integrated sense of self or consciousness (Bromberg, 2011). Trauma can neither be held nor processed as a memory, and talking about it brings no relief because the unbearable and shameful affect is relived through talking.

Working with clients who have developed a dissociative structure of mind suggests that the role of the therapeutic process is to increase the client's confidence in their ability to withstand their overwhelming affect by providing a transitional space (Bromberg, 2011). The clinician must strive to remain as attuned as possible to the client's experience of being unable to hear or experience the therapist's subjectivity, and be aware of the potential for creating dissociative states in the client.

Assessment and formulation for 'Peter'

When Peter self-referred to me for therapy, he was under the care of his GP and the community mental health team as he was considered to be at risk of suicide. I am a chartered Counselling Psychologist in independent practice. Counselling Psychology training in the UK is theoretically pluralistic, and my practice and clinical supervision since qualification has been informed by psychoanalytic psychotherapeutic approaches. He had been prescribed medication for anxiety, which made his experience of symptoms just about tolerable. His suicidality and the severity of his symptoms meant that he was not considered suitable for local primary care counselling, and he refused to consider psychiatric or secondary care. As his military service had not been for the UK, he did not qualify for psychological support from the organizations that provide this to British soldiers and veterans. Peter could tolerate the physical symptoms of panic attacks in the knowledge that they would eventually end. He was however very afraid that he would permanently 'break down' psychically.

At assessment, Peter was experiencing flashbacks, periods of dissociation, panic attacks, low mood and he had clear plans for killing himself if he felt this to be necessary. There was occasional self-harming behaviour by cutting, which had a grounding function when he felt himself to be dissociating. He was very afraid that he would become violent and harm someone during a dissociative episode, though this had never happened. He deliberately abstained from alcohol and drugs but craved the relief that they would have given him. He had used both in the past for this purpose.

In the assessment, he described a recent precipitating incident at work in which he had emailed some incorrect documents to his boss, and had been 'publicly humiliated' for the error. He had admired his boss enormously before this and experienced it a betrayal of trust with a resulting steep rise in anxiety.

From a very young age, Peter's father had beaten him severely and frequently. He described his mother as detached and also abused by her husband, and she was unable to protect Peter. He had one older brother who was reportedly never beaten. His father's violence towards Peter ended abruptly when he was 14 and for the first time retaliated, not in his own defence, but his mother's. After leaving university before graduating, he became an elite forces soldier for five years. The training lasted 18 months and included sadistic and brutal methods, particularly torture, in which recruits took turns at being the victim and then perpetrator. Peter described how he was able to submit to episodes of torture without having to be restrained. He was infamous for his extraordinary capacity to withstand physical pain.

Peter was initially unable to hold in his mind any thoughts or feelings about the emotional and physical pain that he suffered, and struggled to hear my description of his early experience as child abuse. Over a number of weeks, he became gradually more able to consider this possibility, but this meant that he had to confront the awareness and subsequent anger at his mother's failure to protect him.

It became evident through his descriptions that he had developed the capacity to dissociate from painful and frightening experiences as a very young child and that this had been adaptive. As a young adult solider, his dissociative ability earned him his reputation as fearless and able to withstand extreme physical and mental pain, and led directly to him experiencing countless more traumatic situations.

Peter's sense of self hinged on not turning away from danger, but always going towards it, his undying loyalty to his former comrades from his platoon and his willingness to put his own life at risk to fight for others. He experienced himself as living in a different, parallel world to everyone around him. He could see and be seen by other people, but they could not understand what he felt like and he could not feel like them because he was 'different', not 'normal'. I understood this belief in his specialness as a defence against the unconscious phantasy that he was in fact monstrous, a killer, unable to feel remorse and potentially extremely dangerous to others.

In his current life, he experienced overwhelming anxiety when placed in interpersonal situations in which he experienced himself being 'ambushed' and shamed. Situations like this occurred at work, when line managers or bosses either deliberately disregarded his recommendations or explicitly called his competence into question. The experience of anxiety would lead either to panic, or to dissociation.

The course of therapy

In this section, I will try to give a sense of what it was like to experience the therapy with Peter, focusing on the experience of dissociation and subsequent enactments.

Peter was terrified of 'breaking down' into what he imagined would be madness, afraid of the impending 'storm'. He felt as though he was being pulled inexorably towards disintegration, and experienced a dislocation in time through dissociation outside of the therapy. In session, while he was not as starkly dissociative, we both noticed that he would quickly shut off from emerging painful feelings, often using a kind of gallows humour. Peter was afraid and angry at the possibility of being forgotten and unrecognized, and experienced a profound sense of loneliness in the world. At times, it felt to him that he was the last person alive, disconnected entirely from both his own feelings and from others. At work, he struggled to concentrate and was distressed by this as his exceptional professional capabilities had always been an important element of his self-concept. Peter's conscious experience of anger could be experienced only somatically. He recognized the physical symptoms, but believed that if he allowed himself to feel anger purely as an emotion, he might kill the person he was angry with – anger was lethal and therefore in phantasy, intolerable. This made him feel highly anxious around other people and he described how he would become frozen and fearful in everyday situations. At this time, he reported having nightmares that he could not remember.

Peter described coming to therapy as like violating himself. It forced him to re-evaluate his experience entirely, all of the structures that he had created to keep himself psychically safe, everything that he thought he knew about himself and the things that he had done and had done to him were now in doubt. This felt to him overwhelmingly hopeless, and that he was now adrift, unable to see a way back to ever feeling as though he could manage. He described it as a *Catch 22*; he did not want to remember because it felt too awful, but was convinced that unless he remembered there could be no way out of his intolerable pain. I was caught in this double bind with him. His sense of isolation was profound, and critical thoughts about himself – all the criticism he had ever heard – dominated his conscious experience.

Peter was able for short periods able to allow me to feel concern for him, yet he found my concern and that of others frightening, and it had to be closely monitored. He was certain that he did not have feelings like normal people. He believed that he was not like other people, that he was not really 'human'. At these times, he was dissociating less frequently and tentatively seemed to be resolving to live. He began to be able to tolerate for brief periods of time feelings of loss and regret. There seemed to be the a glimmer of a possibility of survival for him, yet this change came hand-in-hand with an increasing sense of dread as well as a deep grief and mourning for the loss of control over his feelings that he had once had and that was now seemingly irretrievably lost.

Remembrance Sunday took place around this time, and recognition of the war dead evoked an intense envy in him. He said that he felt 'lost'. Misrecognition was also experienced at work, where points of difference with colleagues were experienced as intolerably difficult to bear. It made him feel 'hollowed out', unseen, not really there. I thought about how physical danger had provided a way for him to feel acutely recognized and I became more aware of the extent to which he felt cut off from other people, isolated and with no hope or possibility of any alternative existence. This was the defining subjective experience of his trauma. Over the course of therapy, Peter's tendency to dissociate rose and fell, to be replaced by constant, debilitating anxiety, making the dissociation seem preferable.

About half way through the year, the therapy began to be increasingly experienced by Peter as persecutory. He felt more desperate and suicidal. His experience was only just tolerable and I felt he was certain that I would not be able to bear it with him. Although I felt helpless and miserable about his experience, I also believed that his acknowledgement of my recognition of him would have been impossible when he began the therapy and as such represented change.

The tendency to dissociate returned with force, and Peter described periods of 'absence' in which he felt no sense of time passing. He no longer recognized himself and I felt a complementary helplessness. He craved a return to an earlier state of not knowing. Comprehension of the harmful effects of his father's violence was felt to be 'dreadful' because once thought, it could not be changed and he felt himself to be without hope. He began to mourn for himself, and experience regret, an experience that felt only just bearable for us both in sessions. He said that the pain must mean that he was 'normal' and therefore not 'special' any more. I wondered whether along with the horror, that there may be some relief in this too. The possibility of survival began to tentatively exist, but there was a psychic cost to this change with the recognition of what was being lost. His previous ability to perform at consistently high levels had been imbricated with the trauma, but now ordinary failures had to be countenanced. Ambivalence was possible, but the fear of 'something worse' in the unreachable parts of his mind lingered, and once the effects of a new medication settled, time and its dislocation began to be felt again. At this point, there was a scheduled break for the end of the year.

After the break, Peter's persecutory experience of the therapy intensified. His constant anxiety was only just tolerable and he was exhausted. It seemed as though his pain and anguish continued to build with each session, with no hope of respite. He brought a dream of digging a grave in which he became trapped. Any feelings became dangerous, even happiness, which was too closely linked to sadness, and therefore anger. He punished himself relentlessly by thinking about past mistakes. One morning, Peter arrived and told me that he had had a fantasy the day before that I was a spy, and that even while knowing that it was not true, found himself on the brink of panic. I said that he felt that I was dangerous to him. This interpretation had little effect on his anxiety, and he decided that he would take a four-week break from the therapy. I felt that I had no choice but to agree. The therapy itself had become a perversion of care, it seemed that something malignant was being enacted and anything I did would be experienced as persecutory. By leaving, Peter was doing the only thing he could think of to protect the therapy and me.

On return, Peter said that although he experienced the therapy as good, after the sessions would be compelled to undo all of the goodness with relentless criticism of himself. In the final phase, anger began to be felt and he was terrified that this meant that he would become dangerous. Interpersonal situations at work continued to be a source of distress, and everyday conflicts caused him to respond as though he was under serious threat, unable to think. He described a 'chasm' in his mind and how he longed for nothingness, and quiet. At this point, there was an unscheduled break because of a work commitment that had been arranged without his prior knowledge, and we had one more session after this. In the email written almost exactly one year after our first meeting, Peter told me that he feared that if the therapy continued, it would inevitably lead to him killing himself.

Discussion

Peter's goals at the beginning of therapy were the reduction in his experience of anxiety and suicidality. Clearly, this was not achieved, yet much that was therapeutic was. At the end of therapy, he remained alive, which was a considerable achievement on his part. He had been able to tolerate a year of therapy, during which it is impossible to underemphasize the profound changes he underwent in his understanding of his experience, in both his present and past. He had been able to make links, extend to himself some compassion and experience grief for what he had suffered, without his mind disintegrating, or 'breaking down', as he had feared he would. He had gained a new understanding of emotions, and what it meant for him and others to have them. There were brief glimpses of the 'resoluteness' described by Stolorow (2007), in which Peter appeared to be experiencing the desire to go on living with an acceptance of what had happened to him.

In the end though, the therapy itself had to be destroyed because it represented care, and with limited capacity to care for himself, my attempts were experienced as creating the possibility of something that in phantasy was intolerable. Inter-subjective regulation of affect, or attunement, was impossible for Peter to experience at these times, and the therapeutic situation could not be experienced as safe (Bromberg, 2011). Breaks contributed to this difficulty and it was my supervisor who noted that there had been the unscheduled break two weeks prior to Peter ending the therapy, and that furthermore we had begun to discuss the approaching long summer break.

This case study has starkly illustrated how impending and actual breaks seemed to elicit the most disturbing transferential experiences. The persecution Peter experienced in nightmares and fantasies intensified after a break or a scheduled holiday, no matter how longed for it was. It is my contention that had we had sessions more frequently than once a week, it may have been possible to contain Peter's unbearable affect more completely, enabling him to tolerate this experience. Our subsequent joint dissociation from unbearably painful affect can be usefully thought about as enactments in which Peter experienced my subjectivity as shame-inducing, although at the time, I was not able to see this clearly. We both felt helpless. He was in the grip of intolerable shame, and I too was caught in a double bind or Catch-22. I imagined at the time that if I tried to persuade him too forcefully to remain in therapy, I would be intensifying his experience of being attacked, but by letting him go, I was failing to bear his pain. Stolorow (2007) provides an explanation of this inter-subjective dilemma, suggesting that the developmentally traumatized client unconsciously expects their'… emerging feeling states to be met with disgust, disdain, disinterest, alarm, hostility, withdrawal, exploitation … or that they will damage the analysis and destroy the therapeutic bond' (p. 4). I have wondered whether the outcome could have been different if I had been able to find a way to interpret this understanding to him in a way that he could have made use of. Instead, I settled for a compromise, in which I tried to let him know as gently as possible that I believed in the goodness of the therapy as a joint endeavour, and in our capacity to survive it.

Bromberg (2011) suggests that the therapist has to recognize and be able to work with the client's shame or the client will feel worse than they did before, with the part of the self that holds the shame remaining dissociated and unreachable. I believe that this is a useful description of Peter's experience, demonstrated when he spoke of his terror at the possibility of an imminent 'storm' in his mind in which he believed he would disintegrate and 'break down'. Thinking about killing off this experience in suicide was the only possible way to soothe himself. The actual 'safeness' of the therapeutic situation was meaningless to him at this point (Bromberg, 2011). With his very sense of stability of self in danger, it was too dangerous for him to drop his dissociation. It was at these points that I believe I was pulled into the dissociative process.

Through undertaking a close reading of the case, I now believe that I was unable to remain securely enough anchored in the transference to be able to formulate the joint process of dissociation in sessions, and crucially, to be able to represent this understanding of unconscious experience to Peter (Stolorow, 2007). For my own future practice and for clinicians working with this kind of complex trauma presentation, I suggest the need, based on the theoretical approach outlined above, to be acutely alive to the possibility of enactments in which both members of the therapeutic dyad dissociate to avoid affect. On occasion, I became aware that I was colluding with Peter's avoidance of affect and yet counter-transferentially experienced a reluctance to interpret this to him, believing that the therapeutic alliance would be at risk if I did so. Theoretically, it could be argued that at these times, I was unable to give Peter an experience of attunement by letting him know when I recognized the potential for the therapy to become traumatizing for him. Rather than not interpreting at these moments, I now believe that I ought to have made my understanding explicit. In addition to the clinical value this finding has, writing the case study has provided an opportunity to reflect deeply on my own process, acknowledge that the study may represent an attempt to create an ending for work that felt to me to be unfinished and to work through some of the inevitable questions that remain unanswered. It could be interpreted as an attempt to do what I was unable to do in the sessions.

In June, one month after ended therapy, I received the following email:

> ... I wanted to say that I am not doing well, but that I am coping without hopefully being destructive. The anxiety is high and self harm happens more often now, but somehow I feel more me ... You have given me an understanding of myself that I would not have had otherwise. So yes, just saying I am still alive and managing to not slide too far back from where we left it.

Peter continued to send short emails from time to time, letting me know that he was struggling but alive. I received them gratefully and with a tentative, ongoing sense of hope for him.

Note

1. The client's identity has been disguised, some details have been changed in order to maintain confidentiality and he has consented to the use of this material.

Disclosure statement

No potential conflict of interest was reported by the author.

References

Braun, V., & Clarke, V. (2006). Using thematic analysis in psychology. *Qualitative Research in Psychology, 3*(2), 77–101.

Bromberg, P. M. (2011). *Awakening the dreamer*. New York, NY: Routledge.

Cozolino, L. (2014). *The neuroscience of human relationships* (2nd ed.). New York, NY: WW. Norton & Company.

Fishman, D. B. (2005). Editor's introduction to PCSP – From single case to database: A new method for enhancing psychotherapy practice. *Pragmatic Case Studies in Psychotherapy* [Online], *1*(1), Article 2, 1–50. Retrieved from http://pcsp.libraries.rutgers.edu/index.php/pcsp/article/view/855/2167

Flyvbjerg, B. (2006). Five misunderstandings about case-study research. *Qualitative Inquiry, 12,* 219–245.

Habermas, J. (1971). *Knowledge and human interests.* Boston, MA: Beacon Press.

Kohut, H. (1971). *The analysis of the self.* Madison, CT: International Universities Press.

Kudler, H. S., Krupnick, J. L., Blank, A. S., Herman, J. L., & Horowitz, M. J. (2009). Psychodynamic therapy for adults. In E. B. Foa, T. M. Keane, M. J. Friedman, & J. A. Cohen, (Eds). *Effective treatments for PTSD* (2nd ed.) (pp 346–369). New York, NY: Guilford Press.

McLeod, J. (2010). *Case study research: In counselling and psychotherapy.* London: Sage.

Schore, A. N. (2001). The effects of a secure attachment relationship on right brain development, affect regulation & infant mental health. *Infant Mental Health Journal, 22,* 7–66.

Schore, J. R., & Schore, A. N. (2008). Modern attachment theory: The central role of affect regulation in development and treatment. *Clinical Social Work Journal, 36,* 9–20.

Smith, J. A., Flowers, P., & Larkin, M. (2009). *Interpretative phenomenological analysis: Theory, method and research.* London: Sage.

Stern, D. N. (1985). *The interpersonal world of the infant.* London: Karnac.

Stolorow, R. D. (1997). Dynamic, dyadic, intersubjective systems: An evolving paradigm for psychoanalysis. *Psychoanalytic Psychology, 14,* 337–346.

Stolorow, R. D. (2007). *Trauma and human existence: Autobiographical, psychoanalytic and philosophical reflections.* New York, NY: Routledge.

Yin, R. K. (2009). *Case study research: Designs and methods* (4th ed.). Thousand Oaks, CA: Sage.

A shift in narratives: From 'attachment' to 'belonging' in therapeutic work with adoptive families. A single case study

Ferdinando Salamino and Elisa Gusmini

ABSTRACT

This study analyses a one-year family therapy with an adopted adolescent, with regards to its outcome and process.

Method: This study will use Stratton's attribution scheme with Stratton's attribution scheme processes regarding attachment, bonding, and mutual belonging. An analysis of the inference styles (monadic, dyadic, triadic) used by the family during the conversation will also be provided, in order to highlight inference schemes recurring in family discourse and their change throughout the course of therapy. The study will provide a systematic view on how the introduction, by the therapist team, of triadic, relational hypotheses based on present narratives and interactions can promote a semantic shift from the concept of 'attachment' to the alternative concept of 'belonging'.

Aim of the study: Aim of the study is to highlight advantages of adopting a socio-constructionist approach when dealing with the problem represented by mutual belonging in adoptive families.

From a socio-constructionist perspective, creation of emotional and affective bonding within a family is a conversational process, subject to continuous changes and revolutions throughout the individual and family history.

Focusing on resources and ongoing relationships, rather than damage and early trauma, a socio-constructionist approach may represent a powerful resource in strengthening emotional ties within the current family.

UN CAMBIO EN LAS NARRATIVAS: de "apego"a "pertenencia" en el trabajo terapéutico con familias adoptivas. Un estudio de caso individual

Este studio analiza un anño de terapiafamiliar con un adolescente adoptado, en relación con el procso y los resultados. Se usará el esquema de Stratton (2003a; 1003b) para explorar losprocesos de atribución familiar en relación con la vinculación afectiva y la pertenencia mutual. Se usará también un sistema de códigos unificados para atribuciones causales, para destacar los esquemas de interferencia recurrentes en el discurso familiar y sus cambios a través del curso de la terapia.

Como consecuencia, el etudio proporcionará una vision sistemática de cómo la introducción por parte del equipo terapéutico, de hipótesis relacionales triádicas basadas en narrativas presents e interacciones, pueden promover un cambio semántico del concepto de "apego" al concepto alternative de "pertenencia".

El objetivo del studio es destacar las ventajas de adopter un método soio-construccionista cuando se trabaja con el problema que presenta la pertenencia mutual en familias adoptivas.Desde la perspective socio-construccionista, la creació de una vinculación afectiva y emocional dentro de una familia, es un proceso conversacional, sujeto a cambios continuos y revoluciones a través de la historia individual y familiar. Focalizándonos en los recursos y las relaciones continuas en lugar de en el dañ y trauma a temprana edad, un método construccionista puede resultar un poderoso recurso para reforzar los lazos emocionales dentro de la familia.

Un cambiamento nelle narrazioni: da "attaccamento" a "appart-enenza" nel lavoro terapeutico con le famiglie adottive. Uno studio di caso

Questo studio analizza un anno di terapia familiare di un caso riguardante un adolescente adottato, relativamente all'esito e al processo.

Questo studio utilizza lo schema di Stratton (2003a; 2003b) per esplorare i processi familiari di attribuzione relativi all'attaccamento, al *bonding* e alla reciproca appartenenza. Utilizzando il sistema di codifica per attribuzioni causali, viene data evidenza agli schemi di inferenza ricorrenti nel discorso familiare e al loro cambiamento durante la terapia.

Lo studio, quindi, fornisce una visione sistematica relativa all'introduzione, da parte del team terapeutico, di ipotesi relazionali triadiche basate sulle narrazioni attuali e sulle interazioni visione che possa promuovere uno slittamento semantico dal concetto di "attaccamento" al concetto di "appartenenza".

Scopo dello studio è quello di evidenziare i vantaggi di un approccio socio-costruzionista applicato a problemi di reciproca appartenenza in famiglie adottive. Nella prospettiva socio-costruzionista, la creazione di legami emotivi e affettivi all'interno della famiglia è un processo conversazionale, soggetto a continui cambiamenti e rivoluzioni sia nella storia dell'individuo che in quella della famiglia. Concentrandosi sulle risorse e sulle relazioni in corso, piuttosto che su danno e trauma precoci, l'approccio socio-costruzionista può rappresentare una risorsa potente per il rafforzamento dei legami affettivi all'interno della famiglia.

Changement de discours : de « l'attachement » à « l'appartenance » dans le cadre du travail thérapeutique avec des familles adoptantes – une étude de cas

Cette étude analyse une année de thérapie familiale menée avec une famille ayant adopté un adolescent. Ce travail utilise le schéma de Stratton (2003a; 2003b) pour explorer les processus d'attribution de la famille en ce qui concerne l'attachement, le lien et l'appartenance mutuelle. Un système de codes pour les attributions causales est également utilisé pour souligner les schémas d'inférence récurrents dans le discours familial et leur changement au cours de la thérapie. Cette étude fournira donc une vision systématique de la façon dont l'équipe thérapeutique, en introduisant des hypothèses triadiques et relationnelles basées sur les récits et interactions du moment, peut promouvoir un glissement sémantique du concept « d'attachement » à celui « d'appartenance » proposé à la place. Le but de cette étude était de mettre l'accent sur les avantages qu'il y a à adopter une approche socioconstructiviste lorsqu'on est confronté au problème de l'appartenance mutuelle dans des familles adoptantes. Si l'on se réfère à une perspective socioconstructiviste, la création d'un lien émotionnel et affectif effectif au sein d'une famille est un processus conversationnel, sujet à des changements constants et des révolutions tout au long de l'histoire familiale et individuelle. En se concentrant sur les ressources et les relations actuelles plutôt que sur les dégâts et les traumatismes anciens, une approche socioconstructiviste peut représenter une ressource robuste permettant de renforcer les liens dans la famille actuelle.

Μια μεταβολή στις αφηγήσεις: από την «προσκόλληση» στο «ανήκειν» στη θεραπευτική δουλειά με θετές οικογένειες. Μια μελέτη περίπτωσης

Η παρούσα έρευνα αναλύει το αποτέλεσμα και τη διαδικασία της οικογενειακής θεραπείας διάρκειας ενός έτους με μια οικογένεια με έναν υιοθετημένο έφηβο. Θα χρησιμοποιήσει το σχήμα του Stratton (2003a; 2003b) για τη διερεύνηση των οικογενειακών διαδικασιών απόδοσης αναφορικά με την προσκόλληση, το δεσμό και την αμοιβαία αίσθηση του «ανήκειν». Θα χρησιμοποιηθεί, επίσης, το ενοποιημένο σύστημα κωδικοποίησης για τις αιτιώδεις αποδόσεις για την ανάδειξη των επαναλαμβανόμενων συμπερασματικών σχημάτων στο λόγο της οικογένειας και της αλλαγής τους κατά τη διάρκεια της θεραπείας.
Επομένως, η έρευνα θα παράσχει μια συστηματική παρουσίαση του τρόπου με τον οποίο, η εισαγωγή της τριαδικής σχεσιακής υπόθεσης βασισμένης στις παρούσες αφηγήσεις και αλληλεπιδράσεις από την πλευρά της θεραπευτικής ομάδας, μπορεί να προσφέρει μια σημασιολογική στροφή από την έννοια της «προσκόλλησης» στην εναλλακτική έννοια της αίσθησης του «ανήκειν».
Ο στόχος της έρευνας είναι να τονίσει τα πλεονεκτήματα της υιοθέτησης μιας κοινωνικο-κονστρουξιονιστικής προσέγγισης στην αντιμετώπιση του προβλήματος που αφορά την αμοιβαία αίσθηση του «ανήκειν» στις θετές οικογένειες.
Από μια κοινωνικο- κονστρουξιονιστική οπτική, η ανάπτυξη των συναισθηματικών και συγκινησιακών δεσμών μέσα στην οικογένεια είναι μια διαδικασία, που υπόκειται σε συνεχείς αλλαγές και εξελίξεις μέσα από τις ατομικές και οικογενειακές ιστορίες.
Εστιασμένη σε δυναμικά και εξελισσόμενες σχέσεις, παρά στη βλάβη και στο πρώιμο τραύμα, η κοινωνικο- κονστρουξιονιστική προσέγγιση μπορεί να αποτελέσει μια ισχυρή πηγή στην ενδυνάμωση των συναισθηματικών δεσμών με τη συγκεκριμένη οικογένεια.

Introduction

Adoption has always been a challenging subject for family therapists. Its inner nature, suspended between past and present, between the need to acknowledge loss and the aim to build new opportunities, is always at risk of putting families and therapists in a maze where the way out is not easily found. Attachment theory (Ainsworth, 1969; Bowlby, 1969) offers a powerful explanatory structure and a reliable 'map' to orient both therapists and families in front of this maze.

For this reason, several authors (Dallos & Vetere, 2009; Diamond, 2014; Kenrick, Lindsey, & Tollemache, 2006; Moran, Diamond, & Diamond, 2005; Vetere & Dallos, 2008) have suggested to embed core elements from attachment theory within the epistemological framework of systemic thinking, despite some theoretical inconsistencies (for instance, attachment theory's focus on the past, as opposed to systemic therapy prioritizing the *here and now*). As Dallos and Vetere (2009) point out, therapeutic approaches should not be evaluated only on their theoretical soundness, but mainly on their usefulness in addressing the complexity of family situations. What defines 'usefulness' in this context?
According to Anderson and Goolishian (1992), 'the therapeutic system is a problem-organizing, problem-dis-solving system' (p. 27). The goal of therapy is therefore the dissolution of the problem, and the consequent dissolution of the therapy itself. Is attachment-based family therapy a self-dissolving systems?

The 'phantom pain' effect in therapy with adoption.

As previously stated, attachment theory can be quite a useful map in understanding adoption, but what can happen if the map becomes the territory, and we start confusing the real object with the categories we designed to describe it? We might start thinking of 'attachment' as a real organ, which can be broken and may therefore need repairing at some stage. In our experience with adoptive families, we found the goal of 're-building' or 'repairing' attachment, frequently considered as paramount in family therapy with adoption, somehow constraining.

Whilst attachment theory was designed as a therapy of hope, offering a non-pathologizing view of the individual as opposed to Freudian's pessimistic perspective, its translation in the field of family therapy has sometimes taken a different path. Therapeutic processes based on attachment often convey the idea that adoption is '*a lifetime event, that adoption issues may emerge and ree-merge at different points across the lifespan and that all adoptive families may need advice, information and support at some stage*' (Beek, 1999, p. 21). Authors like Vadilonga (2010) and Schofield and Beek (2005) suggest that therapy with adoption is a reparative effort that cannot be dismissed at any time, and families should constantly engage with therapeutic agencies.

This rather non-self-dissolving attitude is not much inherent to attachment theory itself. Sroufe, Carlson, Levy, and Egeland (1999) clarify that early attach-ment is not linearly linked to development of psychopathology. Similarly, recent studies have moved toward a more flexible, less narrow view of attachment process. For instance, Dozier, Stoval, Albus, and Bates (2001) highlight how chil-dren in foster care are able to readjust their attachment style in order to tune up with new caregivers.

Crittenden and Claussen (2003) follow a similar route, describing how contex-tual and cultural variables may add variability to attachment pathways, making the 'attachment' construct wider and more flexible.

Nonetheless, many attachment-based therapeutic approaches seem to translate into practice a very rigid perspective on attachment, strongly linked to the idea that

> once a sequence of behavior has become organized, it tends to persist and does so even if it has developed on non-functional lines and even in the absence of the external stimuli and/or the internal conditions on which it first depended. The precise form that any particular form of behavior takes and the sequence within which it is first organized are thus of the greatest consequence for its future. (Bowlby, 1969, p. 169)

Therefore, controversial treatments arise, with little supporting evidence and the only common denominator of dealing with the attachment wound (Chaffin et al., 2006; Hanson & Spratt, 2000). Considering the building of mutual belong-ing between parents and children as a mostly innate process, many attach-ment-based therapies are at risk of trading a negative and pessimistic view on adopted children's fate (Barth, John, Crea, Thoburn, & Quinton, 2005).

The controversial construct of 'reactive attachment disorder' and its clinical applications (American Psychiatric Association, 2013) are a perfect example of how confusing the map with the territory can turn a deeply relational, non-pathol-ogizing theory into a labeling and rather deterministic therapeutic perspective.

The risks of over-diagnosing attachment disorders, with a negative impact on children and families' well-being, are also stressed by several studies (Woolgar & Baldock, 2015; Woolgar & Scott, 2014). From our perspective, clinical conversa-tion with adoptive families often confronts the therapist with a sort of 'phantom pain' effect. Phantom pain can be described as the suffering caused by a part of ourselves that is irreversibly lost, and yet is perceived as still attached. Although the pain can be perceived as real and perfectly localized, it cannot be soothed as the suffering part cannot be reached. As therapeutic conversation focusses on failed attachment in the child, along with parental infertility, 'phantom pain effect' may crystallize as a family narrative, potentially disrupting the creation of new relational ties within the adoptive family.

Another potentially detrimental effect of attachment-based therapies with adoption resides in its focus on birth family relationships. Both parents and children are engaged to work on their own internal working models, structured during early childhood. As a result, 'this kind of therapeutic setting brings every-one back to his own family, or to the ghost of it' (Salamino, 2016, p. 1).

Making attachment the ultimate center of gravity of a therapeutic inter-vention may generate a conversational 'black hole' (Fellin & Salamino, 2016; Salamino & Gusmini, 2016) that is able to shut down professional curiosity and close any other possible therapeutic pathway.

Are there therapeutic alternatives to attachment, when dealing with the complexity of mutual belonging in adoptive families?

This case study aims at proposing a different approach to family therapy with adoption. Whilst considering attachment a relevant emotional and cognitive dimension involved in mutual bonding between adoptive parents and their children, we decided not to include attachment-based narratives in hypotheses and explanations we shared with the family, focusing therapeutic conversation on current family relationships. We also tried to offer triadic explanations, as opposed to attachment theory's dyadic attributions.

Our aim is to explore how a therapeutic approach focused on current inter-actions and triadic pathways of communication may contribute to change in the family's attribution scheme and mutual perceptions.

Looking for 'the pattern that connects'. A reasonable quest for family therapists?

Bateson (1979) invites us to find 'the pattern which connects all the living crea-tures' (p. 8), and this task still seems crucial when we work with families, espe-cially families in which 'blood ties' are not available. When biology fails and the innate connecting pattern cannot be claimed, we need to promote other forms of mutual belonging, by following different conversational patterns. As Harré, Moghaddam, Cairnie, Rothbart, and Sabat (2009) highlight, 'any encoun-ter might develop along more than one story-line, and support more than one story-line evolving simultaneously' (p. 8). Attachment-related storylines are therefore not the only ones available for re-framing and giving meaning to interactive and relational behaviors among members of an adoptive family.

Our paper proposes a non-attachment based short-term therapy, the goal of which is to promote and strengthen mutual belonging in adoptive families through the use of present-focused narratives. Our therapeutic conversation with families, underpinned by a Post-Milan approach (Campbell, 1999; Hoffman, 1988; Ugazio, 2007), focuses on the generative nature of *hic and nunc* interaction, thus strength-ening emotional ties and perceptions of mutual belonging within the current family.

The intervention we designed, and which is exemplified in this paper, does not aim at repairing the wound of disrupted attachment, but at building new

Table 1. The structure of the therapy.

Period	Phase of therapy	Number of sessions	Setting	Duration (h)
June–July 2012	Initial consultation	2	Parents only	2
September 2012–March 2013	Family therapy	7	Family therapy	2
October 2014	Intermediate follow-up	1	Family therapy	2
January 2016	Definitive follow-up	1	Family therapy	2

relational pathways and opportunities in the present. As such, we accept the possibility that further individual interventions focused on trauma or other past-related issues may still be an option if necessary, but we decided to prioritize the building of new family interactions and well-being.

Method

This study analyses a one-year family therapy with an adopted adolescent, with regards to its outcome and process. Therapy sessions were held 1 per month, for a total of nine sessions, in 2012 (see Table 1). Two subsequent follow-up sessions took place 1 and 3 years after the end of therapy.

We will present a qualitative analysis of parents' causal attributions of child's behavior. The study also analyzes the therapist's hypotheses and explanations, introduced with the strategic purpose of de-constructing and re-framing the family's view of the problem. Stratton's (2003a, 2003b) attribution scheme and unitizing coding system for causal attributions (Ugazio, Fellin, Colciago, Pennacchio, & Negri, 2008) will be used for this purpose. *Verbatim* samples of therapeutic conversations will help the reader get a direct understanding of the case and a deeper emotional connection with the flow of the therapy.

Stratton's scheme aims at identifying core elements of an attribution styles in a family. Specifically, it allows distinction between:

STABLE or UNSTABLE

(Will the cause operate reliably in the future?)

GLOBAL or SPECIFIC

(Has it a range of important outcomes?)

INTERNAL or EXTERNAL

(Does it originate within that person or thing?)

PERSONAL or UNIVERSAL

(Does the attribution differentiate that person or thing from others?)

CONTROLLABLE or UNCONTROLLABLE

(Could the person or thing influence the outcome?). (Stratton, 2003a, p. 165).

Unitizing coding system (Ugazio et al., 2008) allows a distinction between:

Monadic inference – behaviors of a person are explained by an inner variable, like the person's immaturity.

Dyadic inference – individual behaviors are explained by referring to a relationship with another person, e.g. the primary caregiver, like in attachment-based explanation.

Triadic inference – individual behavior is explained as embedded in a pattern of relationships in which at least two other persons are actively involved (for instance, a child's aggression towards mother might be perceived as instigated by father and perpetuated by mother's reaction).

For the purpose of this study, the first two sessions, the 9th session and the first one-year follow-up sessions were fully transcribed.[1] Both Stratton's attribution scheme (2003a, 2003b) and unitizing coding system (Ugazio et al., 2008) were applied to the transcripts to identify the main features of attribution styles of the parents. Unitizing coding system was applied in a simplified fashion, to distinguish between monadic, dyadic and triadic attribution, although the system itself would allow more sophisticated distinction.

Only parents' attributions were considered in this study. This was mainly due to the initial consultation taking place with parents only. Although it would have been interesting to explore the child's attributions, we chose to exclude them from the analysis to ensure longitudinal consistency.

The goal of the study is to explore how the family discourse about attachment, mutual belonging and individual development changed throughout the therapy, and how the therapist uses hypotheses and explanations widely focused on present narratives, rather than past narratives, to lead this change.

For this purpose, we will compare attributions occurring during the initial consultation with those we obtained during the follow-up sessions. We will also provide an overview of some major changes that occurred in individual and family life.

Introducing Organa family[2]: structure and presenting problem.

The Organa family is from Bergamo (see Figure 1). The adoptive parents Marco and Elena requested consultation in June 2012, apparently due to the increasing deviant behaviors and academic issues of their adoptive son Nino. Nino was 15 at the time of consultation. He was adopted under special regulation at the age of 9 (after being in foster care with the same family for two years), therefore he was allowed to keep regular contacts with his birth father and grandmother (the birth mother left home soon after his birth and never tried to get in touch with him).

His adoptive parents felt increasingly threatened by the presence of the birth father, as the social workers were putting a lot of pressure on them to allow more contacts between him and Nino. Nino himself manifested in more than one occasion the intention to stay with the man. Nino's individual psychotherapist, who has seen the child for 6 years, stated that Nino's birth father could be a positive presence for the child, allowing him to connect with his own biological roots. The situation, when we had our first session, was critical. The family felt

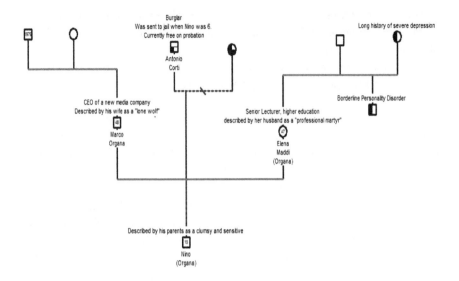

Figure 1. The organa family genogram.

cornered and surrounded by hostile presences, and a deep sense of illegitimacy and unworthiness was palpable in the room.

Results

During the consultation, Nino's parents produced 17 causal attributions regarding their son's behaviors (see Table 2).

All explanations and hypotheses provided by Nino's adoptive parents during the consultation shared some core elements:

(1) They were focused on Nino's past and his blood ties.
(2) They conveyed a view of Nino as inherently childish and immature.
(3) They provided a view of the world outside the family as extremely dangerous and hostile, a place Nino was not fit for (and would possibly never be), highlighting the necessity of protection.
(4) They resorted to a monadic or dyadic inference field (Ugazio et al., 2008).

The initial explanation of the problem is provided by Elena (attribution n° 1):

Elena: We are very concerned about Nino. I would dare saying we're scared. He is displaying all these deviant behaviors. He gets in touch with his father without telling us, he drinks and smokes too much. It is like a scheme: every time he has to choose between the right thing and the wrong one he is like compelled to follow the more deviant path. He is clearly scared too about all these things he does. But he simply cannot stop. I think there is something inside him, something that he is scared of. He is like crying for help, for our attention. It's like him telling us he is not ready to act as an independent person.[3]

Table 2. Attributions in the first two sessions of consultation.

Number	Session	Attributor	Stable vs. unstable	Specific vs. global	Internal vs. external	Personal vs. universal	Controllable vs. uncontrollable	Inference field
1	1st	Elena	Stable	Global	Internal	Personal	Uncontrollable	Dyad
2	1st	Marco	Stable	Global	Internal	Personal	Uncontrollable	Dyad
3	1st	Elena	Stable	Global	Internal	Personal	Controllable	Dyad
4	1st	Elena	Stable	Global	External	Personal	Uncontrollable	Dyad
5	1st	Elena	Stable	Specific	Internal	Personal	Controllable	Monad
6	1st	Marco	Stable	Global	Internal	Universal	Uncontrollable	Monad
7	1st	Marco	Stable	Global	Internal	Personal	Uncontrollable	Dyad
8	2nd	Elena	Unstable	Global	Internal	Universal	Uncontrollable	Dyad
9	2nd	Elena	Stable	Global	Internal	Personal	Uncontrollable	Dyad
10	2nd	Marco	Stable	Global	Internal	Personal	Controllable	Dyad
11	2nd	Elena	Stable	Global	Internal	Personal	Uncontrollable	Monad
12	2nd	Marco	Unstable	Global	External	Personal	Controllable	Monad
13	2nd	Elena	Stable	Specific	Internal	Universal	Uncontrollable	Monad
14	2nd	Elena	Stable	Global	Internal	Personal	Controllable	Dyad
15	2nd	Marco	Stable	Specific	External	Personal	Controllable	Dyad
16	2nd	Marco	Unstable	Global	External	Universal	Controllable	Dyad
17	2nd	Elena	Stable	Global	Internal	Personal	Uncontrollable	Monad

This attribution can be described as 'stable' (it is a 'scheme' recurring in every similar situation), global (it is likely to affect multiple areas of Nino's life and relationships), internal (originated inside Nino, with no external influence, it is 'something inside him'), and personal (makes him different from others). It is apparently uncontrollable (Nino himself is scared by his behaviors but cannot control them), and originated into a unidirectional dyadic (Ugazio et al., 2008) inference field (Elena states he is unconsciously crying for their help and attention by displaying these behaviors). When asked to give his opinion about it, Marco (attribution n°2) added an interesting piece of explanation, as he says:

Marco: I think that in some ways he shares something with his father. His father is a sort of stray cat, he used to live on the streets, making his money as a burglar until he was jailed. He has serious problems with alcohol, he is trying to recover but you know, when you have this thing you never get really rid of it. I think it is something in your blood. It is like a legacy.

Therapist: A legacy of stray cats?.

Marco: Something like that, yes.

Marco's attribution confirms a stable, uncontrollable variable, which originates from the inside and makes Nino inherently different from other boys. He links this to blood ties with his father, adding a 'genetic flavor' to the explanation. The 'legacy theory' is accepted by Elena (attribution n°3), although she adds a more relational factor:

Elena: I have a different idea. Nino's father is more of a black cat[4] rather than a stray one. He is so unlucky that everyone getting too close to him is doomed to suffer. Nino wants to save his father. But like everyone he will suffer if he gets too close to him. Add to this that Nino never had a positive role model he could cling to, and for all his first seven years he had no reliable attachment figure, no secure base. His personality is not strong enough to stay away from bad influences.

Elena's integration of Marco's previous attribution enlighten us about the strong presence of a psychological discourse about attachment and construction of identity, which possibly originates from the long relationship this family had with Nino's individual therapist.

As this explanation introduces a principle of intentionality in Nino's actions (he is trying to save his father) it contains a potentially positive and non-pathologizing view of the child, but this is immediately counteracted by the idea that Nino is too fragile due to disrupted attachment, and therefore defenseless against bad influences. This vulnerability to bad influences comes back during the second session, with regards to Nino's relationship with his peers group (attributions n° 8 and 9).

Elena: we are also rather worried about his new friends, they are all kids with a bad reputation. In fact his old friends from the Parish are avoiding him now. My fear is that he can throw himself away. Because of course he has this emotional dysregulation, due to his story, and also maybe because he is growing up. He is so eager to cut this umbilical cord he has with me… I am scared he could get into alcohol, that's it! Or drugs. As he smokes so much, so uncontrollably. Since his father already has a story with alcohol I am scared he will end like him. His father is not a bad person. He is just someone who is not able to say 'no' to anyone. I see the same trait in Nino, he never learnt to say no.

Here the attribution scheme dances between a phase-related explanation (connecting the behavior to a sort of adolescent crisis, and therefore less stable and personal) and one more rooted into Nino's internal working models, constructed within his relationship with his birth father. However, the trait of immaturity and vulnerability is confirmed. Elena is also blaming her husband's selfishness, which is driving Nino away from them (attribution n° 15).

Elena: I think he needs a father figure. He never had a reliable one. All these behaviors … Also, the fact he continues to say he wants to get back to his father …

Marco: he said he wants to see him more, not that he wants to stay with him.

Elena: No, forgive me Marco, he clearly said he is planning to stay with him. I think he is telling us he wants Marco to be more present with him. Problem is, my husband is a lone wolf, he is so self-centered. He lets you in his own world, but only at his own conditions. If you want to stay with him, you need to share his interests, he never shares yours. This is wrong. We cannot ask Nino to do this, he already went through so much, he is entitled to have a father who wants to spend time with him regardless.

In this attribution, Elena connects Nino's behavior with current family relational patterns, but does so relying on a dyadic matrix (*he needs a father*) based on what Verrier (1994) could have arguably described as Nino's "primal wound" ("since he never had one"). As a result, Nino is still in the 'needy child' position, and Marco is blamed for not being able to meet his needs. This kind of hypothesis is dangerous in family therapy as it makes both the co-parental sub-system and the marital sub-system vulnerable to conflict.

Stray cats, black cats, tabby cats: re-framing the problem.

Our strategic goal is to introduce a degree of dissonance (Hester & Adams, 2014; Selvini, Boscolo, Cecchin, & Prata, 1980; Ugazio, 1989), enabling a shift in narratives around the problem. Therefore, we privileged hypotheses:

(1) Focused on current family relationships.
(2) Positioning Nino as a competent member of the family, promoting a non-pathologizing view.
(3) Re-framing the concept of 'protection', enabling a different relationship between family and the outside world.
(4) Resorting on a triadic inference field (Ugazio et al., 2008).

When we addressed the 'need for a father' theory in the second session, we embraced Elena's idea that there was an element of intentional provocation in Nino's behavior, but we introduced a triadic matrix of hypothesizing (see Figure 2), suggesting Nino's behavior could have a different, and less self-centered, purpose.

Therapist: What you say, Elena, is very interesting, because we are used to see young boys trying to get rid of their parents the more they can. We need to understand where all this extra need for a father may come from, because, from our perspective, Nino had plenty of father. His father was Nino's only caregiver for the first years. We may question the quality of the caregiving, nonetheless, it was a strong bonding. They were together all the time, they were two stray cats surviving together on the streets.

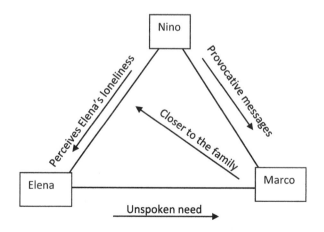

Figure 2. A triadic hypothesis about Nino's behavior.

Now, it is very unlikely for a stray cat to have all these extra needs.

Elena: I never saw it that way.

Our choice to 'raise a comparison with a developmental norm' (Tomm, 1987, p. 177), has the purpose of introducing a degree of reflexivity in the parents' idea that Nino's position is the only possible for an adopted child. Our intention was to re-frame Nino's behavior as an intentional (although not necessarily conscious) move in the triadic game of the family.

We were aware of the difficult relationships Elena had with her own family, in which she is a sort of outcast, and her persistent, yet unsuccessful attempts to involve Marco in this conflict. She would like to have Marco 'on my side', as she repeated more than once in the session, but her husband seemed to avoid any sort of call to arms. As a result, Elena's sense of loneliness and exclusion increased.

Therapist (talking to Marco):   Do you think it would be possible that Nino perceives Elena's loneliness? His vulnerability to others' expectations, that you both described, is likely to have also made him very receptive to others' needs as well, especially with Elena that is so close to him.

Marco: It is true that Elena is cornered by her family, don't know … possibly she would like me to be on her side but, you know, it's her family, what role could I play in?

Elena: I did not choose them, I chose you. You should simply choose me.

Curiously, Marco proposed the 'blood ties' explanation again, when it comes to the couple. This explanation privileges vertical relationships (parent-child) over horizontal ones (husband-wife). Conversely, Elena displayed a more distrustful attitude over blood ties, recalling the dimension of mutual choice.

This discrepancy offers interesting therapeutic options, as Nino represents both a vertical relationship (being their son), and a horizontal one (as adoption strongly relies on choice). We then invited the couple to take our alternative explanation into consideration.

Therapist: You see how Nino is provoking Marco, using his own explanations against him. I mean, who lives by blood ties, dies by blood ties. Marco has to face the competition with another father, who has an advantage over him, so he has to be more involved to bridge the gap. By doing this, Nino is forcing Marco back to the family, and back to you, Elena, in the end.

Elena: He is doing it for me? I never thought he could do something like that. It is true that Marco is irritated by the competition with Antonio, though. I have to think about it.

Marco (laughing):   Sons are always on the mother's side, it seems!.

We were promoting a main shift in narratives, from a narrative about 'blood ties' – irreversibly related to attachment and biological legacy – toward a narrative about 'co-construction of a choice', where belonging occurs as a result of mutual acknowledgment. We were also aware that our previous hypothesis was putting Marco in a difficult position, as we acknowledged Elena's loneliness and that was at risk of blaming him. We had to regain neutrality, intended as 'the generation of a state of curiosity in the therapist's mind' (Cecchin, 1987, p. 405).

Possibly, one of the more crucial passages toward this desired outcome is displayed during the fifth session. The 'cats metaphor', already used in the second session, is taken a step forward, including Nino as a competent observer.

Therapist:	Your mum says you are a stray cat who likes cuddles like a tabby cat.
Nino:	I love cuddles.
Therapist:	And what cat is Marco?.
Nino:	He is a European cat. The kind of cat you see on the streets. He is independent and does not like cuddles.
Therapist:	Your mom thinks Antonio is a black cat instead.
Nino:	He is. But it is not his fault. He is just unlucky.
Therapist:	Your mom thinks it's dangerous for you to care so much for this black cat, not because he's bad, but because this bad luck can be contagious somehow. She thinks that if you try to save him you can go down with him. Would you agree?
Nino:	I just want to see him. I don't want to forget about him.
Therapist:	Nino has a strong sense of loyalty, not only with Antonio. He did not want to come here because he did not want to betray his therapist. Usually cats are described as loyal to houses, whilst dogs are loyal to people. Where do Nino's canine traits come from?
Elena:	I think I am a very loyal person.
Nino:	She is 100% altruistic.
Marco:	She is a professional martyr.
Therapist:	So, if there was a poor black cat on the street, wounded and hungry, mom would try to save him, despite the danger, much like you do?
Nino:	Much more than me. Mom is fond of black cats.
Therapist:	She has some black cats to take care of?
Nino:	Both her mom and brother are black cats. They make her cry all the time, nonetheless she keeps them close.

Therapist:	What does dad think of it?
Nino:	He gets mad at her because she is wasting lots of money and time and energies. He says they are never going to give he what she wants.
Therapist:	What does she want?
Nino:	Don't know. Love, I guess.
Therapist:	So, your altruism may cause you trouble, according to mum. And mum's altruism will cause her trouble, according to your father. Altruism is a disease running in the family!.
Marco (laughing):	I am immune.

Marco's immunity to Elena's altruistic attitude towards black cats was the final piece of the triadic hypothesis we were co-constructing with this family. In the family's attribution style, Nino's behaviors were mainly described as stable, global traits of personality, originated by his damaging history of disrupted attachment.

In the piece of conversation above, we started introducing a different idea: Nino was carrying on a sort of 'reductio ad absurdum' (Boscolo & Bertrando, 1996; Ugazio, 2013) of Elena's principles of loyalty and altruism. Showing her how dangerous it could be to stay so close to 'black cats', he was helping Marco.

Therapist:	Nino, it seems all these behaviors that make you not independent force your mum to be involved with you all the time. What do you think could happen if you were a bit more independent?
Nino:	She would have more time for herself, I think.
Therapist:	Are you sure? Because you told me that there are black cats all around the house that crave mum's attention. What would they do if she had a little less to do with you?
Marco (laughing):	They would eat her alive.
Nino:	Grandma would like to have her all day.
Elena (smiling at Nino):	Now that you say it, I think the only thing that keeps her from calling me every hour is that she does not want to talk about Nino and his problems.

Both parents acknowledged that, with his behavior, Nino protected Elena both from her mother's pressure and her husband's wrath. This was a strong moment of mutual connection and a shift in narratives seemed forthcoming, as we reached a non-individual, non-innate triadic way of understanding Nino's issues (see Figure 3).

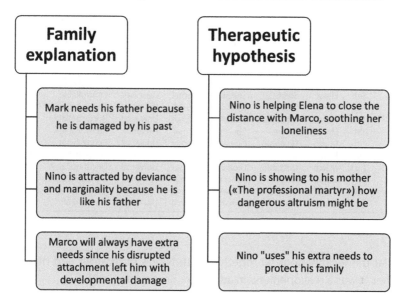

Figure 3. Shifting from monadic/dyadic, past focused narratives to triadic, present focused ones.

Our final reframing was very distant from the original attributions, yet the family seemed ready to consider this, as we were able to match dissonance with plausibility (Ugazio, 1984):

Therapist: Nino was enigmatic for us, as we saw a smart stray cat who seemed to have lost his whiskers. He presents himself as clumsy, immature and needy, but this is inconsistent with his story. Now, what if Nino did not lose his whiskers? What if he simply traded them in exchange for something more precious? What if those whiskers were the price he wanted to pay, in order to belong to you? As a member of this family, he is altruistic and a bit blind when it comes to loyalty, like his mum. But he is also sensitive to his father's needs for independence. He is the perfect product of this family. Would it be possible for us to help him staying connected to this family without having to give up his whiskers entirely?

The reaction of the family was very positive, as Elena said it was 'a really encouraging perspective' and Marco added 'we can learn to protect each other in a different way'.

These positive signs were confirmed by the intermediate follow-up session. Elena and Marco reported that they decided not to renew the request for Nino's special needs teaching assistant (who used to help Nino in class since he arrived in the new family), and Nino was able to complete the academic year along with the rest of the class, gaining a boost in self-confidence.

The family also identified a possible strategy to let Nino increase his contacts with his birth father, without giving up protection. They decided to organize

Table 3. Attributions in the last therapy session and the one year follow-up.

Number	Ses-sion	Attrib-utor	Stable vs. unstable	Spe-cific vs. global	Inter-nal vs. external	Personal vs. uni-versal	Controllable vs. uncontrol-lable	Infer-ence field
1	9th	Elena	Unstable	Specific	External	Universal	Controllable	Dyad
2	9th	Elena	Stable	Specific	External	Personal	Controllable	Dyad
3	9th	Elena	Stable	Global	Internal	Universal	Controllable	Triad
4	9th	Marco	Unstable	Global	External	Universal	Uncontrollable	Dyad
5	9th	Elena	Stable	Specific	Internal	Personal	Controllable	Monad
6	9th	Marco	Unstable	Global	External	Universal	Controllable	Monad
7	9th	Elena	Stable	Specific	Internal	Personal	Controllable	Dyad
8	FU1	Marco	Unstable	Global	Internal	Universal	Uncontrollable	Dyad
9	FU1	Elena	Stable	Specific	Internal	Personal	Uncontrollable	Triad
10	FU1	Elena	Unstable	Global	External	Universal	Controllable	Monad
11	FU1	Marco	Stable	Specific	External	Universal	Controllable	Dyad

regular dinner meetings all together, with Nino's birthfather and his grand-mother. It was a real openness in adoption (Brodzinsky, 2005)!

Both parents reported during our first follow-up that they were all enjoying these meetings, and Nino seemed to have lost any interest for secrecy when getting in touch with his father.

Our final follow up confirmed the progress that had been made. Nino completed his studies and started working as a mechanic, a field in which his 'stray cat' dexterity was an added value. Meetings with his biological father continued regularly. Social workers significantly decreased their pressure on the family, with a consequent increase in systemic well-being.

Family attribution style also changed toward a less pathologizing view of Nino's behavior, which is described both as less individual and more controllable (see Table 3). Elena was able to summarize the journey of her family, and the shift in narratives they achieved:

> Elena: We were so concerned about Nino and his desire to save Antonio, but I think we were wrong. As a family, we have always been inclusive. We are helpful and altruistic. That's who we are, that is why we are together in the first place. Nino is part of us, and we shall not be worried by recognizing he acts like us.

Discussion

This case study highlighted some positive aspects of family therapy for adoption, based on a post-Milan approach. The dramatic change in attribution styles and explanatory models (see Figure 4), achieved in a relatively short time, supports the idea that focusing on current relationships and patterns of mutual connection in the present can be a valuable strategy when dealing with crystallized perspectives like those often encountered in adoptive families.

A post-Milan approach frees the therapist from the constraining goal of restoring normality, thus allowing the child and his/her family to engage in

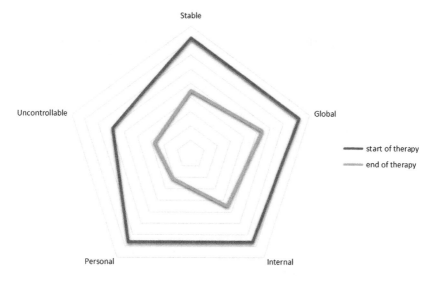

Figure 4. Changes in attributions between the start and the end of therapy.

a constructive process, rather than a repairing one. For this reason, our team focused on issues and problems related to the current family situation.

In some respects, it is a less ambitious therapeutic process, since it does not aim at healing the wound of disrupted attachment. Nonetheless, it presents the advantage of empowering legitimacy and mutual belonging, thus promoting a sense of hope within the family.

There are of course limitations of this study. Primarily, its 'single case' nature does not allow us to draw any conclusions about translation of this approach to other families and contexts, although our recent practice with adoption in two different countries (Italy and UK) is giving promising results.

Second, a three years follow-up does not tell us enough about further development of Nino's relational skills. For instance, we were not able to explore how is internal working models could affect long-term emotional relationships.

On a methodological level, the mixed structure of settings (consultation with parents, therapy with the whole family) poses some question about our material, as we can assume some of the core themes and narratives emerging during the family sessions would have possibly been expressed differently in a couple setting.

However, there is an encouraging consistency between our strategies and the predicted outcomes, as the family seemed to respond positively to our attempt to re-frame the presenting problem within a different matrix. Further research with larger and more reliable samples could hopefully confirm viability of this approach in adoption family therapy.

Notes

1. Parents allowed the recording of sessions and the use of transcripts for research purposes, by individually signing a written consent before the start of the consultation.
2. All names, places and sensitive data were modified in compliance with confidenciality policy.
3. Dialogues are translated from Italian.
4. Black cats are regarded as bearers of bad luck' in the Italian tradition. Although this superstition only survives to its full extent in very underdeveloped areas of the country, it is often used as a metaphor in common language.

Acknowledgments

We would like to thank the University of Northampton, for supporting us in our clinical and research project.
A heartfelt "thank you!" goes to the European Institute of Systemic-relational Therapies and to its founder Valeria Ugazio, for providing such a challenging, exciting and creative arena, where we could share ideas and build new perspectives.
Thanks to Prof. Lisa Fellin of University of East London, a great friend and amazing researcher, whose tireless scientific curiosity and generosity represented an unceasing encouragement in the process of sharpening our idea.
Our last acknowledgement goes to our patients, who gave approval for this research and were with us, tolerating the pain and uncertainty of the intense journey we described in our paper. Hopefully, we caused them some benefit, surely they enriched us greatly, as professionals and human beings.

Disclosure statement

No potential conflict of interest was reported by the authors.

References

Ainsworth, M. D. S. (1969). Object relations, dependency, and attachment: A theoretical review of the infant-mother relationship. *Child Development, 40*, 969–1025.

American Psychiatric Association. (2013). *Diagnostic and statistical manual of mental disorders* (5th ed.). Washington, DC: Author.

Anderson, H., & Goolishian, H. (1992). The client is the expert: A not-knowing approach to therapy. In S. McNamee & K. Gergen (Eds.), *Therapy as social construction* pp. (25–39).

Barth, R. P., John, K., Crea, T. M., Thoburn, J., & Quinton, D. (2005), Beyond attachment theory and therapy: Towards sensitive and evidence-based interventions with foster and adoptive families in distress. *Child and Family Social Work, 10*, 257–268. doi:10.1111/j.1365-2206.2005.00380.x

Bateson, G. (1979). *Mind and nature: A necessary unity.* New York, NY: Dutton.

Beek, M. (1999). Parenting children with attachment difficulties: Views of adoptive parents and implications for post-adoption services. *Adoption & Fostering, 23*, 16–23. doi:10.1177/030857599902300104

Boscolo, L., & Bertrando, P. (1996). *Systemic therapy with individuals.* London: Karnac Books.

Bowlby, J. (1969). *Attachment and loss. 1. Attachment.* London: Hogarth.

Brodzinsky, D. M. (2005). Reconceptualizing openness in adoption: Implications for theory, research, and practice. In D. M. Brodzinsky & J. Palacios (Eds.), *Psychological issues in adoption: Research and practice* (pp. 145–166).

Campbell, D. (1999). Family therapy and beyond: Where is the Milan systemic approach today? *Child Psychology and Psychiatry Review, 4*, 76–84. doi:10.1017/s1360641799001896

Cecchin, G. (1987). Hypothesizing, circularity, and neutrality revisited: An invitation to curiosity. *Family Process, 26*, 405–413. doi:10.1111/j.1545-5300.1987.00405

Chaffin, M., Hanson, R., Saunders, B. E., Nichols, T., Barnett, D., Zeanah, C., & LeTourneau, E. (2006). Report of the APSAC task force on attachment therapy, reactive attachment disorder, and attachment problems. *Child Maltreatment, 11*, 76–89. doi:10.1177/1077559505283699

Crittenden, P. M., & Claussen, A. H. (2003). *The organization of attachment relationships: Maturation, culture, and context.* Cambridge, UK: Cambridge University Press. doi:10.1002/casp.861

Dallos, R., & Vetere, A. (2009). *Systemic therapy and attachment narratives: Applications in a range of clinical settings.* London: Routledge. doi:10.1111/j.1467-6427.2010.00497_1.x

Diamond, G. M. (2014). Attachment-based family therapy interventions. *Psychotherapy, 51*(1), 15–19. doi:10.1037/a0032689

Dozier, M., Stoval, K. C., Albus, K. E., & Bates, B. (2001). Attachment for infants in foster care: The role of caregiver state of mind. *Child Development, 72*, 1467–1477. doi:10.1111/1467-8624.00360

Fellin, L. C., & Salamino, F. (2016, July). Who is to blame? Causal attributions and foster families: a content and discourse analysis. In L. C. Fellin (chair) (Ed.), *Steps beyond broken attachments in systemic work with adoption and foster care.* Symposium conducted at the CAMHS Conference, Northampton, UK.

Hanson, R. F., & Spratt, E. G. (2000). Reactive attachment disorder: What we know about the disorder and implications for treatment. *Child Maltreatment, 5*, 137–145. doi:10.1177/1077559500005002005

Harré, R., Moghaddam, F. M., Cairnie, T. P., Rothbart, D., & Sabat, S. R. (2009). Recent advances in positioning theory. *Theory & Psychology, 19*, 5–31. doi:10.1177/0959354308101417

Hester, P. T., & Adams, M. G. (2014). *Systemic thinking: Fundamentals for understanding problems and messes.* New York, NY: Springer.

Hoffman, L. (1988). A constructivist position for family therapy. *The Irish Journal of Psychology, 9*, 110–129. doi:10.1080/03033910.1988.10557709

Kenrick, J., Lindsey, C., & Tollemache, L. (2006). *Creating new families: Therapeutic approaches to fostering, adoption, and kinship care*. London: Karnac Books.

Moran, G., Diamond, G. M., & Diamond, G. S. (2005). The relational reframe and parents' problem constructions in attachment-based family therapy. *Psychotherapy Research, 15*, 226–235. doi:10.1080/10503300512331387780

Salamino, F. (2016). *Towards a systemic-relational alternative to attachment therapies with adoption and foster care: The Kintsugi strategy*. Manuscript submitted for publication.

Salamino, F., & Gusmini, E. (2016, May). Beyond repair: Therapeutic strategies with an adopted adolescent and his family. In L. C. Fellin (chair) (Ed.), *Disrupted attachment, disrupted families? Systemic pathways for change in adoption and foster care*. Symposium conducted at the 6th Qualitative Research in Mental Health Conference, Chania, Greece.

Schofield, G., & Beek, M. (2005). Providing a secure base: Parenting children in long-term foster family care. *Attachment & Human Development, 7*, 3–26. doi:10.1080/14616730500049019

Selvini, M. P., Boscolo, L., Cecchin, G., & Prata, G. (1980). Hypothesizing – Circularity – Neutrality: Three guidelines for the conductor of the session. *Family Process, 19*, 3–12. doi:10.1111/j.1545-5300.1980.00003.x

Sroufe, L. A., Carlson, E. A., Levy, A. K., & Egeland, B. (1999). Implications of attachment theory for developmental psychopathology. *Development and Psychopathology, 11*(1), 1–13. doi:10.1017/s0954579499001923

Stratton, P. (2003a). Causal attributions during therapy I: Responsibility and blame. *Journal of Family Therapy, 25*, 136–160. doi:10.1111/1467-6427.00241

Stratton, P. (2003b). Causal attributions during therapy II: Reconstituted families and parental blaming. *Journal of Family Therapy, 25*, 161–180. doi:10.1111/1467-6427.00242

Tomm, K. (1987). Interventive interviewing: Part II. Reflexive questioning as a means to enable self-healing. *Family Process, 26*, 167–183. doi:10.1111/j.1545-5300.1987.00167.x

Ugazio, V. (1984). Ipotizzazione e processo terapeutico [Hypothesizing and therapeutic process]. *Terapia Familiare, 16*, 27–45.

Ugazio, V. (1989). L'indicazione terapeutica: una prospettiva sistemico-costruttivista. [The therapeutic indication: A systemic-constructivist perspective] *Terapia familiare, 31*, 27–40.

Ugazio, V. (2007). Le psicoterapie sistemico-costruzioniste: specificità e recenti evoluzioni. In E. Molinari & A. Labella (Eds.), *Psicologia clinica* (pp. 81–102). Milan: Springer.

Ugazio, V. (2013). *Semantic polarities and psychopathologies in the family: Permitted and forbidden stories* [Systemic-constructionist therapies: Specificity and recent developments]. London: Routledge. doi:10.4324/9780203552384

Ugazio, V., Fellin, L., Colciago, F., Pennacchio, R., & Negri, A. (2008). 1 to 3: From the monad to the triad. A unitizing and coding manual for the fields of inference of causal explanations. *Testing, Psychometrics, Methodology in Applied Psychology, 15*, 171–192.

Vadilonga, F. (Ed.). (2010). *Curare l'adozione: modelli di sostegno e presa in carico della crisi adottiva* [Curing adoption: Support and taking charge models for the adoptive crisis]. Milano.

Verrier, N. (1994). *The primal wound*. Cortina, MD: Gateway Press Inc.

Vetere, A., & Dallos, R. (2008). Systemic therapy and attachment narratives. *Journal of Family Therapy, 30*, 374–385. doi:10.1111/j.1467-6427.2008.00449.x

Woolgar, M., & Baldock, E. (2015). Attachment disorders versus more common problems in looked after and adopted children: Comparing community and expert assessments. *Child and Adolescent Mental Health, 20*, 34–40. doi:10.1111/camh.12052

Woolgar, M., & Scott, S. (2014). The negative consequences of over-diagnosing attachment disorders in adopted children: The importance of comprehensive formulations. *Clinical Child Psychology and Psychiatry, 19*, 355–366. doi:10.1177/1359104513478545

Critical incidents in mental health units may be better understood and managed with a Freudian/ Lacanian psychoanalytic framework

Gerard Patrick Moore (iD)

ABSTRACT
This paper explores critical incident management in an Irish adult public mental health services with a population catchment area of approximately 245,000 people. Data were collected by non-participant observation, informal opportunistic interviews and formal psychoanalytic interviews. The amassed data were analysed using a Freudian/Lacanian framework. Findings indicated that due to the unconscious influence of the group, some critical incidents arise from staffs' lack of consistent engagement with patients and failure to recognise or tolerate overwhelming levels of anxiety. Some critical incidents were managed by the imposition of restrictions or pseudo-treatment reflecting impatience, guilt, hatred and despair which compromises care. Incidents of acting out by service occupants were a consequence of the failure to work with transference. Staff interventions mirror patient and their family's behaviours resulting in rejection, dismissal and banishment. Critical incidents may be more manageable if staff were provided with appropriate supports enabling them to operate differently: by better accepting negative feeling towards patients and learning transference management skills. The patient–staff relationship needs to be reconsidered in the light of two conclusions: firstly, that all staff are suffering from a constitutional lack to utilise their natural qualities to manage transference or more likely, membership of the group unconsciously prohibits the use of this natural skill.

LOS INCIDENTES CRITICOS EN LAS UNIDADES DE SALUD MENTAL PUEDEN SER MEJOR COMPRENDIDOS Y MANEJADOS DENTRO DE UN MARCO DE TRABAJO PSICOANALITICO FREUDIANO/LACANIANO

Este artículo explora el manejo de incidentes críticos en servicios públicos irlandeses de salud mental para adultos, en un población de 245.000 personas, los datos fueron recogidos mediante observación no participante, entrevistas informales de oportunidad y entrevistas psicoanalíticas formales. Se analizaron los resultados obtenidos utilizando un marco de trabajo Freudiano/Lacaniano. Estos resultados indicaron que, debido a la influencia del inconsciente del grupo se originaron algunos incidentes críticos por falta de un compromiso consciente del personal con respecto a los pacientes y su falla para reconocer o tolerar

extremos niveles de ansiedad. Algunos incidents se manejaron por imposición de restricciones o por medio de un pseudo-tratamiento que perjudicaba el cuidado a los pacientes.La falla en trabajar con la transferencia trajo como consecuencia incidentes de 'acting-out' por parte de los ocupantes en servicio. Las intervenciones del personal reflejan las conductas de los pacientes y sus familias, resultando en rechazo, despido o prohibición. Se espera poder manejar major estos incidents si el personal recibe el apoyo adecuado que les permita operar de manera diferente; por ejemplo, aprendiendo a aceptar sus sentimientos negativos hacia los pacientes y proporcionarles habilidad para trabajar con la transferencia. La relación pacientes-personal necesita ser reconsiderada a la luz de dos conclusions: que el personal adolece de una falta constitucional para utilizar sus cualidades naturales en el manejo de la transferencia y que probablemente, ser miembro del grupo prohibe esta habilidad natural.

Incidenti critici nelle unità di salute mentale, una cornice concettuale lacaniana/psicoanalitico-freudiana per meglio comprenderli e gestirli

Questo contributo prende in esame la gestione critica di incidenti occorsi in servizi pubblici di salute mentale per adulti irlandesi, con una popolazione di circa 245.000 persone. I dati sono stati raccolti tramite osservazione non partecipante, colloqui opportunistici informali e colloqui formali ad orientamento psicoanalitico. I dati raccolti sono stati analizzati utilizzando una cornice concettuale freudiano/ lacaniana. I risultati indicano che, a causa della influenza inconscia esercitata dal gruppo, alcune situazioni critiche sono originate dalla mancanza di un impegno coerente verso i pazienti e dall'incapacità di riconoscere o tollerare livelli di ansia personale straordinari. Alcuni incidenti critici sono stati gestiti con l'imposizione di restrizioni o pseudo-trattamenti che compromettono la cura. Episodi di acting-out dagli occupanti dei servizio erano una conseguenza del mancato lavoro sul transfert. Alcuni interventi rispecchiano i comportamenti del paziente e della sua famiglia con conseguente rifiuto, revoca e espulsione. Gli incidenti critici potrebbero essere meglio gestiti se al personale fosse fornito adeguato supporto che permetta di operare in modo diverso; ad esempio accettare i sentimenti negativi sperimentati nei confronti dei pazienti e apprendere come gestire il transfert. Il rapporto paziente-personale ha bisogno di essere riconsiderato alla luce di due considerazioni: in primo luogo che tutto il personale è incapace di valorizzare le proprie qualità naturali nella gestione del transfert o, più probabilmente, l'appartenenza al gruppo vieta inconsciamente l'uso di questa abilità.

Mieux comprendre et mieux gérer les incidents critiques au sein d'unités de santé mentale à l'aide d'un cadre de référence psychanalytique Freudien/lacanien

Cet article explore la gestion d'incidents critiques survenus dans des services de santé mentale irlandais couvrant une population d'environ 245 000 personnes. Les données ont été collectées à l'aide d'observations, d'entretiens informels menés sur le vif et d'entretiens psychanalytiques formels. Les données collectées ont été analysées en utilisant un cadre de référence théorique Freudien/Lacanien. Les résultats indiquent qu'à cause de l'influence inconsciente du groupe, certains incidents critiques sont la résultante du manque d'engagement consistant du personnel avec les patients et d'un échec à reconnaitre ou tolérer des niveaux d'anxiété trop élevés. Certains incidents critiques sont gérés par l'imposition de restrictions ou de pseudo-traitements compromettant le soin. Certains passages à l'acte de la part d'occupants du service sont une conséquence du manque de travail avec le transfert. Les interventions du personnel apparaissent en miroir

avec les comportements du patient et de sa famille avec pour résultante le rejet, l'exclusion et le bannissement. Les incidents critiques pourraient être mieux gerés si l'on fournissait au personnel un soutien adéquat leur permettant d'opérer différemment: en acceptant mieux les émotions négatives envers les patients et en apprenant à manier le transfert. La relation patient-soignant doit être reconsidérée a la lumière de deux conclusions: premièrement que le personnel souffre d'un manque constitutionnel d'utilisation de leurs qualités naturelles pour gérer le transfert ou plus probablement que l'appartenance à un groupe interdit inconsciemment l'utilisation de ces compétences naturelles.

Τα κρίσιμα περιστατικά σε μονάδες ψυχικής υγείας μπορούν να γίνουν καλύτερα κατανοητά και διαχειρίσιμα σε ένα φροϋδικό/ λακανικό ψυχαναλυτικό πλαίσιο

Το παρόν άρθρο διερευνά τη διαχείριση κρίσιμων περιστατικών σε μια Ιρλανδική δημόσια υπηρεσία ψυχικής υγείας ενηλίκων με πληθυσμό περίπου 245.000 κατοίκους. Η συλλογή των δεδομένων πραγματοποιήθηκε μέσω μη συμμετοχικής παρατήρησης, ανεπίσημων ευκαιριακών συνεντεύξεων και επίσημων ψυχαναλυτικών συνεντεύξεων.Τα δεδομένα που συγκεντρώθηκαν αναλύθηκαν με τη χρήση ενός Φροϋδικού/ Λακανικού πλαισίου. Τα αποτελέσματα έδειξαν ότι εξαιτίας της ασυνείδητης επίδρασης της ομάδας, ορισμένα κρίσιμα περιστατικά εγείρονται από την απουσία σταθερής σχέσης του προσωπικού με τους ασθενείς και την αποτυχία αναγνώρισης και ανοχής υψηλών επιπέδων άγχους.Η διαχείριση ορισμένων κρίσιμων περιστατικών έγινε με την επιβολή περιορισμών ή με ψευδοθεραπείες, οι οποίες θέτουν σε κίνδυνο τη φροντίδα. Τα περιστατικά εκδραμάτισης ήταν η συνέπεια της αποτυχίας του προσωπικού να εργαστεί με τη μεταβίβαση. Οι παρεμβάσεις του προσωπικού καθρεφτίζουν τις συμπεριφορές του ασθενή και της οικογένειας τους που οδηγούν σε απόρριψη, αποβολή και εκτόπιση. Η διαχείριση των κρίσιμων περιστατικών μπορεί να είναι πιο επιτυχής αν το προσωπικό είχε την κατάλληλη υποστήριξη που θα επέτρεπε να δράσει διαφορετικά μέσα από την καλύτερη αποδοχή των αρνητικών συναισθημάτων προς τους πελάτες και την εκμάθηση δεξιοτήτων διαχείρισης της μεταβίβασης. Η σχέση ανάμεσα στον πελάτη και στο προσωπικόχρειάζεται να αναθεωρηθεί μέσα από δύο συμπεράσματα. Πρώτον ότι όλα τα μέλη του προσωπικού υποφέρουν απόconstitutional έλλειψηχρήσης των φυσικών ποιοτήτων για τη διαχείριση της μεταβίβασης ή πιθανότερα από το ότι η συμμετοχή στην ομάδα ασυνείδητα παρεμποδίζει την αξιοποίηση αυτής της φυσικής δεξιότητας.

Introduction

A process of change has been imposed on the Irish Mental Health Services with an overt purpose of reformation and quality improvement. This paper which focuses on critical incident management in one Irish public mental health service with a catchment population of approximately 245,000 people living in a mix of urban and rural settings is extracted from a larger study (Moore, 2012) of transference enactment. It views critical incidents through 'a lens informed by specific aspects of psychoanalysis' (Bicknell & Liefooghe, 2005, p. 9) mainly Freudian and Lacanian approaches and demonstrates that the constituting nature of an institution influences the dynamic between individuals, suggesting that change is unlikely to occur without recognition of the impact of the unconscious (Menzies Lyth, 1989). Denial and suppression of the realities of the organisation often go unidentified by its members resulting in stagnation in relation to development and a reduction in effectiveness. Once an institution has been established, it becomes extremely difficult to change its essential structure, which modifies the personal structure of the individual for a short or permanent period of time. 'Social institutions arise through the efforts of human beings to satisfy their needs, but they become external realities comparatively independent of individuals that never the less affected the structure of the individual' (Fenichel, 1946).

Relationships in the mental health services and society in general are understood as an ego-to-ego interactive process. Psychoanalysis takes an alternative perspective by accounting for the influence of the unconscious in intra and interpersonal encounters. Psychoanalytic research is concerned with the functioning of the unconscious. Service transformation is rarely concerned with intra and interpersonal encounters and when interpersonal encounters are considered, the concentration is on ego-to-ego relationships. This disavows the unconscious of service occupants; consequently, service policy transformation enables stagnation and the style of subject–Other relationships enables regression in service occupants. This ensures a steady supply of people seeking mental health care and generates sufficient jouissance (pleasure that contains a threat of annihilation) (Evans, 2005, p. 91) for service delivery personnel to flourish. A paradox of intentionality exists between a conscious overt agenda of improvement and an unconscious covert agenda of stagnation and regression, maintained by shared social fantasy and exhibited via transference in the social reality of service delivery. The demise of physical institutions does not guarantee a demise of institutional practices which are a reflection of group behaviour (Freud, 1921) supported by the institution of the law.

Methodology and method

Links between research methods and the use of psychoanalysis to explore group behaviour can be found in the early foundations of the qualitative approach (Wallace, 1983) commencing with Freud's earliest anthropological texts which investigate the unconscious structure of the human mind in the development of social structures. Psychoanalysis gathers empirical evidence and questions it in a focused investigation based on a belief in the unconscious. The evidence from psychoanalysis is constructed from the speech and actions of partici-pants, verified against external reality, inclusive of shared cultural assump-tions, sociological and psychoanalytic knowledge (Hollway & Jefferson, 2007). Psychoanalysis privileges the unique discourse of the individual, as does the qualitative researcher in their transcription and analysis of all the utterances of their subject. For this study following a review of relevant literature, and ethi-cal approval, data were collected in acute inpatient settings, day hospitals and community services during a 12-month period by interviews and non-partici-pant observation, informal opportunistic conversations and formal interviews. Non-participant observation involved being present and observing, listening to, recording and reflecting on events as they unfold without physically engaging in them. Observing but not engaging in group's activities causes elements of reactivity from participants both conscious and unconsciously. Fieldwork in this study included non-participant observation and interviews which imply an additional level of engagement. Interviews require engagement and even maintaining quite presence and floating attention, techniques of psychoanal-ysis, implicating the researcher in the process. The researcher and participants are subject to projections and introjections of ideas and feelings.

> It also means that the impressions that we have about each other are not derived simply from the "real" relationship, but that what we say and do in the interaction will be mediated by internal fantasies which derive from our histories of significant relationships. (Hollway & Jefferson, 2007, p. 45)

For example, when conducting observation in a unit area, where different activ-ities and conversations may occur simultaneously, why would the researcher choose to listen more attentively and report on one over another? Pragmatically, one conversation is louder, easier to hear and report accurately or arguably a particular incident appeared more dramatic and draws the researcher's atten-tion. Alternatively, what was being related referred to something on which the researcher already has some knowledge and therefore they are drawn to the opportunity to expand or extend information. These choices alert the researcher to analyse their motivation by including and recording their thoughts and responses to the data. In other words, transference and countertransference are liable to colour the observation and interview process. 'This analysis would also require a reflexive analysis of the position of the analyst, something Lacanian's insist upon in the argument that there is no other resistance to analysis that that of the analyst' (Parker, 2005, p. 173).

The data were analysed with a Freudian/Lacanian theory of the subject and guided by Parker's (2008) assertion that psychoanalysis is concerned with questions of form rather than content focusing on the disjunction between consciousness and the unconscious. Additionally, the amassed data were verified by establishing a correspondence with external reality (Glynos & Stavrakakis, 2002, p. 32). This validation against external reality, part of the process of normal science, is identified by Hollway and Jefferson (2007) as integral to a psychoanalytic method.

The primary intent of the application of psychoanalytic theories to organisations is to offer the opportunity to alter key relationships between and amongst organisational members, staff and patients (Diamond, 1993, p. 20). The evidence that group psychology is an extension of individual psychology allowed Freud and later researchers (Bion, 1990; Bicknell & Liefooghe, 2005; Burkard, 1999; Comerford, 2010; DeBoard, 2005; Erlich-Ginor & Erlich, 1998; Long & Newton, 1997; Main, 1957; Menzies Lyth, 1988; Vanheule & Verhaeghe, 2003) to put organisations on the couch. In psychoanalysis, the analysand on the couch free associates in the presences of the analyst's floating attention. In this study, the mental health services speak on a metaphoric couch and the researcher/ analyst utilises floating attention offering an interpretation of a specific aspect of the unconscious life of the organisation. 'One analyses patterns of relationships (intersubjectivity) and individual perceptions of organisational experience' (Menzies Lyth, 1989, p. 33). The identity of the organisation is analysed. The researcher adopts an analytic position and is mindful to the history of the organisation, particularly in relation to managing critical incidents.

Critical instances, transference and acting out

The World Health Organisation (WHO) defines a critical incident as 'an event out of the range of normal experience – one which is sudden and unexpected, makes you lose control, involves the perception of a threat to life and can include elements of physical or emotional loss (WHO, 2006). Intra and interpersonal encounters may present as critical incidents which when explored with a psychoanalytic lens may lead to improve communication. Consciously recognised critical incidents make the subject stop, think and raise questions on an aspect of beliefs, values, attitude or behaviour, and may increase awareness or challenge understanding of social justice issues or may involve conflict, hostility, aggression or criticism (Fook & Cooper, 2003). Many critical incidents go unnoticed or unexplored and this may relate to unconscious issues of communication, culture, relationships, affects or beliefs and have the potential as they are unacknowledged, unrecognised, unreported and unexamined to lead to acting out. Acting out equals transference without analysis, staff respond to incidents of acting out and are as prone to acting out as patients (Harari, 2001; Main, 1957). Previous researchers concerned with the homogenous quality of social institutions have found a reciprocal nature in the unconscious fears and primitive fantasies evident in mental health units (Main, 1957; Menzies Lyth 1988, 1989; Reggio & Novello, 2007; Shur, 1994). Critical incidents evoke omnipotence and aggression in staff, managed by the imposition of treatment, often the administration of medication when staff can no longer tolerate the anxiety, impatience, guilt, hatred and despair evoked by patients (Main, 1957; Shur, 1994). Acting out is the demand for love, an attempt to avoid anxiety (Freud, 1914, 1917a, Harari, 2001; Rowan, 2000; Shur, 1994). Three critical incidents drawn from the larger study (Moore, 2012) are analysed below to demonstrate the unacknowledged unconscious elements that influence care. Direct quotes from study participants and the researcher's field notes are presented in italic.

Incident 1 – the tobacco pouch

Observation of staff's approach to a critical incident in an acute admission unit contained elements described by Freud (1917a), Lacan (1960–1961), Main (1957), Shur (1994) and Harari (2001) relating to unconscious attempts to manage anxiety provoked by the work. On arrival, I noted what I considered to be a series of additional defences to create distance between staff and patients had been put in place, signs on the office door, a sense of urgency in staff activity and curtness in their responses to patients. The cause was not apparent but an incident occurred shortly afterwards confirmed my belief that staff were experiencing elements of work as overwhelming and guarding against this. The notice, the urgency and curt responses were understood by the researcher as unnamed and unacknowledged negative transference and anxiety, activities designed to keep the patients at bay, staff's unconscious defences. *I was not in the office long when a student nurse came in and whispered something to a senior nurse. I could not catch all that was being said but managed to pick up that a patient was doing something in the unit toilet. She is looking for trouble again.* This critical incident placed a negative locus of control with the patient, had to be reported, but due to its sensitive nature, as a whisper. The staff acted immediately leaving the office equipped with disposable gloves. *In the background I became aware of a loud distressed inarticulate babbling and shouting coming from the bathroom area. After this settled down, a number of nurses returned and discussed the incident. The patient had told the student she had inserted a pouch of tobacco into her vagina the night before and was now in pain and without cigarettes. The senior nurse put the patient in the bath, notified the duty doctor and decided that the patient should be sent to the local general hospital accident and emergency unit.*

This incident lead to an immediate action by the staff. The inserted tobacco pouch was intolerable for patient and staff, too much to articulate so action in the guise of treatment was imposed. The patient unable to speak can only act out and regress to inarticulate babbling and shouting. The staff's defences against the anxiety provoked by the work are over saturated and they opt to remove the patient from the scene that they cannot abandon. However, the actual dismissal, the plan to send the patient away was reduced to a dismissal of the truth of their story by the intervention of another nurse who announced that the patient had now removed the tobacco pouch and returned to bed. The doctor and possible transfer to the accident and emergency unit were no longer required and summed up in the words of a participant, *She took it out herself. It's all in a day's work. Now she is looking for a pain-killer. She only did it this morning. I saw the pouch on her locker this morning.*

This incident reflects Main's (1957) observations on nurses' reactions to increased levels of anxiety. The decision to transfer was made quickly without discussion and as quickly reversed. The patient's story, inserting the tobacco pouch the previous evening, refuted and the request for analgesia ignored. In this critical incident, transference, master discourse and the power of the leader are observable. Staff certainty that the patient lied about the timing of the insertion, their unconscious response to the tense atmosphere and the anxiety the incident created went unanalysed. Power is used to delay responding to the request for analgesia, it is unquestioned by everyone present. Lacan (1960–1961) identified that if transference is not analysed, the analyst fallen from his or her place sends the analysand directly towards acting out and the message that could not be heard returns abruptly in a manner that can be seen, 'Acting out equals transference without analysis, transference equals acting out without analysis' (Harari, 2001, p. 84).

Combining Harari's (2001) statement with the ubiquitous nature of transference and Freud's (1912) contention that transference is in place prior to analysis demonstrates that staff unconsciously contribute to incidents of acting out. Acting out is presented by Lacan as having a greater power of demand than the symptom; the subject is so overwhelmed by their anxiety that they take action (Rowan, 2000). Additionally, the lack of demand towards the patient contributes to acting out more than the symptoms that drove them into care, indicating the potentially destructive or negative nature of admission. Freud emphasises the emergence of negative transference in the institution particularly when the treatment regime is non-analytic, naming it as 'nothing less than mental bondage' (Freud, 1912, p. 101). Manifestations of transference in the institution are attributable to the neurotic condition; patients overwhelmed by anxiety take action. They are not asking for something, not seeking attention, they are demanding something to be demanded of them, this is unconsciously resisted by staff.

Incident 2 – the vomit stain

Resistance needs to be lifted to explore transference; repression is linked to resistance. The symptom par excellence of resistance is retaining the idea that standard mental health interventions, a one size fits all approach, can be applied to patients and those who do not respond favourably are resisting opportunities for recover. Staff experienced some patients as critical complaining that, *Some patients will just criticise. Some of them might not be compliant to anything but you take the steps to try and encourage them.*

Symptoms provoke staff anxiety and a standard way of dealing with the otherwise overwhelming sense of powerlessness is evoked by recognising that the interventions are useless and managed by dismissal of the patient instead of the intervention, throwing out the baby but retaining the bathwater. Staff were constantly concerned with bed occupancy levels including the number of involuntary admissions. An observed discussion on the highest number of involuntary admission experienced since the change in mental health legislation (Government of Ireland, 2001) had the explicit purpose of changing patients' legal status or discharging them from care is summarised here in the words of the treating doctor, '*I am sending her home, she is no better*'. This decision to discharge the patient with no apparent improvement went unquestioned by the five staff present. Literature indicated that difficult and recalcitrant patients are transferred, discharged or scapegoated (DeBoard, 2005; Freud, 1915; Menzies Lyth, 1988; Miller & Gwynne, 1972). The conversation shifted seamlessly to

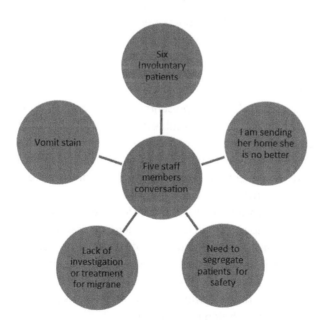

Diagram 1. Unconscious aspects of staff discourse.

removing a vomit stain from a carpet and another patient being cared for in the high observation area to protect her from the patient being considered for discharge that she had a disagreement with (Diagram 1).

In the staff discussion, the recalcitrant patient appears to be unconsciously connected to a vomit stain that needs to be erased, it is as if she does not deserve care or segregation for safety, her presence could be understood as a reminder of failure in the system. Following the decision to discharge the discussion shifts to writing her a prescription. The doctor asks why she had a regular prescription for migraine medication and decides to exclude it. There appeared to have been no investigation of a possible link to having a migraine and requiring admission to services or any discussion relating to the intervention of admission to hospital having failed. The failed intervention leads to a decision to dismiss the patient, its quality is unquestioned and the locus of control for the failure is attributed to the patient.

Incident 3 – the sinking ship

During a patient's review in a day hospital, the staff debated a patient requesting discharge and referral to a community clinic. The patient's request did not match the staff plan so the first thing discussed was a justification for excluding patients in general from the review process, *I don't know whether the team meeting with the patients sitting in is necessary a good thing, sometimes it's more stressful for the patient's than the illness itself*. The patient requesting discharge is putting himself in the place of subject who knows (Lacan, 1993), is excluded from the meeting and labelled as uncooperative. Staff refer the decision to the consultant, the big Other (Kanter, 2007; Vanheule & Verhaeghe, 2003), who if he supports staffs' recommendation will be lavished with unconscious love and if he rejects it will be subject to disapproval alongside a deepening dislike for the patient. In this incident, Lacan's big Other is symbolically represented as the Consultant who as lead clinician represents conscious and unconscious ideas of authority, power and knowledge, a subject who has expertise and knowledge about the patient than they themselves lack. Perceiving patients, who evoke anxiety, as troublesome is repetition of a pattern in the social world. Transference of feelings onto the patient not justified by the situation is due to the readiness for feelings derived from somewhere else to emerge; the patient merely provides opportunity for their expression. Transference appeared in the findings as a desire to keep the patient in hospital where love can be lavished on him. Transference can have a welcoming or positive quality or appear hostile and negative, a reversal into the opposite occurs (Freud, 1914). The declaration that the patient who has a history of repeated admissions and has migrated across Europe is seeking discharge is *'showing his true colours'* is presented here as a defence against overwhelming transference.

This case management illustrates repetition of abandonment by staff, and anticipated 'passage a l'acte'[1] (Evans, 2005, p. 136) by the patient, the team is complicit in a desire that the symptom would be repeated. There is no review of their desire expressed at a multidisciplinary team meeting that the patient emigrates and only vague recognition of repetitive action. 'Untamed instincts can assert themselves before there is time to put the reigns of transference on them, or that the bonds which attach the patient to the treatment are broken by him in a repetitive action', (Freud, 1912, p. 154). The work of the analyst to keep the analysand in analysis as 'one cannot overcome an enemy who is absent or not within range' (Freud, 1912, p. 152) is reversed in mental health. Staff do not put the reins of transference on the patient and actively encourage the repetitive action of abandonment. This hope for passage a lacte' has a paradoxical quality as an action of this kind is spontaneous; here, it appears as an unconscious team wish that has the potential to be transmitted to the patient. This warrants exploration from the perspective of the patient's history of being abandoned and abandoning, alongside staff's complicity. There is repetition of the past in the present and the quality of the intervention is unquestioned; instead, the patient's commitment is considered questionable.

Lacan cautions against just seeing transference as a repetition, reminding us that if something cannot be remembered, it is repeated in behaviour. 'This behaviour in order to reveal what it repeats, is handed over to the analyst's reconstructions', (Lacan, 1994, p. 194). The patient has handed over something to the team to reconstruct. Transference is the transference of power from the patient/subject to staff/Other described as follows by a patient, *Each nurse is allocated so many patients so that they would speak to them during the course of the day and they would write up notes. Observe them like how are they feeling, their mood, if they are eating, if they are getting involved in things and that. They would write up the notes and they would be given to the doctor. The doctor would then review you, so that nurse is responsible for you all the time.*

The patient, seeking truth, assumes its location in the staff. *The nurse is responsible for you* is the point at which the locus of power to provide the answer containing the truth of the subject shifts from the patient to the nurse. There is a struggle between the staff and the patient, 'between intellect and instinctual life, between understanding and seeking to act' (Freud, 1912, p. 108). This struggle is played out in the transference and 'it is on this field that the victory must be won' (Freud, 1912, p. 108). The data evidence this shift in the locus of control and an attempt from at least one member of the team to reconstruct what is happening in relation to the sinking ship critical incident: *he has gained insight since I first met him. We should provide everything – leave everything open to him.* In the ensuing team conflict, one member argues for exploration of the patient's unconscious and ongoing engagement in psychotherapeutic work: *he needs containment, some kind of movement to changing things internally.* Another carries the hope that he will leave, *we hope to move him along quickly* and a third maintains the position that he is already lost, *the ship is sinking quickly – he sees the crisis all around him*. The patient has needs and longings which (Freud, 1917b) should be kept active in order to impel him to do the necessary work to make changes, but his needs and longings are resisted. This patient's actions and stories have brought staff resistance to the fore, resistance to the recalcitrant patient and each other's ideas. My analysis is that they are unable to trust each other enough to speak about failing; therefore, they hope the patient will leave, allowing them to ignore what is happening at a team level.

> Transference is essentially resistance. The transference is the means by which the communication of the unconscious is interrupted, by which the unconscious closes up again. Far from being the handing over of powers to the unconscious, the transference is, on the contrary, it's closing up. (Lacan, 1994, p. 130)

It is effectively closed up by staff resistance with simultaneous displays of identification with the leader and contagion of affect. (Freud, 1921; Leader & Groves, 1995)

Discussion

The tobacco pouch, the vomit stain and the sinking ship are all critical incidents where patients provide staff with opportunities to operate either at the lowest common denominator imposed by the group or to rise above it (Freud, 1921). The patients are demanding a demand be made of them. The critical incidents presented in this paper were not managed by opening a dialogue with the patient; instead, they were managed by the imposition of restrictions or pseudo-treatment reflecting the challenges imposed by the work when staff supports and appropriate supervision are unavailable. Incidents of acting out by service occupants are a consequence of the failure to work with transference (Harari, 2001; Main, 1957; Shur, 1994). Acting out is the demand for love and the attempt to avoid anxiety and was observed in patients and staff's response to the system. Staff activities, attending to bureaucratic tasks, are designed to keep the patients at bay and can only be tolerated for so long; eventually, there is no choice but to act out, to demand a libidinal response to reduce anxiety. The findings indicated that staff interventions with critical incidents mirror patient and their family's behaviours resulting in repetition rather than resolution. The management of critical incidents by evoking a Master discourse (Fink, 1995) and the power of the leader evidenced unrecognised and unmediated transference. The lack of any consistent coordinated clinical supervision for the mental health staff confines retrospective analysis of critical incidents to a bureaucratic reporting system. This ensures that critical incidents are not subjected to any consistent exploration of the conscious or unconscious processes that are influencing patient and staff interactions. Instead, analysis is confined to a University discourse (Foucault, 2006; Loose, 2002) which seeks material rather than psychical evidence to elucidate what has occurred. Consequently, the only solutions that can be brokered are based in tangible physical and procedural changes such as rules, protocols, policies and the physical environment, all of which maintain the status quo.

Critical incidents need topographical exploration, an exploration for the place where something became unconscious, enabling the lifting of repression (Freud, 1912). Instead, what is promptly re-established is an earlier experience of the Other and the associated repression is represented in the transference. Symptoms are a route to the unconscious and carry meaning. The symptom may have undergone several displacements, but has at its root a formation that needs uncovering and understanding, the 'replacing of what is unconscious by what is conscious' (Freud, 1917b, p. 486). This enables the lifting of repressions, removal of the preconditions for the formation of symptoms and allows pathological unconscious formations to be transformed into normal formations; then, it is possible to find solutions. This is a significant difference between a psychoanalytic and a psychiatry understanding of the symptom. While psychiatry remains dominant in the mental health services, other professions such as mental health nursing and psychology will struggle not to be overshadowed by its powerful influence. Psychoanalysis does not initially seek to remove symptoms; the emphasis is on finding meaning, whereas psychiatry aims to remove or contain them. The finding that patients and staff who act out are not encouraged to speak is central to this study. It demonstrates that study participants regardless of their role (patient or staff) were limited by the service structure built around a single model of care. This leads to an unconscious resistance to change transmitted by becoming being part of the group. The lack of opportunity to engage in psychotherapy, open dialogue or clinical supervision to counter balance the toll of occupying a demanding anxiety-provoking environment ensures the continuation of a system where transference has a negative colouration. The response to critical incidents is a rush of activity to reduce or remove the object/subject, the placement of the patient in a place of safety and a shutting down of the incident. The staff member is rarely removed or transference and remains unanalysed, staff fail as subjects supposed to know and the patient is unconsciously directed to additional incidents of acting out which feeds staffs' misplaced belief in their worth. The unspoken becomes an unavoidable observation which returns us to Harari's (2001) equation on the outcome of the absence of analysis where acting out equates to absent transference management.

This indicates that patients experience the demand to act out as more powerful than the symptoms they first experienced. Critical incidents are misunderstood as a demand for attention rather than a demand for demand. Patients and staff who act out are bypassing the Other; it is a virtual transference. The Other has symbolically failed the subject. Being with and providing a framework for symbolic work is absent and the subject regresses to a primitive or pre-symbolic way of acting.

Critical incidents are reducible if staff operated differently on two levels; firstly, learning the skills to manage transference; however, knowledge alone is insufficient. Therefore, secondly, additional learning to better accept negative feeling towards patients who act out by developing awareness of the mechanism of transference is required. This does not imply that all staff should be psychoanalysts; rather, they should reconsider the importance of the subject–Other relationship's contribution to patients and their own unconscious structures. Lacan argues that the model by which transference is used in analysis is not that different from how we manage it naturally and the model of analysis which gives transference a structural quality could be used to introduce the 'universality of the application' (Lacan, 1994, p. 125). This is particularly important for consideration in services from which two conclusions can be drawn; firstly, and most unlikely, all staff are suffering from a constitutional lack to utilise their natural qualities to manage transference. Or, secondly, and more likely, membership of the group unconsciously prohibits the use of this natural skill. This power of the group to inhibit therapeutic work was identified as *a tendency to be influenced* by staff new to the system.

To demand is not the same as to ask for. If demand is not met, the Other is bypassed by the subject, the Other is no longer the subject supposed to know and virtual transference is demonstrated in savage acting out. Harari's (2001) signifier 'savagery' evokes Klein's (1952) object relations theory, Freud's (1921) identification of regression to primitive states, Menzies Lyth's (1988) commentary on defence mechanisms and the savage attacks that patients commit on themselves. This is frequently met with a countertransference response from staff leaving the overwhelmed patient Otherless in directing their libidinal energy. The subject supposed to know becomes the subject who does not know, a direct consequence of failure in responding appropriately or providing an analytic discourse. Main (1957) noted that when staff learnt how to better accept negative feeling to patients who acted out, the need to rely on medication to manage critical incidents dropped dramatically. If the demand in services shifts from a demand for demand to a demand to follow routine, obey rules and accept treatments, the destructive negative nature of admission emerges and creates a situation where intense transference occurs but in unworthy forms, or, paraphrasing Freud, it amounts to nothing less than mental bondage with erotic colouring (Freud, 1912, p. 101). The patient accepts or rejects the rules to gain a libidinal response from staff. For staff, the issue is built around a conflict; a choice has to be made between the unconscious influence of the group which is built around the lowest common denominator and the rules set out by society for service delivery (Freud, 1921). However, the element of choice may go unrecognised under the powerful unconscious group influence. Lacking analytic discourse and unconscious aspects of critical incidents remain unexplored; the meaning of the symptom can only be speculated on and understood at the level of behaviour; when understood as a symptom, the jouissance for patient and staff becomes discernible.

Conclusion

In this paper, I am advocating the use of 'natural skills' around managing the subject–Other relationship, not rebuilding the service to deliver psychoanalysis to patients as the reader might expect. The initial place for psychoanalysis in services is with the staff rather than patients, as psychoanalytic practice in the form of supervision has the potential to free staff from the bondage of the social dynamic created by the group in which they operate. If staff were de-incarcerated, if the system was, as desired by one participant, *much more pluralistic kind of equalised kind of thing where you would have different perspectives cohering in some useful fashion*, they would be positioned to demand a demand from the patient. Reflection on the nature and conduct of work is required. Reflection is a problematic word indicative of looking at an image of the self, a reversed fixed image that is captivating and narcissistic. Beyond reflection analysis is required, a deconstruction of the imaginary (Fotaki, 2010, p. 704) in which services are psychically deconstructed alongside analysis of their component parts, the occupants. A process of clinical supervision is required for staff that enables analysis of their needs and society demands. Broad societal questions need to be superimposed on the specific situation so that national, local and individual unconscious beliefs are examined. This could be facilitated via a psychoanalytic-orientated supervision which does not require the participants to have a psychoanalytic training (Balint, 1957). If we demand something of ourselves, we can demand something of the subject who is the patient.

The findings concur with the literature that in the study site transference is omnipresent, unacknowledged and unmanaged in subject–Other relationships leading to a powerful negative effect on therapeutic alliances (Freud, 1912; Lacan, 1960–1961). Refusal to recognise what is being projected from the past exhibits resistance and repression and a disavowal of failures of the current situation that staff and patients operate in. This inhibits opportunities for productive therapeutic work and promotes the status quo which is of scant benefit to the patients and prevents any progresses towards a practice focused on the provision of an enabling environment for the emergence of truth and recovery. In the study site, the system fails its inhabitants primarily through the non-action and non-engagement of staff exhibited in their efforts to keep patients at bay. Distorted use of transference allowed subjects to repeat and fail to work through the structure created by primary relationships. Participants in this study failed to recognise the unconscious equating to the primary object of the (m)Other and the later imposition of the name of the father (Lacan, 1993, p. 22). When there is no controlled interpretation of transference which could be achieved by the provision of appropriate clinical supervision, there is a subsequent lack of transference management and interpretation. The study site and occupants had the potential but not the opportunity for growth, development and change, it is troublesome for all its occupants.

Note

1. Passage a l'acte denotes an exiting from the scene which differentiates it from acting out where the person remains in the scene; the difference here is that acting out is a symbolic message to the big Other and 'passage a lacte' is an exit from the symbolic order to the real, a flight from the Other.

Disclosure statement

No potential conflict of interest was reported by the author.

ORCID

Gerard Patrick Moore ⓘ http://orcid.org/0000-0002-2717-433X

References

Balint, M. (1957). *The doctor, his patient and the illness*. New York, NY: International Universities Press Inc.

Bicknell, M., & Liefooghe, A. (2005). *Jouissance in an evermore stressful world*. Paper presented at the 22nd Annual Meetings of the International Society for the Psychoanalytic Study of Organizations Baltimore, Maryland, USA. Retrieved from http://library.ispso.org/library/jouissance-evermore-stressful-world

Bion, W. R. (1990). *Experiences in groups and other papers*. London: Rathbone Books.

Burkard, S. (1999). Psychotic organization as a metaphoric frame for the study of organizational and interorganizational interorganizational dynamics. *Administration and Society, 5*, 588–615.

Comerford, H. (2010). *'Creatures of each other'? Reflections on the mutuality of the construction of boundaries/barriers between society and the mentally Ill* [Online]. Retrieved from May 15, 2016, from http://www.isop.org/Symposia/Melbourne/Comerford.htm

DeBoard, R. (2005). *The psychoanalysis of organizations*. London: Routledge.

Diamond, M. A. (1993). *The unconscious life of organizations. interpreting organisational identity*. London: Quorum Books.

Erlich-Ginor, M., & Erlich, S. (1998). Mental health under fire: Organizational interventions in a wounded service. Retrieved from http://www.isop.org/Symposia/Jerusalem/1998erlich-ginor.htm

Evans, D. (2005). *An introductory dictionary of lacanian psychoanalysis*. London: Routledge.

Fenichel, O. (1946). *The psycho-analytic theory of neurosis*. London: Routledge & Kegan Paul.

Fink, B. (1995). *The Lacanian subject between Language and Jouissance*. Princeton, NJ: Princeton University Press.

Fook, J., & Cooper, L. (2003). *Bachelor of social work fieldwork manual*. Monash, UP. Dept. of Social Work, School of Primary Health Care. Print.

Fotaki, M. (2010). Why do public policies fail so often? Exploring health policy making as an imaginary and symbolic construction. *Organisation, 17*, 703–720.

Foucault, M. (2006). *History of Madness*. (J. Murphy, & J. Khalfa, Trans.). London: Routledge.

Freud, S. (1912). *The Dynamics of Transference* (J. Strachey, Trans.) Case History of Schreber, Papers on Technique and Other Works (Vol. XII, pp. 97-108). London: Vintage Hogarth Press. (Reprinted from: 2001).

Freud, S. (1914). *On Narcissism: An Introduction* (J.F. Strachey & A., Trans.) An Infantile Neurosis and Other Works (Vol. XVII). London: Vintage Hogarth Press. (Reprinted from: 1995).

Freud, S. (1915). *Observations on Transference-Love* (J. Strachey, Trans.) Case Histories of Schreiber, Papers on Technique and Other Works (Vol. XII). London: Vintage Hogarth Press. (Reprinted from: 2001).

Freud, S. (1917a). *Transference* (A. F. James Strachey, A. Strachey, & A. Tyson, Trans.) Introductory Lectures on Psychoanalysis (Part III) (Vol. XVI, pp. 431–447). London: Vintage The Hogarth Press. (Reprinted from: 2001).

Freud, S. (1917b). *A difficulty in the path of psychoanalysis* (J. Strachey, A. Freud, A. Strachey, & A. Tyson, Trans.) An Infantile Neurosis and Other Works (Vol. XVIII). London: Vintage Hogarth Press. (Reprinted from: 2001).

Freud, S. (1921). *Group psychology and the analysis of the Ego* (A. F. James Strachey, A. Strachey, & A. Tyson, Trans.) Beyond the Pleasure Principle Group Psychology and Other Works (Vol. XVIII). London: Vintage Hogarth Press. (Reprinted from: 2001).

Glynos, J., & Stavrakakis, Y. (2002). *Lacan and science*. London: Karnack.

Government of Ireland (2001). *Mental health act*. Dublin: The Stationary Office.

Harari, R. (2001). *Lacan's Seminar on 'Anxiety'*. (J. Lamb-Ruiz, C., Trans., 1st ed.). New York, NY: Other Press.

Hollway, W., & Jefferson, T. (2007). *Doing qualitative research differently, free association, narrative and the interview method*. London: Sage.

Kanter, J. (2007). Compassion fatigue and secondary traumatization: A second look. *Clinical Social Work Journal, 35*, 289–293.

Klein, M. (1952). The origins of transference. *The International Journal of Psycho-analysis, 33*, 433–438.

Lacan, J. (1960–1961). Transference unedited (ed.) The seminar of jacques Lacan book VIII. Retrieved from http://www.lacaninireland.com/web/wp-content/uploads/2010/06/THE-SEMINAR-OF-JACQUES-LACAN-VIII-Draft-21.pdf

Lacan, J. (1993). *ECRITS a selection*. London: Routledge Press.

Lacan, J. (1994). *The four fundamental concepts of psycho-analysis*. (A. Sheridan, Trans., 1st ed.). London: Penguin Books.

Leader, D., & Groves, J. (1995). *Lacan for beginners*. Cambridge: Icon Books.

Long, S., & Newton, J. (1997). *Collaborative action research in an organisation: Can psychoanalytically informed thinking deepen the collaboration?* Paper presented at the 14th Annual Meeting of the International Society for the Psychoanalytic Study of Organizations, Philadelphia, PA. Retrieved from http://library.ispso.org/library/collaborative-action-research-organisation-can-psychoanalytically-informed-thinking-deepen-c

Loose, R. (2002). *The subject of addiction*. London: Karnac.

Main, T. (1957). *The ailment*. New York, NY: New York University Press.

Menzies Lyth, I. (1988). *Containing anxiety in institutions selected essays* (Vol. 1). London: Free Association Books.

Menzies Lyth, I. (1989). *The dynamics of the social selected essays* (Vol. 2). London: Free Association Books.

Miller, E. J., & Gwynne, G. V. (1972). *A life apart*. London: Tavistock Publications.

Moore, G. (2012). *A psychoanalytic investigation of transference management in the Irish adult public mental health services* (PhD thesis). Dublin City University. Retrieved May 15, 2016, from http://doras.dcu.ie/17515/1/

Parker, I. (2005). Lacanian discourse analysis in psychology: Seven theoretical elements. *Theory & Psychology, 15*, 163–182.

Parker, I. (2008). Psychoanalytic theory and psychology: Conditions of possibility for clinical and cultural practice. *Theory & Psychology, 18*, 147–165.

Reggio, D., & Novello, M. (2007). An interview with Dr. Jean Oury. *Radical Philosophy, 143*, 32–46.

Rowan, A. (2000). The place of acting out in psychoanalysis: From Freud to Lacan. *Psychoanalytic Perspective, 41*, 83–100.

Shur, R. (1994). *Counter-transference enactment how institutions and therapist actualize primitive internal worlds* (1st ed., Vol. 1). London: Jason Aronson INC.

Vanheule, S., & Verhaeghe, P. (2003). *'Slave labour and mastery': A psychanalytic study of professional burnout* (Doctor in der Psychologische Wetenschappen), University of Ghent, Ghent. Retrieved from http://lib.ugent.be/fulltxt/RUG01/000/774/608/RUG01-000774608_2010_0001_AC.pdf

Wallace, E. R. (1983). *Freud and anthropology* (1st ed., Vol. 1). New York, NY: International University Press, INC.

World Health Organisation. (2006). *Stress management in emergency deployment*. Geneva: World Health Organization.

The impact of professional role on working with risk in a home treatment team

Maxine Sacks and Maria Iliopoulou

ABSTRACT

The purpose of the Home Treatment Team (HTT) is to respond rapidly and appropriately to those experiencing a mental health crisis. This has been found to be effective in reducing hospital admissions and is popular with patients who value the option of being offered home visits instead of hospital admission. Most staff in mental health work with high-risk situations but this is the main focus of the HTT. The authors used interpretative phenomenological analysis to explore how the staff of a well-established HTT experience risk. Twenty-four staff attended five focus groups over a two-month period. Invited to talk about risk in general all of the groups focused on unusual risk events; aggression and violence and challenging suicidal behaviour. The discussions revealed the different ways that professional identity can impact on risk management. The findings have the potential to help staff to work in a more self-aware way and to help teams develop more effective procedures.

EL IMPACTO DEL ROLE PROFESIONAL EN EL TRABAJO DE UN EQUIPO DE TRATAMIENTO EN EL HOGAR, EN SITUACIONES DE RIESGO

El objetivo del Equipo de Tratamiento en el Hogar (ETH), es responder rápida y adecuadamente a las personas que experimentan crisis de salud mental, lo cual ha sido efectivo. De esta manera se reduce el número de admisiones hospitalarias y los pacientes valoran la opción de ser vistos en sus hogares en lugar de ser hospitalizados. La mayoría del personal de salud mental trabaja aen situaciones de alto riesgo siendo éste el principal objetivo del ETH. Los autores usaron análisis interpretative fenomenológico (AIF) para explorar cómo el personalde un bien establecido ETH experimentó riesgo durante sus labores. Venticuatro integrantes del equipo asistieron a cinco grupos durante dos meses. Al hablar de su experiencia todos los participantes enfocaron situaciones de riesgos no commumes: agresión y violencia y conducta suicida. Las discusiones revelaron las marcadas diferencias en las cuales la identidad professional impacta el manejo del riesgo. Se espera que los resultados puedan ayudar al personal a estar más consciente de estas sitauciones de manera que puedan ayudar a otros equipos a desarrollar procedimientos efectivos en este campo.

L'impatto del ruolo professionale sulla percezione del rischio nel lavoro di una squadra di trattamento domiciliare che opera in favore della salute mentale

Lo scopo del team di trattamento domiciliare (HTT) è rispondere in modo rapido e adeguato a coloro che presentano critiche condizioni di salute mentale. Si tratta di un trattamento di comprovata efficacia nel ridurre i ricoveri ospedalieri ed è comune con i pazienti che apprezzano la possibilità di avere visite a domicilio in sostituzione del ricovero ospedaliero. La maggior parte di coloro che lavorano nell'ambito della salute mentale incontra situazioni ad alto rischio, ma gestire queste situazioni è l'obiettivo principale del HTT. Gli autori hanno utilizzato l'analisi fenomenologica interpretativa (IPA) per esplorare le percezioni del rischio del personale con consolidata esperienza HTT. Ventiquattro persone hanno preso parte a cinque gruppi di discussione per un periodo di due mesi. Invitati a parlare di rischio, in generale, tutti i gruppi si sono concentrati su eventi di rischio inusuali, quali l'aggressione, la violenza e il comportamento suicidario. Le discussioni hanno evidenziato le modalità in cui l'identità professionale ha un impatto sulla gestione del rischio. I risultati emersi potrebbero aiutare i professionisti della salute mentale a lavorare in modo più consapevole e a sviluppare procedure di intervento più efficaci.

L'impact du rôle professionnel au sein d'une équipe de soin à domicile travaillant avec des situations à risque

L'objectif d'une équipe de soin à domicile (HTT) est de répondre rapidement et de manière adéquate à ceux qui traversent une crise psychiatrique Il a été démontré que ce type d'intervention peut réduire les admissions à l'hôpital et est populaire auprès des patients qui préfèrent l'option de traitement à domicile comme alternative à une hospitalisation. La plupart des équipes travaillant dans le champ de la santé mentale travaillent avec des situations à haut risque qui constituent cependant l'axe principal du travail des HTT. Les auteurs de cet article ont utilisé la méthode IPA (analyse interprétative phénoménologique) pour explorer l'expérience que le personnel d'une équipe HTT bien établie a du risque. Vingt-quatre membres de l'équipe ont pris part à cinq groupes de discussion sur une période de deux mois. Invités à parler du risque en général, tous les groupes se sont concentrés sur des évènements inhabituels présentant un risque ; sur l'agression et la violence et les comportements suicidaires difficiles à gérer. Les discussions ont révélé les différentes façons dont l'identité professionnelle peut avoir un impact sur la gestion du risque. Les résultats peuvent potentiellement aider le personnel à travailler de manière plus réflexive et aider les équipes à développer des procédures plus effectives.

Η επίδραση του επαγγελματικού ρόλου στην εργασία με συνθήκες επικινδυνότητας σε μια ομάδα περίθαλψης στο σπίτι

Στόχος της Ομάδας Περίθαλψης στο Σπίτι (ΟΠΣ) αποτελεί η άμεση και κατάλληλη ανταπόκριση στα άτομα που βιώνουν μια κρίση ψυχικής υγείας. Έχει βρεθεί ότι αυτή η προσέγγιση είναι αποτελεσματική όσον αφορά τη μείωση του αριθμού των εισαγωγών σε νοσοκομείο και είναι δημοφιλής ανάμεσα σε αυτούς τους ασθενείς που εκτιμούν το να έχουν την επιλογή για κατ' οίκον επισκέψεις αντί της νοσοκομειακής εισαγωγής. Οι περισσότεροι επαγγελματίες που εργάζονται στο χώρο της ψυχικής υγείας αντιμετωπίζουν περιπτώσεις υψηλής επικινδυνότητας, αλλά στην περίπτωση της ΟΠΣ αυτό αποτελεί το βασικό στοιχείο. Οι συγγραφείς χρησιμοποίησαν την Ερμηνευτική Φαινομενολογική Ανάλυση (ΕΦΑ) για να διερευνήσουν τον τρόπο με τον οποίο βιώνει την επικινδυνότητα το προσωπικό μιας καλά εδραιωμένης ΟΠΣ. Είκοσι τέσσερα μέλη του προσωπικού συμμετείχαν σε πέντε ομάδες εστίασης σε διάστημα δύο μηνών. Με βάση την πρόσκληση των ερευνητριών να μιλήσουν γενικά για την επικινδυνότητα, όλες οι ομάδες εστίασαν σε ασυνήθιστα περιστατικά επικινδυνότητας, στην επιθετικότητα και στη βία, και στην προκλητική αυτοκτονική συμπεριφορά. Οι συζητήσεις αποκάλυψαν τους διαφορετικούς τρόπους με τους οποίους η επαγγελματική ταυτότητα του προσωπικού μπορεί να επηρεάσει τη διαχείριση των κρίσεων. Τα ευρήματα μπορεί να βοηθήσουν το προσωπικό να εργάζεται με αυξημένη αυτεπίγνωση και τις ομάδες να αναπτύξουν πιο αποτελεσματικές διαδικασίες.

Context

The Home Treatment Team (HTT) offers treatment in their own homes to people suffering a mental health crisis. HTTs were rolled out across the UK in line with Department of Health (2001) which offered guidelines for setting up teams to meet the standards set out in Department of Health (1999) to provide effective mental health services within the NHS. Short-term funding was provided to establish the teams, once running it was anticipated that the HTTs would be funded by the savings generated by reduced hospital admissions.

Hospital admission can be stressful and disruptive. On leaving the ward people are frequently faced with the same difficulties that led to the admission, triggering a relapse that eventually leads to another admission. In addition, hospital stays are expensive and health services in the UK are facing increasing financial pressures.

Aim

The HTT works with those people at risk of self-harm or suicide who are judged to be capable of managing in their own homes with the right support. About 40% of patients attending the City and Hackney HTT have a diagnosis of depression or bipolar affective disorder, 35% have a diagnosis of psychosis and about 25% have a diagnosis of personality disorder. The local HTT also provides psychiatric liaison to the Accident and Emergency (A&E) service at the general hospital on the same site.

The success of the team depends on the ability of staff to deal with risk in the community on a daily basis. A number of authors have written about client attributes that influence the risk of suicide or violence. (Douglas et al., 1997; Joiner, 2007) but very little has been written about the experience of staff who work with these issues, although there is a literature on staff burnout (e.g. Miller, 1999). It was therefore appropriate to use a qualitative approach to begin to understand this area. We hoped that an understanding of the team experience of dealing with risk would prove helpful to the team by helping them to understand more about how they manage risk.

Method

We chose to use interpretative phenomenological analysis (IPA) because we wanted to understand the experience of the team. IPA is designed to 'explore in detail how participants are making sense of their personal and social world' (Smith & Osborn, 2008, p. 53). As described by Palmer, Larkin, De Visser, and Fadden (2010) 'The aim of IPA is to understand and make sense of another person's sense-making activities, with regard to a given phenomenon, in a given context'. As psychologists we were interested in how staff employed in an HTT experience working with risk. IPA appeared to be the right approach for this task because we were asking people to talk about events with a high level of salience, the kind of events that IPA is designed to investigate because they elicit rich responses from participants.

We chose to interview the staff in groups because we wanted to include all of the staff in the team and the use of groups would draw a 'larger sample into a smaller number of data collection events' (Palmer et al., 2010). We were confident that the discussions would provide rich data because the staff team is a 'naturally occurring group' (Palmer et al., 2010). It was anticipated that the staff would encourage each other to talk about their experience of risk. This is consistent with the IPA approach of encouraging people to 'speak about the topic with as little prompting from the interviewer as possible' (Smith & Osborn, 2008, p. 61).

The team consisted of 27 clinical staff including a team manager, a psychologist, nurses, social workers, OTs, two support workers, two consultant psychiatrists and two junior doctors. The focus of the groups was explained to the team and everyone was given a letter inviting them to participate. Participants were invited to sign a consent form which explained the process including that the discussions would be taped and quotes would be anonymised. In the event 24 staff participated in five focus groups; four groups consisted of five participants and one consisted of four. The focus group discussions were taped and transcribed verbatim.

Focus groups

The groups were facilitated by the researcher external to the team. The first question in the schedule was 'What are the risks that are managed by the team?' The facilitator had prepared further questions but in the event these were not used. Staff prompted each other to supply details of events and provided validating comments. The facilitator offered summaries and asked clarifying questions.

There were a range of experiences that could have been discussed in response to the opening questions but all five groups focused on two areas, aggression and violence and challenging suicidal behaviour. People brought some difficult events to the discussions including experiences from time when the team was first established, twelve years previously.

Analysis

For the purpose of analysis each of the five groups was treated as a participant. Each comment was coded in the conventional IPA manner then labelled with name of the group in which the comment had been made. In terms of the double hermeneutic of the IPA approach we, the researchers, were attempting to make sense of how the team experiences risk. The results were presented to the HTT for discussion and a subset of the data was presented to the London Regional IPA Group for validation.

Results

The analysis yielded 69 subthemes which fell into six main themes: Professional role and responsibility, Challenging presentations, History and current situation, Policies and procedures, Difficult emotions and Team culture. We organised the six main themes into two meta-themes. The first four themes were included in the meta-theme 'Managing risk in the context of caring for the client' and the final two themes were included in the meta-theme 'Managing the impact on ourselves' as shown in the Table 1. All of the themes were present in all of the groups but to differing extents.

Themes and Meta-themes.

Meta-themes	Themes
Managing risk in the context of caring for the client	• Professional role and responsibility • Challenging presentations • History and current situation • Policies and procedures
Managing the impact on ourselves	• Difficult emotions • Team culture

The purpose of the project was to help the team to understand how they manage risk. It was hoped that this might generate ideas to help the team to manage risk better in the future. Of the six themes that emerged the themes that offer the team the best opportunities for change are Professional role and responsibility, Policies and procedure and Team culture. This paper will discuss the impact of Professional role and responsibility.

Professional role and responsibility

We identified four subthemes within this main theme. Each of the four sub-themes appeared in all five focus groups:

(1)   Professional role.
(2)   Responsibility.
(3)   It's part of the job.
(4)   Understanding the client's perspective.

Professional role

The groups revealed that professional role is perceived as limiting how you can behave in a range of contexts. One participant felt that you cannot ask for an apology when you have been insulted at work. She had been racially abused by a patient but: 'At that point you need to be a professional person you can't reply – you have to act in a professional way'. This left her feeling bad because: 'They have taken my rights away – I was – I wasn't able to respond the way I wanted'. In another context she would have asked for an apology 'and that makes you feel better because you have responded and tell them that that's not nice' (Gp5).

Another member of staff cited the requirement to act professionally as her reason for meeting with the police before she had started to recover from an incident: 'I need to still face the police even though I was still scared – I still need to be like a professional – a professional person'. For this member of staff recovery did not start until the following day: 'At the end of the day – that night I didn't cope – I was quite upset' (GP1).

Three of the groups provided examples of patients taking minor overdoses. In all three instances staff felt that their professional role obliged them to deal with the event as if it was a significant overdose. They felt that the service was being used in an unhelpful way but felt that their role gave them no choice.

'Some of them will say they have taken four paracetamol tablets which is – I mean – slightly overdose – but the fact that he has taken it – as a professional I can't just go …' (Gp2).

Finally in this subtheme, a member of staff described his feelings when a patient took an overdose in front of him. His impulse was to intervene physically but his professional role did not allow this:

I was like confused – you know what. My heart said you I should stop this person from doing it – but then I thought – professionally – am I supposed to get involved and – um – I literally had to – kind of – go outside and say – look he has taken an overdose we need to call an ambulance. (Gp3)

Responsibility

Staff expressed a sense of responsibility for the actions and behaviour of patients and also expressed the converse, that patients were not responsible for their own actions. This had the effect of reducing the impact when patients were abusive because the behaviour could be seen as part of the illness rather than a personal attack. If 'you could attribute it to somebody being really genuinely ill it was a lot easier to deal with' (GP5). The alternative was 'if you felt that the person was well or didn't have mental health problems at the time then it's very difficult to justify why you have been exposed to violence' (Gp5).

Possibly related to the belief that patients could not be held responsible for their actions was the belief that staff are responsible for everything that takes place.

> I wasn't probably as observant and – or as receptive to what was happening at the time. So then … she…and – probably because I did have an agenda – she got quite frustrated. And it resulted in her trashing her flat … which … was very violent. (Gp1)

This staff member felt that her sense of being culpable for the client's behaviour could have been mitigated by debriefing but this event dated from the early days of the team when debriefing was not standard: 'So you are sort of left feeling quite responsible … for what had happened. Because there had been no debriefing' (Gp1).

Another colleague in the same group contributed his own similar experience:

> Because like (my colleague) I was – like – feeling maybe I had done something wrong, probably like my body language or the way that I spoke to her. Probably I was not… I started to think that probably I was maybe not very clear what I was saying. (Gp1)

Then a third participant expressed a similar perspective: 'And I thought, did I make this happen? Would he have reacted this way if I was a little more clear?' (Gp1).

Staff also expressed a sense of responsibility for mental health issues outside of their direct responsibility. The opening discussion in Group 5 was about an incident in which a patient started shouting in the waiting room in A&E. Everyone was frightened but the HTT staff member in psychiatric liaison felt that she had to deal with it: 'Because I am psych'. No one else stepped forward and she understood that they wanted to avoid risk. 'One of the A & E nurses was quite helpful but obviously everybody has to think of their safety'. She was also thinking of her safety but competing with that she was thinking of 'my role'. She added that she was 'trying to be helpful as well' (Gp 5).

A participant in another group felt that it was part of his job to reduce stigma by making sure that that people with mental problems were not perceived as dangerous. This could lead to a lack of attention to risk:

> I basically find myself in this split personality position where, even though I know it might be difficult or dangerous, or risky working with somebody, I cannot let the general public believe that the person I'm going to be seeing could be that. And from that position – yes – sometimes you can be going there with your guard a little bit lower than if I wasn't in that professional position. (Gp4)

Finally in the same group there was a participant who put himself at risk by intervening in an incident in the street. There was no obvious mental health involvement but he saw someone in difficulty and stepped forward to help. This then became a work incident when he had to complete an incident form. This reminds us that our colleagues are often strongly motivated to help others even when it is not part of their job:

> We saw a young girl we felt she had been intimidated by somebody else in the street and then we wanted to intervene by calling the police and this guy turned on me (laughter) – you remember I had to do the incident reporting. (Gp4)

It's part of the job

There was a sense that it was not acceptable to complain about or experience difficult emotions about stressful events that occurred in the course of the job. Staff felt that; 'a level of risk is part of the job' and 'you have to deal with it' (Gp5). 'It's much a part of what we do but obviously that doesn't make it any easier or any safer' (Gp5).

In another group a participant felt that she should not be upset by difficult events: 'It does not make me feel anything because I know it is – it is actually expected when we are working in this kind of client group' (Gp 2).

Understanding the client's perspective

A number of statements reflected attempts to see things from the client's point of view. This contained an element of risk management as staff described trying to assess risk by judging what the client was thinking and feeling. Staff also stated that developing good rapport could relax the client and avoid provoking paranoia. On the other hand there were statements which revealed that seeing things from the client's perspective can lead to risky situations.

An example of the latter was a participant in Group 5 who described going into a flat with a colleague despite their misgivings because the patient was begging them: 'We just felt uncomfortable – he was crying and very, very insistent that we came in – and he really wanted to talk to us'. Their discomfort proved well-founded when they were confronted by a machete on the kitchen table. In retrospect, despite the anxiety this provoked, she tried to see this from the client's point of view: 'Maybe he had the machete there because of – you know – he had no choice …' (Gp5).

Another participant in the same group reported a similar experience when a client: 'Started lifting – you know – raising up – his voice – so I had no choice'. He entered the flat knowing that it was risky and commented that: 'Fortunately nothing happened' (Gp5).

Similarly a participant said he would not ask more than one colleague to accompany him on a home visit, even when this was indicated by the risk, because of the possible impact on the client:

If you going to be saying – I can't see that one until four or five of us going – then you start thinking about – well – how is the patient or the service user going to feel if you are the professionals coming to see me – you come almost like the police – such a massive number. (Gp 4)

Another staff member pointed out that there could be a direct conflict between awareness of risk and building rapport: 'You become too focused on things – and then obviously that kind of affects your rapport' (Gp5).

Examples of using this perspective to manage risk include another participant in the same group speaking about the importance of building rapport to keep the patient calm: 'Good communication – whatever – I suppose it could make the patient more relaxed and stuff' and their awareness that trying too hard could backfire because: 'The patient may feel patronized and even – you know – aggravated' (Gp5).

Discussion

The focus groups revealed that the areas of risk that HTT staff find difficult are aggression and violence and challenging suicidal behaviour including self-harm executed in front of staff. The staff did not use the focus groups to talk about the mainstream work of the HTT, managing suicidal feelings and behaviours. The focus groups revealed the importance of debriefing. This was routine within the HTT at the time of the study but had not been when the team first started, and some staff had not had the chance to process difficult events from those years.

Elliott Jaques points out that while much of the decision-making in our jobs is dictated for us by rules and procedures other aspects are discretionary and require on-going decision-making. The compulsory rules and procedures are important because they 'limit uncertainty within manageable bounds' (Jaques, 1990, p. 126). Where the rules are unclear staff are responsible for decision-making. The material from this study invites us to consider the extent to which behaviour is dictated by rules and how decisions are made outside of the rules in relation to the management of risk.

The 'Professional role' subtheme reveals how staff perceive limits on their behaviour due to the job. This meant not asking for an apology and prioritising procedure over debriefing. It also meant following procedures for an overdose even when the overdose was unlikely to cause harm and not physically restraining a client from taking an overdose. The latter issues are policies but it is unclear whether the former are policies or whether this is an interpretation of what the role requires.

The 'Responsibility' subtheme illuminates some of the ways that decisions are made by this staff group. The decision to help the patient who was shouting in A&E (Gp5) appears to have been dictated by a sense of responsibility for anyone with mental health problems. However another member of staff states that 'all the medical teams expect us to deal with the clients' (Gp5) in A&E. This is consistent with the literature on the treatment of patients with mental health problems in A&E. Crowley (2000) found that general staff working in A&E find people with mental health problems hard to manage and are often unsympathetic to them. Perego (1999) found that A&E staff can feel unskilled and unconfident in dealing with mental health issues. This suggests that additional support and education for staff in A&E might take some of the pressure off the liaison staff to step forward whenever a mental health issue might be involved.

The 'Responsibility' subtheme shows that removing responsibility from the client because they are ill makes the aggression and violence easier to bear. However this leaves staff with a sense that they are responsible for everything that happens. One staff member mentioned that debriefing can help to mitigate this.

The subtheme 'Understanding the client's perspective' illustrates the importance of empathy in mental health work. The HTT staff talk about the importance of building rapport to reduce the client's feelings of anger and paranoia, thereby helping to manage risk. They also use their ability to understand the client's point of view as an on-going risk assessment. During a home visit staff try to work out what the client is thinking and feeling and what the implications of that might be. It is possible that this element of the work could be made more explicit in a way that could help staff to manage risk more effectively.

The 'It's part of the job' subtheme illustrates that staff do not feel justified in feeling upset or complaining about being subjected to violence and aggression by patients because it is part of their role.

Before starting the project the researchers met with an external advisor who highlighted the relevance of one of the researchers being embedded in the team. The researchers agreed that the external staff member would lead the focus groups and take responsibility for maintaining an external perspective throughout the project. The importance of this was highlighted during the analysis when the theme discussed in this paper emerged. The embedded staff member admitted that she found it hard to examine themes which might be perceived as revealing problems within the team. This illustrates the difficulty, in practice, of achieving Husserl's 'bracketing' of individual experience (Smith, Flowers, & Larkin, 2009). In the context of this project this was facilitated by the researchers maintaining a dialogue about the work from two different perspectives.

Conclusion

This project was designed to make the experience of managing risk explicit and help staff to think about how to make better use of their skills and resources. Locke (1976) suggests that job satisfaction is the result of appraising one's work in terms of the needs and values one has, and the possibilities for meeting these. The possibility for stress and burnout arises when this drive leads the professional to ignore other needs and community staff have been found to be particularly vulnerable to stress and burnout, in particular the emotional exhaustion component (Prosser et al., 1996).

The material from this study shows some of the ways that this can happen. Our staff have a strong sense of responsibility and are motivated to help others. Their interpretation of their role can encourage them to take risks and fail to look after themselves emotionally, including not acknowledging when they feel upset. This could be an area where understanding their own responses could help staff to look after themselves better.

Other strategies suggested by this study include improved education about mental health for colleagues in A&E, regular debriefing after difficult or stressful events, explicit rules about the limits of the job and reflection on the circumstances in which staff might be tempted to compromise their safety.

Acknowledgements

The authors would like to thank the City and Hackney Home Treatment Team whose skilled work inspired this research and who gave their time to the focus groups and subsequent discussions.

Disclosure statement

No potential conflict of interest was reported by the authors.

References

Crowley, J. J. (2000). A clash of cultures: A&E and mental health. *Accident and Emergency Nursing, 8*, 2–8.

Department of Health. (1999). *Mental health national service framework*. London: Department of Health.

Department of Health. (2001). *The mental health policy implementation guide*. London: Department of Health.

Douglas, K. S., Ogloff, J. R. P., & Nichols, K. L. (1997, August). *Violence by psychiatric patients: Validity of the HCR-20 scheme and psychopathy checklist: Screening version*. Paper presented at the annual convention of the American Psychiatric Association, Chicago, IL.

Jaques, E. (1990). *Creativity and work*. Connecticut: International Universities Press.

Joiner, T. (2007). *Why people die by suicide*. Cambridge: Harvard University Press.

Locke, E. A. (1976). The nature and causes of job satisfaction. In M. D. Dunes (Ed.), *Handbook of industrial and organisational psychology* (pp. 1297–1349). Chicago, IL: Rand McNally.

Miller, D. (1999). *Dying to care: Work, stress and burnout in HIV/AIDS*. London: Routledge.

Palmer, M., Larkin, M., De Visser, R., & Fadden, G. (2010). Developing an interpretative phenomenological approach to focus group data. *Qualitative Research in Psychology, 7*, 1–22.

Perego, M. (1999). Why A&E nurses feel inadequate in managing patients who deliberately self-harm. *Emergency Nurse, 6*, 24–27.

Prosser, D., Johnson, S., Kuipers, E., Szmukler, G., Bebbington, P., & Thornicroft, G. (1996). Mental health, 'burnout' and job satisfaction among hospital and community based mental health staff. *British Journal of Psychiatry, 169*, 334–337.

Smith, J. A., & Osborn, M. (2008). Interpretative phenomenological analysis. In J. A. Smith (Ed.), *Qualitative psychology: A practical guide to methods* (pp. 214–224). London: Sage.

Smith, J. A., Flowers, P., & Larkin, M. (2009). *Interpretative phenomenological analysis: Theory method and research*. London: Sage.

From victimhood to sisterhood part II – Exploring the possibilities of transformation and solidarity in qualitative research

Leah Salter

ABSTRACT

This paper will build on 'From Victimhood to Sisterhood', previously published in this journal; to answer some of the questions posed to and by the author relating to the complexities of being a practice-based/insider researcher. The paper provides a context to the inter-related practices of the author as a psychotherapist, a group facilitator and a doctoral researcher; with particular reference to her work (as both a practitioner and researcher) with women who have been sexually abused. The (potentially isolating) context of practising in an island community alongside stories of connection is offered within a frame of 'solidarity'. Developing ideas from the first paper, which as a reflective piece, featured a first person, auto-ethnographic account of the author's practice, this paper positions itself more firmly as aligned with research as social action.

EXPLORANDO LAS POSIBILIDADES DE TRANSFORMACION DESDE LA VICTIMIZACION A LA SOLIDARIDAD ENTRE MUJERES

Este artículo se construirá a partir de uno previamente publicado en esta revista para responder a las preguntas de la autora en relación a las complejidades de ser una investigadora que trabaja con base en la práctica y a la vez dentro de una institución. El artículo proporciona un contexto a las prácticas inter-relacionadas de la autora como psicoterapeuta, como facilitadora de grupos y como investigadora para su tesis doctoral, con una referencia particular a su trabajo con mujeres que han sufrido abuso sexual. El contexto potencialmente aislador al trabajar en una comunidad que funciona en una isla, permite hilvanar hstorias de conexion dentro de un marco de solidaridad. El artículo anterior, como una pieza reflexiva escrita en primera persona y dando cuenta auto-etnográfica de la práctica de la autora, por una parte ha permitido el desarrollo de las ideas que presento ahora, y por otra, contribuye a establecer un enlace entre la investigación y la acción social.

Da vittimismo a sorellanza parte II - Esplorare le possibilità di trasformazione e di solidarietà nella ricerca qualitativa

Questo documento si baserà sul contributo "Da vittimismo a Sorellanza", già pubblicato in questa rivista, cercando di rispondere ad alcune delle domande poste all'autore in relazione alla complessità dell'essere un ricercatore dall'interno, che si basa sulla pratica. Il documento costituisce un'esperienza di pratiche interconnesse, poiché l'autore opera come psicoterapeuta, facilitatore di gruppo e ricercatore, con particolare riferimento al suo lavoro (sia come praticante che come ricercatore) con le donne che hanno subito abusi sessuali. L'ambito (potenzialmente isolato) è una comunità ove storie di legami sono presentate entro una cornice di "solidarietà". Il presente paper sviluppa idee a partire dal primo articolo, considerato come strumento di riflessione e caratterizzato da riferimenti auto-etnografici della pratica degli autori in prima persona, tuttavia si posiziona in modo più saldamente allineato alla ricerca quale azione sociale.

Du statut de victime à la solidarité féminine – seconde partie : Exploration des possibilités de transformation et de solidarité dans la recherche qualitative

Cet article se référera à l'article 'Du statut de victime à la solidarité féminine' publié dans un volume précédent de ce journal ; il tente de répondre à certaines des questions posées à et par l'auteur concernant les complexités associées au fait d'être une chercheuse 'de l'intérieur', ancrée dans la pratique. Cet article fournit un contexte aux pratiques associées de psychothérapeute, facilitatrice de groupe et doctorante avec une référence particulière faite au travail de l'auteur (en tant que praticienne et chercheuse) avec des femmes ayant subi des abus sexuels. Le contexte (potentiellement isolant) de pratique sur une île ainsi que des histoires de connexion sont proposés en référence à un cadre de « solidarité ». Développant des idées du premier article, écrit à la première personne pour refléter le travail de réflexion auto-ethnographique sur la pratique de l'auteur, le présent article est plus fermement aligné sur l'idée de recherche comme action sociale.

Από θυματοποίηση στην αδελφότητα μέρος II - Διερεύνηση των δυνατοτήτων του μετασχηματισμού και της αλληλεγγύης στην ποιοτική

Το παρόν άρθρο θα επεκτείνει το άρθρο «Από τη θυματοποίηση στην αδελφότητα» που είχε εκδοθεί παλαιότερα σε αυτό το περιοδικό, για να απαντήσει σε κάποιες ερωτήσεις που τέθηκαν προς και από την συγγραφέα σχετικά με τα σύνθετα ζητήματα που προκύπτουν όταν κανείς είναι «εκ των έσω» κλινικός ερευνητής. Το άρθρο προσφέρει ένα πλαίσιο για τις αλληλοπλεκόμενες πρακτικές της συγγραφέως ως ψυχοθεραπεύτριας, διευκολύντριας ομάδας και διδακτορικής ερευνήτριας με ιδιαίτερη αναφορά στην εργασία της (ως κλινικού και ερευνήτριας) με γυναίκες που έχουν κακοποιηθεί σεξουαλικά. Το (πιθανώς απομονωτικό) πλαίσιο εργασίας σε μια νησιωτική κοινότητα παράλληλα με τις ιστορίες προσφέρονται μέσα στο πλαίσιο της «αλληλεγγύης». Αναπτύσσοντας ιδέες από το πρώτο άρθρο το οποίο ως μια αναστοχαστική εργασία, περιέλαβε μια προσωπική αυτοεθνογραφική αφήγηση από την πρακτική των συγγραφέων, αυτό το άρθρο τοποθετείται απόλυτα ευθυγραμμισμένο με την έρευνα ως κοινωνική δράση.

Introduction

When I presented the beginnings of this research paper at a conference in Crete (May 2016) I presented some themes, feedback and personal reflections from my research into how women have 'gone on' following abuse and oppression, and following on from their involvement in a group for women who have been sexually abused. Inquiring into my practice as a Systemic Psychotherapist and group facilitator sits alongside the learning experience of being with the women who were part of the group. I conducted (what I have named as) 'conversational inquiries' with women I have co-facilitated groups with and women who have attended/been part of those groups. This is within a wider methodological frame of a narrative inquiry. Conversational inquiry is so named to mark out the dialogues that I am part of as different to a traditional interview. The tone is more conversational and pays attention to pre-existing relationships. What I am inquiring into is as much about the process of the inquiry as it is about the content of the dialogue.

At the time of the presentation, I had begun to make wider connections with the themes emerging from these conversations as they relate to the transformative nature of therapeutic group work practices and the dual process of research as a transformative practice in its own right. This paper demonstrates in many ways how this additional layer of dialogue has helped me to go on and develop those ideas.

The process of 'talking again' with women who had been part of a community of practice such as a therapeutic group was enabling new stories to emerge for the women who had been part of the group, and for myself; offering a new community context and a new layer of 'transformation' and 'solidarity'. Some of the questions that the presentation invoked focused on my role as a researcher-practitioner. As insider research, some questions were raised about validity and objectivity. These are important questions. Did my dual role affect the direction of the inquiry and the content of the conversations? Absolutely. Does this make the research less valid? I think this needs a longer dialogue, which hopefully this paper will offer a contribution to.

Insider research offers a voice from within practice, with the inquiry taking place within the organisation or group that the researcher is a member of. It is often criticised as being subjective and biased. It *is*, and as a researcher, I *am* biased, I have my own experiences and my own prejudices that shape the questions I ask, how I ask them and how I hear any response to them. But I also hold biases as a therapist, and I would as a researcher whether I was researching from within my own practice or not. Is it possible for research to be objective and unbiased when researchers are human beings with their own experiences and worldview that shape who they are, how they relate and how they go about the business of inquiring?

Insider research

If postmodern research 'accepts the inevitability of bias' in research (Van Heutgen, 2004) then insider research, I would suggest, helps to make bias visible (and potentially useful) by recognising the inevitability of bias in practice as well as in research. Patti Lather takes this further and highlights the 'inevitability of failure' of feminist research that is concerned with research as 'praxis'. Lather has written of feminist research as a doubled science, inextricably connected with experiences of loss and of being lost. It also, for me though, speaks to the dual role of an insider researcher, where we are engaged in researching our practice, critiquing our practice *and* critiquing the methods with which we inquire into/ use in our practice. Within such a 'minefield' of complexity, not least because of the multiple roles and relationships we are engaged in, getting lost, or at least losing our way at times, does feel inevitable. In naming failure though, Lather goes further to suggest that those researchers who are informed by feminism and social justice who are looking at the 'intersection of research, theory, and politics' are bound to fail in their intent to 'produce different knowledge, and to produce knowledge differently' (Lather, 2007).

> Always already swept up in language games that constantly undo themselves, we are all a little lost in finding our way into ethnographic practices that open to the irreducible heterogeneity of the other as we face the problems of doing feminist research in this historical time. (Lather, 2007, p. 149)

In this paper then, as a follow on from earlier work, I am positioning myself more firmly as an insider-researcher and as a feminist researcher concerned with the dual processes of practice and research and the inevitability of getting lost within the movement between the multiple relationships and multiple positions I take up.

> [I]nsiderness or outsiderness are not fixed or static positions, rather they are ever-shifting and permeable social locations ... (Naples, 1996, p. 140).

Going on

As a systemic psychotherapist and group practitioner I have become interested in, perhaps almost preoccupied with, ideas around how we 'go on' in our lives and make sense of our own stories of 'going on'. In my research I have been talking with women who have experiences of oppression and abuse, talking with them about how they go on in their lives following those experiences and how they go on following the end of a group work programme that has been part of their story. One of the questions I ask women in my conversational inquiry is 'what did/do we think we were/are making together (and how)?', followed on by 'what were/are we becoming?' and 'how were/are we contributing to better social worlds?'. The notion of 'going on' requires more than a nod to Wittgenstein (1953), who might suggest that there are multiple ways of 'going on'. John Shotter develops Wittgenstein's ideas of going on as a grounding for 'an inexhaustible source of new possibilities' (Shotter, 1994) that can be viewed as fluid and impermanent. It speaks therefore to movement and emergence which, for me, connects with the nature of insider research as both emergent and inherently relational.

The notion of (co)creating better social worlds also requires a reference point. I have used the frame of Co-ordinated Management of Meaning (Pearce & Cronen, 1980) to talk with women about how they/we have 'gone on' after the group(s) we have been part of and how we feel we have been/are 'contributing to better social worlds' (Pearce, 2007). I had thought of this as quite an abstract idea and one for which I imagined I would need to offer both a bridging explanation and an example. However, without exception, all of the women I spoke with responded positively to the question, in a way that suggested that this had immediate resonance for them, without the need for further explanation.

For example, in a group conversation I had with the group I facilitate for women who had experienced sexual abuse, in an island community one of the responses was …

Laura: I think we're able to speak out. I went to the paper with my story to help others to come forward. We're able to raise awareness and support others … You've taken a group who were mere shells of ourselves and turned us in to whole people.

Anna: (it's like) a butterfly effect. People don't stop (growing). We are always evolving, so the group may not grow (physically) but we will (go on). So our 'world' may be just this group of people but it will still grow and get bigger.

Laura has spoken out publicly about her experiences and anonymously shared her story of injustice with the local paper. She is one of the women who is most actively involved in getting the group set up as a community network and her commitment to that has been unwavering. In particular, she hopes to support women going through court cases and going on in their lives following court processes that often leave women still feeling unheard and invalidated. Laura experienced sexual abuse as a child and marital rape as an adult. She has fought for justice without the outcomes she has hoped for and remains understandably frustrated at the system. She has successfully used that energy to help to set up this support group for other women, to support others and to speak out against injustice. Anna also continues to support the cause of enabling women to speak out about their experiences and the energy generated in our conversations about the future direction of the group has been inspiring. Lucy, my co-facilitator of the group, named it in our group conversation as a 'Mexican wave', the energy from one person encouraging the next person, and so on. You might also call this 'solidarity' or 'social action'. This island community group have met with politically motivated support groups from other parts of the UK and made connections that have enabled them to feel part of a bigger movement through which they have experienced the unity that comes from women joining together in this way.

Feminist informed research has the same possibility to connect people across different cultures and communities to create new social worlds and new 'communities of practice', which speaks to research as 'joint enterprise' (Wenger, 1998) or what Shotter might call 'joint action'.

> In our living contacts with an other or otherness, then, our mere surroundings are transformed into 'a world', or at least, into a partially shared world that we sense ourselves as being in along with the others and othernesses around us. (Shotter, 2011, p. 1)

I have also been influenced by Laurel Richardson (1990), who suggests, as Patti Lather does, that research can and should go beyond a desire to impartially convey 'a truth' or 'truths' but should also be concerned with social justice, providing a 'sociological community' that helps form a 'shared consciousness' inviting social action on the part of the collective and creating the possibility for 'social transformation'. This has been one of the cornerstones of my research to date and is inextricably linked with my own experiences, my own stories of injustice and my own frustrations with hearing the stories of women who have experienced the double abuse of not having their experience validated at the level of relationship, community or society. Women's experiences of abuse continue to be unheard because they are unpalatable and difficult to hear. In the specific context of an island community they are also in direct opposition to the dominant discourse of island life as being safe, harmonious and idyllic. Women learn sophisticated ways to 'go on' living when the people who abused them are likely to be family members, members of the community and people they need to continue to have some form of relationship with. Of course, women who live in different communities also experience these kinds of issues; and the complexity of familial abuse is part of that story also. In a small and isolated community though the risks of telling have an additional meaning because the 'victim's' identity and personal story is likely to become public knowledge as much as that of the abuser.

The women I work with are also members of another kind of community as they are all women who access mental health services. The double stigma of being a 'victim' of abuse and a mental health service user is closely felt. Some women have also had the doubly injurious experience of having their experiences of abuse unheard and/or invalidated by the legal system because of their history of mental health difficulties. This is a painful and dangerous double-edged sword and one that I also feel as a systemic psychotherapist working in mental health services where practices become defined in a particular way.

There is continued tension for me in working within a system that has the potential to further oppress people by pathologising their social experiences and 'treating' the 'problem' as if it is one that is located within the person who has experienced the abuse; rather than looking outside at the systems that allow the abuse and the silencing of the abuse to continue. However, I have to balance my discomfort with the transformation I observe within and between women who attend these groups. I have come to see group processes as part of both working with, and challenging from within, the systems that can hold people paralysed in a position of blame and shame. A group context enables stories of pathology to be questioned, challenged and back-grounded whilst other stories of collective resistance and competence are brought to the fore. I see this as part of my role as facilitator *and* researcher, to maintain a position of solidarity within practice and research despite the tensions that abound.

In the predecessor of this paper (Salter, 2015), I spoke about the importance of my leanings towards Narrative Therapy as being one of the key ingredients in challenging the dominant discourse of the medical model and co-creating a space where 'preferred futures' (White, 1995) can be co-constructed, told and lived. This shows itself, I believe, in the excerpt earlier where Laura and Anna are speaking to a shaping of new identities for themselves but also a collective identity. Laura and Anna are part of a combined community stemming from three different groups that my colleague Lucy and I have now facilitated have built a strong community of practice that goes beyond the referred mental health service-based support group. These women have forged out a new identity for themselves and for their group, re-naming it in order to mark it out as something different to the initial group they were part of. They now hold three meetings per month. One meeting is for them to continue to offer support for (and listen to) each other, one meeting is a planning meeting with an eye to the potential future developments of such a group, and the other offers a 'drop-in' for women in the community who might want to disclose, share or talk about their experiences of abuse with other women who share their experience. Women who come to the drop-in do not have to be users of mental health services and so the context is already shifting to one that is non-pathologising. The women from the original groups who facilitate the drop-ins are accessing training in listening and support skills and are further developing their own resources as they do so. This has been an important development and one that is unlikely to have happened if the women who were part of the groups had not experienced the group as a transformative 'agent of change'.

Here, one of the founder members of the support group, Anne, is sharing her experience of transformation. As a child, Anne experienced sustained physical and sexual abuse from both of her parents where she was raised in Asia. Her feelings of isolation, she feels, contributed to the potential for a fixed story of 'victimhood' that has shifted to a more flexible story of 'sisterhood' through being part of a collective story of change within and beyond the group.

> Anne: ... I think from my experience of meeting women who have gone through this we are all very insecure and we're not sure if the decisions we are making are the right ones and we're not sure ... basically we are unsure about everything because whatever power we had was basically RIPPED from us when we were you know sexually abused ...
>
> ... at the meetings that we had when people started sharing some of our experiences or thoughts or achievements ... that helped us get stronger ... SO much oh God ... the quality of my life is SO much better now than it used to be ... mentally, emotionally and its yeah. And that's why I don't feel like I need to hide my name or who I am because no-one ... cos I think more people who can achieve this need to speak out to say you can achieve this otherwise how are people going to know?

Anne has spoken publically about her experiences of being abused. In the previous 'Victimhood to Sisterhood' paper, I did something somewhat similar, with the intention of deliberately moving away from objectifying language and also to contribute to a discourse of transparency about a subject that is so often unspoken or indeed actively silenced.

Anne's story is not a static one, by naming sexual abuse I am not suggesting that this one experience defines women. Anne is a successful businesswoman and in her spare time is energised to help other women who have had similar experiences and has a particular passion for promoting better understanding of the way previous sexual abuse can impact on women's experiences of pregnancy, birth and parenting. She positions herself purposefully, as have I and others, in solidarity with other women, encapsulated in this quote.

> Every time I was raped, everything I felt as a woman disappeared and all I was left with was fear and pain, and a woman in childbirth whose (had) this (experience) should be ... not supported, that's not the right word ... they need gentler, kinder, listening and more options. Natural childbirth is not the right option for most women who have been raped because this in itself causes trauma. This is what I have been thinking a lot about ... I want to help be the voice of people who cant speak ...

Solidarity

Vikki Reynolds (2014) uses the language of 'imperfect alliance' in her community and activist work as a means to pay attention to what could be categorised as 'outsider' vs. 'insider' positions. Solidarity that names and respects imperfect alliances allows me, as a therapist, to make good use of my insider and outsider positions. I am not from the British island where I work (I am from mainland Wales) but I am part of this particular community of women in a different way. I am an insider researcher by definition of being a researcher-practitioner but I do not pretend to share all of the same experiences of the women I am talking with. I do, though, need to make visible in my research the pre-existing relationships I have with those I am talking with, and my own experiences that shape how we do that talking. Melanie Greene (2014) suggests that *despite* the recognition of the importance of cultural and theoretical reference points; experiences of the researcher and the acknowledgement that researchers need to name their own biases, people rarely address the issue of 'positioning' themselves in their research. In 'From Victimhood to Sisterhood' (Salter, 2015) I made the decision to name my position in relation to this group as a woman who has some experience of childhood sexual abuse. I do not feel that my experience is the same or has been as life impacting for me as it has for other women in the group but I do think as a researcher I have to make known my experience and how that has shaped how I practise as both a therapist and researcher. My own experience was limited by the fact that I was believed by my family and other children were courageous enough to go to the police, so a prosecution was successful; but obviously this has shaped my viewpoint, as have other experiences in life. The most significant impact for me has been in an aversion to language which holds people in a particular position, whether that be 'victim', 'survivor' or even 'expert by experience'. The potential for any such language, however noble the intent, can obliterate or at least temporarily render invisible other important narratives including stories of movement/flexibility. They have the potential to sound fixed and permanent. Most women I speak with have different responses to the legacy of sexual abuse at different stages in their life. It is not a fixed position. Women often talk about pregnancy or becoming a mother as one of those 'trigger' experiences. Talking with other women can also trigger strong memories and emotions. Most women have, at some point, also experimented with ways of avoiding, shutting out or ignoring their past and it is often after those methods have become less useful that they experiment with talking with other people about their experiences. This represents significant risk as any person speaking out publically about issues of identity and stigma will know. It is particularly risky for people living in small communities who are likely to know other women in the group and are thus automatically 'outing' themselves as 'victims' of sexual abuse simply by being present.

The question of neutrality

> Washing one's hands of the conflict between the powerful and the powerless means to side with the powerful, not to be neutral. (Freire, 1985, p 122)

When working with sexual abuse, as either a psychotherapist or as a group facilitator, bringing ideas of neutrality and bias in to the foreground has been an important thread for me. The concept of neutrality can be seen as a contentious and challenging issue for many Systemic Psychotherapists and systemically informed practitioners. Selvini and colleagues (1980) and Cecchin (1987) offered this as a way of being when working with couples and families; and I have found it a helpful one in many areas of my practice, especially in working with couples. In this context though I find I am more influenced by those who have challenged the language of neutrality when working with abuse and oppression. For example Elsa Jones (1993) and Imelda McCarthy (1995, 2001, 2006), have been vocal in questioning this position. Imelda McCarthy (2001) invites us to think about resisting neutrality and oppression, by bringing stories of oppression in to the public space.

> The private and the public cannot be separated when one works with the poor; otherwise we are in danger of creating yet another arena for their silencing and further oppression. (McCarthy, 2001, pp. 271, 272)

Freire (1970, 1985) was perhaps a forerunner in challenging ideas of neutrality when working with people who have experienced oppression, whether that be from a form of direct abuse or other more insidious forms of oppression such as poverty and social exclusion.

Connecting with practices informed by narrative approaches and social justice helps me to move my own practices forward to continue to question my own biases in my therapy practice *and* in my research practice. Challenging neutrality in my practice is, therefore, inherently connected with challenging ideas around objectivity in research. It also connects me to a collective voice and movement of social action that speaks to solidarity.

> In coming to the group, the unique part was that I stopped just thinking of myself as an individual and started thinking wider about what people feel/need. (Anne, 2016)

Issues of power and knowledge in research – A social constructionist lens

Within social constructionist informed research, the concept of knowledge as being co-constructed is often privileged. Gergen and Gergen (2000) suggest that the division between researcher and subject is 'blurred', and that control/power is shared. In the examples of text in this paper, I have already suggested that themes of identity are being co-constructed. I would also argue that this is a co-construction of knowledge between the women in the group and myself as both practitioner/researcher and as part of this group. Whilst I am aware of the potential for power imbalance in me asking questions that I have pre-designed as a starting point, I am also part of the flow of conversation that veers away from those four questions and I allow myself to become part of that movement. I am not though without power and I do not think that my methods are flawless. In my conversation with Anne, for example, I am aware when listening back in our conversations that I missed opportunities for me to ask questions about her views of power. My pre-existing relationship with her, which has been for nearly four years, was probably the biggest factor in this. I was less curious about her remarks because we had had similar conversations previously and my knowledge of her and my own biases/experiences were influencing me. I accepted much of what she said at 'face value', using lots of affirming statements such as 'yes', 'right' etc., and less 'what do you mean when you say …? etc'. This, I am sure, would have been a very different type of dialogue if Anne were taking with someone who had never met her before, or did not have pre-existing knowledge of the experiences she talks about. But then what else might have been lost in that process? And how does my relationship to power and her relationship to power shape our conversation at this one given moment?

Many qualitative researchers working in the health field highlight issues of equality in the research relationship within (what Karnieli-Miller, Strier, and Pessach (2009) call) the 'macrosetting of dominance and authority'. The context of the health setting, they note demonstrates that 'distribution of power is unequal and hierarchical'. (Karnieli-Miller et al., 2009). As a practitioner researcher in a mental health setting, I am very mindful of this. Where possible I try to arrange to meet with the women in my inquiry in a community setting that is familiar to them to at least partially address the potential for the hierarchical clinical setting to be felt as a power differential.

If we take the social constructionist view that knowledge is constructed by dominant discourses, then we may view power, as well as knowledge, as socially constructed. Foucault's (1980, 1991) position that power is 'meta' to, rather than 'held' by a person or group questions the perspective that there are groups in society who have power and those who do not. For women who have experienced sexual abuse, their narrative about power is often a perspective that power was 'taken' from them (or 'ripped' from them to use Anne's words) by more powerful people in society or in their community. This power differential may be in the adult/child relationship, a position of authority within the family or community but also speaks to the groups with authority in society who are charged with protecting us from abuse. If those systems are experienced as a secondary source of abuse because the people they represent are under-represented in their make-up and/or because people do not experience justice, this could be seen as a further demonstration of withheld power. In a research context we also need to pay attention to people's experience of power. Whether we hold the view that power is 'out there' rather than held, or whether we actively work to shift the power differential, it is still likely to be felt by those involved. Whilst *I* may view those I am in conversation with as 'co-researchers' from a post-modern perspective, I am conscious that they may experience *themselves* as 'participants' in a modernist frame, as set by the context of this thing we call research. Postmodernist research questions the nature of research itself. Researchers such as Tuhiwai Smith (1999) also critically challenge Western, colonial ideas of 'knowledge' and 'knowing'. This is an important and highly relevant debate and maybe one of the biggest challenges for the insider researcher. How do we critically deconstruct the processes and practices that we are part of whilst simultaneously speaking out of and in to them? I think we probably do so with the words of Patti Lather in mind that inevitably we will get lost along the way, and if we are lucky we will be able to notice that we are lost and stop to read a map. In so doing we may also choose to pay attention to/question who wrote the map, who commissioned it and how it has become validated as a 'true representation' of the terrain we see before us.

Conclusions

I have offered, in this paper, some further exploration of my role as a practitioner-researcher within the field of mental health and from the broad framework of qualitative research. I have positioned myself as an insider researcher and highlighted some of the challenges and nuances of such a position without the intention of this being a comprehensive review. Speaking from within practice, I have illustrated some themes with direct quotes from women I have been speaking with, and have paid attention to my own position within those conversations and within my research.

The emphasis on social justice and solidarity is reflective of my bias and of the emerging themes from the conversations I have been having. I am aware that this frame privileges a certain discourse and as such is likely to marginalise others. These have though been extremely important concepts in my practice which has, in turn, shaped my research. Working with women who have been sexually abused has been a focus of this paper and my research which intentionally offers a platform for narratives that might otherwise be subjugated or silenced. Voicing my own story has been intentional and certainly not without discomfort, but has been an important marker in my inquiry and in understanding myself as a researcher as well as a practitioner.

Other women who have shared their stories have also done so with thought and intent and it probably goes without saying that I respect them hugely and am deeply appreciative of their contributions to my research and to this paper.

Disclosure statement

No potential conflict of interest was reported by the author.

References

Cecchin, G. (1987). Hypothesizing, circularity, and neutrality revisited: An invitation to curiosity. *Family Process, 26*, 405–413.

Foucault, M. (1980). *Power/knowledge: Selected interviews and other writings 1972–1977.* Brighton: Harvester Press.

Foucault, M. (1991). *Discipline and Punish: the birth of a prison.* London: Penguin.

Freire, P. (1970). *Pedagogy of the oppressed.* New York, NY: Herder and Herder.

Freire, P. (1985). *The politics of education: Culture, power, and liberation.* Westport: Greenwood Publishing.

Gergen, M. M., & Gergen, K. J. (2000). Qualitative inquiry: Tensions and transformations. In N. K. Denzin & Y. S. Lincoln (Eds.), *The handbook of qualitative research* (2nd ed.). (pp. 1025–1046). Thousand Oaks, CA: Sage.

Greene, M. (2014). On the inside looking in: Methodological insights and challenges in conducting qualitative insider research. *The Qualitative Report, 19*(15), 1–13.

Jones, E. (1993). *Family systems therapy: Developments in the Milan-systemic therapies.* New York, NY: Wiley.

Karnieli-Miller, O., Strier, R., & Pessach, L. (2009). Power relations in qualitative research. *Qualitative Health Research, 19*(279), 279–289.

Lather, P. (2007). *Getting lost: Feminist efforts toward a double(d) science.* Albany: State University of New York Press.

McCarthy, I. (Ed.). (1995). *Irish family studies: Selected papers.* Dublin: Family Studies Centre.

McCarthy, I. (2001). Fifth Province re-versings: The social construction of women lone parents' inequality and poverty. *Journal of Family Therapy, 23*, 253–277.

McCarthy, I. (2006). From Milan to the Fifth Province; The legacy of Gianfranco Cecchin. *Human Systems: The Journal of Systemic Consultation and Management, 17*, 257–263.

Naples, N. (1996). A feminist revisiting of the insider/outsider debate: The "outsider phenomenon" in rural Iowa. *Qualitative Sociology, 19*, 83–106.

Selvini, M. P., Boscolo, L., Cecchin, G., & Prata, G. (1980). Hypothesizing-circularity-neutrality: Three guidelines for the conductor of the session. *Family Process, 19*, 3–12.

Pearce, B. (2007). *Making social worlds: A communication perspective.* Oxford: Blackwell.

Pearce, W. B., & Cronen, V. (1980). *Communication, action, and meaning: The creation of social realities.* New York, NY: Praeger.

Reynolds, V. (2014). A solidarity approach: The rhizome and messy inquiry. In G. Simon & A. Chard (Eds.), *Systemic inquiry: Innovations in reflexive practice research* (pp. 127–154). Farnhill: Everything is Connected Press.

Richardson, L. (1990). *Writing strategies: Reaching diverse audiences.* New York, NY: Sage.

Salter, L. (2015). From victimhood to sisterhood – A practice-based reflexive inquiry into narrative informed group work with women who have experienced sexual abuse. *European Journal of Psychotherapy & Counselling, 17*, 402–417.

Shotter, J. (1994). Making sense on the boundaries: On moving between philosophy and psychotherapy. *Royal Institute of Philosophy Supplement, 37*(55), 37–55.

Shotter, J. (2011, March 5–9). *Language, joint action, and the ethical domain: The importance of the relations between our living bodies and their surroundings.* Plenary paper, III Congreso De Psicología Y Responsabilidad Social, Campus San Alberto Magno. Downloaded 22 March, 2016.

Tuhiwai Smith, L. (1999). *Decolonizing methodologies: Research and indigenous peoples.* London: Zed Books.

Van Heutgen, K. (2004). Managing insider research: Learning from experience. *Qualitative Social Work, 3*, 203–219.

Wenger, E. (1998). *Communities of practice: Learning, meaning, and identity*. New York, NY: Cambridge University Press.
White, M. (1995). *Re-authoring lives: Interviews and essays*. Adelaide: Dulwich Centre.
Wittgenstein, L. (1953). *Philosophical investigations*. Oxford: Blackwell.

'Let me in! A comment on insider research'

Helen Ellis-Caird

ABSTRACT

This issue of *EJPC* foregrounds the work of insider researchers investigating clinical practice in an array of contexts including one-to-one work with trauma, group work with those who have been abused, adoptive family work and work with a home treatment team and inpatient team. In this comment piece, I consider the papers from an outsider's perspective and apply a quality lens to gain a surer hold of what the papers can offer. I've highlighted the rich resonance of many of the accounts, but also the specialist language in which most are written, and the lack of space for discussion of the process of research or analysis of data conducted. I argue that this creates barriers in the way of these papers being consumed, understood and applied by a wider audience, which may mean that the impact and implications of the work are not fully realised.

DEJENME ENTRAR..! Comentario acerca de la investigación dentro del campo desde la perspectiva de quien está fuera de él.

Este número de la Revista Europea de Psicoterapia y Orientación Psicológica, pone en primer plano el trabajo del investigador dentro del campo trabajando en la práctica clínica, en un despliegue de contextos incluyendo: trabajo individual con trauma; trabajo de grupo con pacientes que han sido abusados; trabajo con familias adoptivas; con un equipo de trabajo en el hogar y con un equipo con pacientes hospitalizados. En este comentario considero los artículos desde la perspectiva exterior y aplico un lente cualitativo para asegurarme de la comprensión del material presentado en ellos. He destacado la riqueza de la resonancia de muchas de las presentaciones, pero también el uso de un lenguaje especializado en el cual la mayoria de los artículos se presenta y la falta de espacio para la discusión del proceso de investigación o de la conducción del análisis de los datos.

Se discute que ésto crea barreras en la manera en que estos artículos han sido leídos, comprendidos y aplicados por una audiencia amplia, lo cual puede significar que el impacto y las implicaciones del trabajo no han sido realizados en su totalidad.

Fammi entrare! Un commento sulla ricerca privilegiate dal punto di vista di un estraneo

Questo numero di EJPC in primo piano il lavoro dei ricercatori insider indagare la pratica clinica in una vasta gamma di contesti, tra cui 1–1 lavoro con il trauma,

il lavoro di gruppo con quelli che sono stati abusati, lavoro famiglia adottiva e il lavoro con una squadra di trattamento a casa e la squadra del ricoverato. In questo commento pezzo, ritengo le carte dal punto di vista di un estraneo e si applica un obiettivo di qualità per ottenere una presa più sicura di quello che i giornali possono offrire. Ho evidenziato la ricca risonanza di molti dei conti, ma anche il linguaggio specialistico in cui sono scritti più, e la mancanza di spazio per la discussione del processo di ricerca o analisi dei dati condotta. Io sostengo che questo crea barriere nel modo di queste carte di essere consumato, capito e applicato da un pubblico più ampio, il che può significare che l'impatto e le implicazioni del lavoro non sono pienamente realizzati.

Laissez-moi entrer! Un commentaire sur la recherche 'de l'intérieur' à partir d'une perspective 'de l'extérieur'

Ce numéro présente le travail de chercheurs 'de l'intérieur' investiguant la pratique clinique dans divers contextes incluant: le travail individuel avec le traumatisme, le travail de groupe avec des personnes ayant subi des abus, le travail avec des familles adoptantes ainsi que le travail d'une équipe de soins à domicile. Dans ce commentaire, je considère ces articles à partir d'une perspective extérieure et leur applique un prisme qualitatif ce qui permet d'avoir une prise plus ferme quant à ce qu'ils offrent. Je souligne la force des récits présentés mais également le langage spécialisé qui est utilisé dans la plupart des cas et l'absence de discussion quant au processus de recherche ou quant à l'analyse des données. J'estime que cela crée des barrières dans la façon dont cet article peut être utilisé, compris et mis à profit par un public plus large, ce qui peut signifier que les objectifs d'impact des travaux ne sont pas entièrement atteints.

Άφησε με να μπω! Ένα σχόλιο στην έρευνα από την άποψη ενός εξωτερικού

Το παρόν τεύχος του EJPC φέρει στο προσκήνιο το έργο των ερευνητών «εκ των έσω» που μελετούν την κλινική πράξη σε μια σειρά πλαισίων, όπως είναι η ατομική δουλειά με το τραύμα, η ομαδική δουλειά με άτομα που έχουν υποστεί κακοποίηση, η δουλειά με θετές οικογένειες και η δουλειά με μια ομάδα περίθαλψης στο σπίτι και μια ενδονοσοκομειακή ομάδα. Σε αυτό το σχόλιο, προσεγγίζω τα άρθρα από μια εξωτερική οπτική και εξετάζω την ποιότητα τους αναφορικά με τις δυνατότητες που προσφέρουν. Έχω τονίσει την πλούσια συγκίνηση που προκαλούν οι περισσότερες αφηγήσεις, αλλά και την εξειδικευμένη γλώσσα στην οποία τα περισσότερα είναι γραμμένα και την απουσία χώρου για συζήτηση για την ερευνητική διαδικασία και την ανάλυση των δεδομένων. Υποστηρίζω ότι αυτό παρεμποδίζει τον τρόπο με τον οποίο αυτά τα άρθρα μπορούν να αξιοποιηθούν, να κατανοηθούν και να εφαρμοστούν από το ευρύτερο κοινό, το οποίο σημαίνει ότι ο αντίκτυπος και οι συνέπειες του έργου δεν αναγνωρίζονται πλήρως.

Positioning myself on the outside

As a qualitative researcher I set much importance on the explicit positioning of the researcher, taking a reflexive stance from which to set the context of the research which follows. In order to practice what I preach, I thought it would be equally relevant in a comment piece like this one to say a little about me and where I'm coming from in order to fully situate the remarks which follow. To start, I feel something of an outsider to this journal: I am a clinical psychologist, but I'm not currently engaged in clinical practice in an adult mental health setting, and the qualitative research I have conducted has been explorations of experience in physical health settings rather than the examination of an element of my clinical practice. I also position myself as an outsider to some of the methodologies discussed in the five papers; I haven't taken a psychodynamic or action research perspective to my own research and so feel somewhat naïve to both approaches. "I'm writing this at the beginning of 2017, a time of global unease with what appear to be growing divisions between insiders and outsiders. This makes me realise the importance of engaging, of entering debate, of getting a different perspective across, and doing so in a non-specialist forum in order to influence public debate. The response that follows I believe has been informed by all these facets of my experience.

The insider approach

Four of the five papers come from an 'insider researcher' perspective, examining the clinical work or context of the researchers themselves. It was fascinating to get a snap shot of four clinicians working using psychodynamic, systemic and narrative means in an array of different contexts including one-to-one work with trauma, group work with those who have been abused, adoptive family work and work with a home treatment team. Each has used innovative and inventive research methods in their attempt to gain a meaningful and in-depth insight into some aspect of their or their team's practice. Without meaning to patronise, I think this is a huge achievement in itself. I know how incredibly hard it is to weave a research element into my clinical practice, and yet these clinicians have found the time and can now present some of what they found to a wider audience. In our era of evidence-based practice, ensuring that accounts of work not so easily able to be submitted to traditional outcome measures have a voice seems incredibly important.

The fifth paper is not written by a member of the clinical team, but presents a psychodynamic analysis of a mental health service observed over a year. However, I think it shares the broad aim of better understanding the workings of an aspect of clinical practice.

Finding my way in

All the papers present detailed, nuanced analyses, and are complex and specialist in their language, at times prohibitively so for someone in the outsider position I inhabit. This made it difficult for me to make a comment on the value of the papers, particularly in areas which were further from my own practice or expertise. I therefore decided to apply an external structure in the form of Tracy's (2010) eight markers of high quality in qualitative methodological research to get more of a grip on what these papers can say or contribute. These eight markers include (a) a worthy topic, (b) rich rigour, (c) sincerity, (d) credibility, (e) resonance, (f) significant contribution, (g) ethics and (h) meaningful coherence. They demand much of the researcher and, it could be argued, leave little room for the inevitability of 'getting lost' (from victimhood to sisterhood) in the complexity of roles, aims and practices explicit in insider, clinically focused research. I take this point, but Tracy's criteria are designed to be applied flexibly and sensitively, to incorporate the 'big tent' diversity of array of qualitative research methods used today. And rather than applying a straight-jacket to the vivid accounts in these papers, I hope they are one way to highlight what the papers do brilliantly, as well as to offer some suggestions for what they could do even better.

Applying a quality lens

Below I've talked about each paper in turn, highlighting for each the quality markers that seem pertinent.

'Not dead ... abandoned'

This paper presents a clinical case study of psychodynamic work over a 12-month period conducted with a veteran with symptoms of significant trauma. The work ends prematurely due to the client's withdrawal from treatment. The researcher states that their aim in presenting this case study is to examine 'some key relational processes' with a particular focus on understanding the ending of therapy. A significant portion of the paper is focused on giving a detailed theoretical account of the psychoanalytic concepts which informed the work. This was very complex and not entirely accessible to me as someone with only a cursory training in psychodynamic theory and practice. This was followed by a formulation and then a chronological account of the work undertaken. This was fascinating – a rich and moving account of the progress and difficulties encountered in working with a man deeply traumatised by his past and struggling to keep going in his life. I felt real empathy for both the practitioner and the client, and found myself relating it back to similar cases in my own clinical practice. Tracy uses the term resonance to capture this ability of a qualitative paper to move the reader, with my application of the material back to my experience an example of naturalistic generalisation (Stake & Trumbull, 1982) which can occur when qualitative research generates this personal feeling of knowing and experiencing.

In prioritising the rich description of the work, there were other markers of quality which were less centred. The paper lacked a consistent rigour – there was much depth and richness to the theoretical underpinnings, but only brief details of the data collection and analysis strategy. The researcher states that a psychoanalytically informed deductive thematic analysis was conducted and we know that process notes, supervision and self-reflection were data points, but no detail is given on how an analysis was conducted or what themes emerged. I believe that by prioritising the clinical frame rather than the research frame, the analysis that was conducted was lost in the write up. This was problematic for me as it meant the account lacked transparency, which impacted another quality criterion, that of credibility. Without already having an in-depth understanding of psychodynamic practice, I was not willing or able to accept fully the interpretations offered, without the 'back up' of rigour in the analytic process, which left me unconvinced by the conclusions drawn.

To summarise, it seemed to me that the insider researcher frame gave the work a deep resonance, but also meant that it was pitched at quite a specialist level, with clinical material taking precedence over research material. This limited the paper's contribution – resonance alone is unlikely to change practice, resonance with rigour and credibility has more of a chance.

A shift in narratives

This single case study provides a qualitative evaluation of a non-attachment based short-term therapy with the goal to 'promote and strengthen mutual belonging in adoptive families'. The approach was developed by the authors based on their clinical practice over 15 years in the field of adoption. The first of the markers of quality in qualitative research referred to by Tracy is that of having a worthy topic of research. This paper certainly hits this marker for me: it seems only logical that innovation in practice should emerge first and foremost from clinicians who have lived and breathed the field and that research should then test out these innovations. The researcher's goal to examine family discourses, see how these changed over time, and how the therapist influenced this change seems a clear first step to gain an in-depth understanding of the impact of this new approach to family work.

The method itself is very briefly introduced, stating that Stratton's (2003a, 2003b) attribution scheme and unitizing coding system for causal attributions will be used. No explanation of what this is or how data were gathered and analysed is given. Similar to the first paper, this compromised the results presented as the process to get there was not transparent, thus lacking rigour. The paper goes on to give an interesting account of the process of therapy as it unfolded over the year, framing this by the attributions of family members and the interventions of the therapists. It's unclear from the account if these therapists were the researchers themselves. Space may have precluded a self-reflexive voice, which would have better met the marker of sincerity in qualitative research. Use of verbatim text from the therapy sessions was very useful in illustrating the causal attributions. Interpretations are offered to demonstrate the way in which attributions shifted over time, but without an in-depth understanding of the Stratton method, the marker of credibility was not quite met for me.

I feel quite mean in writing this critique, because as you will see as reader of this paper, the approach seemed to be really impactful, leading to long-term change for the family and understandably, the authors prioritised the telling of this story over the more technical details of how they carried out the analysis. But, again, as an outsider who doesn't know the hows and whys, it makes it very difficult to judge what one can take from the work.

The impact of professional role on working with risk in a home treatment team

This paper considers staff experience of working with risk in a home treatment team. The researchers report holding a series of focus groups, including the majority of the clinical team, before an Interpretative Phenomenological Analysis (IPA) was conducted to identify pertinent themes. The detail reported here supported the marker of rigour in data collection, but little information about the data analysis is included, simply stating that a 'conventional' IPA coding strategy was followed. It is therefore difficult to know the rigour of the analytic process. Such an interpretative analysis is at its foundation influenced by the researchers' position, but this was left a little under-explored. I wasn't clear what role both researchers played in the team, and what particular lens this may have lent to the research aims, process and analysis. Some self-reflexive comment is considered at the end in terms of the difficulty to one researcher of identifying a theme potentially critical to their team, but without this woven throughout, the marker of 'sincerity' was only partially met.

In combination, the credibility of the emerging themes were somewhat compromised. Despite this, the theme presented, that of 'professional role and responsibility', had immediate resonance for me and there was an 'aha' moment as I related to the double bind of the constraints of professional role, with the responsibilities this entailed. I felt intuitively that this could be applied to other teams that I have worked in and could go some way to help understand the phenomenon of high burnout rates in mental health teams (Morse, Salyers, Rollins, Monroe-DeVita, & Pfahler, 2012). It made me turn to literature on the implicit psychological contract (George, 2009) between staff and the organisation, and how and why this is constructed and maintained. I certainly thought there was the opportunity here for the work to make a significant contribution to understanding and changing staff experience of work with risk. Perhaps because of the insider frame, the authors focused more on what it meant for their particular team rather than fitting findings into a larger theoretical frame or drawing out the wider implications – this felt like a lost opportunity to me.

Critical incidence in mental health units

This is the only paper which is not conducted by an insider researcher, but instead forms part of a wider study conducted for a PhD. This paper focuses in on critical incidents in mental health units in an Irish public mental health service. A combination of observation and interviews are used to gather data over the course of a year. A psychodynamic/Lacanian framework is then utilised to analyse five critical incidents, highlighting a failure to manage overwhelming levels of anxiety and to work with transference as being culpable in such incidents arising and in the restrictive management strategies imposed.

There was rigour in the theoretical underpinnings and multiple sources for data collection and an interesting discussion of the lens of psychoanalysis used to frame the research, which was helpful to contextualise what came next. However, as was the case for all three studies above, it was hard for me to understand fully and get underneath the skin of the analysis and presentation of results. Perhaps much of this is my lack of familiarity with psychodynamic research methods, but without greater description of the process or verification procedures undertaken, there was little transparency for me on how the incidents presented were selected and analysed. The in-depth detail given of each incident supported the resonance of the account, but a self-reflexive voice from the researcher would have helped here to see how the reporting of these incidents may have been impacted by the researcher's position. The interpretation which follows is fascinating, looking at the role of transference in acting out incidents. This was mainly 'told' rather than 'shown' to the reader, so although there was some face credibility, I certainly felt that understandings from a different lens seemed equally plausible. Some interesting implications and suggestions for service improvement are raised, but the inaccessibility of the account overall to a non-specialist reader may make it difficult to implement. I felt that further 'translation' is needed, with greater focus on showing the reader how the account holds credibility.

From victimhood to sisterhood part II

The paper is a more reflective piece, looking back on research undertaken with women who had experienced sexual abuse. The author describes the research focus on how women had 'gone on' following the completion of a systemic group facilitated by the researcher, grounding this in the Coordinated Management of Meaning model to support such a focus to 'co-create better social worlds'. The author describes how the research allowed a 'talking again' conversational inquiry which enabled new stories to emerge for the women about being part of the group and for the author as facilitator of that group, thus positioning research as a 'transformative practice' for those involved. There was a real rigour in the depth of context, theoretical positioning and research process presented, allowing me to enter the world of the research. Far less information and 'guidance' is provided on the actual process of analysis undertaken or on the detail of the results of that analysis, but as primarily a reflective piece, this felt appropriate.

The paper talks directly to the insider research frame and the way in which this can make inevitable bias more visible, and getting lost a part of the journey. It also holds a reflexive stance throughout, holding a dual lens of both reporting findings from the research, and at the same time reflecting on the doing of that research. For this reason, for me the paper is a gold standard for the reporting of the quality marker of sincerity, the researcher being honest and open about their own position and influence on the research taking place, allowing the researcher's journey to become an explicit and fascinating part of the story.

The paper goes on to reflect on the role of research as concerned with social justice, being part of a collective and creating the possibility of social transformation, as well as reflecting on issues of neutrality and the power of the researcher. These ideas are illustrated in the text by the stories of developing community that came out of the group, giving direct quotations and details of the women's lives to talk to the transformative impact of this kind of insider research. The telling of these stories was deeply resonant but also credible, as the co-creation of the narrative with the research participants was evident throughout.

This paper was better able to meet many of the quality markers that were de-centred by the reporting of clinical content in the other papers. It's important to point out however, that this paper was a companion piece to an earlier account (Salter, 2015) published in this journal. Much of the heavy work of the reporting of the content of research was therefore already completed, allowing the possibility of opening up other aspects of the work more fully. This makes me think about the word constraints of journals and whether this is fair and reasonable for the reporting of qualitative work. This journal advises authors to submit papers no greater than 5000 words and states 'Manuscripts that greatly exceed this will be critically reviewed with respect to length'. Is this fair or a legacy of a reporting system suited for quantitative papers? Is conciseness always best? Certainly not in the case of Salter's paper.

Why let outsiders in?

In reviewing the papers through the lens of quality that I've utilised above, one thing that emerged for me was the emphasis most gave to providing resonant accounts, full of rich, vivid content. The only paper that didn't do this was the one explicitly positioned as a reflection on the research process and so without the need to include this content so fully. I'd argue that this resonance is a fundamental marker, and one that I wonder is particularly emphasised by insider researchers, where the whole reason for embarking on research is to shed more light on a clinical concern. This is also the bit so often missing from quantitative papers – it's much harder to be moved by numbers.

But my assertion is that some of the papers raised resonance without the more staid markers of rigour and sincerity being equally prioritised. This is not problematic if you are already within the world of the researcher, and if you already have an in-depth understanding of the methods used or the clinical approach utilised. But I believe that it is a problem if you're an outsider to these worlds. On my first reading of the papers, I blamed myself, feeling culpable for my difficulty in accessing the material, feeling my relative inexperience as a researcher would be plain to see – and perhaps it is. But as much as I'm inexperienced and non-specialist, so are the majority of the potential readers of these papers. If there are barriers in the way of these papers being consumed, understood and applied by a wider audience, then doesn't it mean that the chances of the work being heard are reduced, limiting the contribution they can make?

I think my focus on accessibility talks to the current climate in which we find ourselves at the beginning of 2017. There is no longer the comfort of assuming that others will think like I do, that the march of a liberal and open democracy will continue necessarily ad infinitum. In such a climate it seems so important that we engage with outsiders, ensuring we are not just talking to other insiders of our own field who will see and get what we mean. I realise this is a very big point to make, and it is hardly the responsibility of hard-working qualitative clinician/researchers that the world has turned a worrying corner, but I do think the macro-context should have relevance to all of our practices. In an age where the expert is down valued or mistrusted, don't we have to do more to reach out? As Tracy (2010) states in her commentary on quality in qualitative research, 'part of making scholarship powerful is talking in ways that are appreciated by a variety of audiences' (p. 838). Does this inevitably mean a 'dumbing down' of researchers' work? I don't think so, there's a difference between being transparent and accessible and being simplistic (Reicher & Haslam, 2017). I believe that as long as researchers focus on talking only to others intimately connected to their worlds, the impact and implications of their work will not be fully realised.

Disclosure statement

No potential conflict of interest was reported by the authors.

References

George, C. (2009). *Psychological contract: Development and management of professional workers*. (Work and Organizational Psychology). Open University Press. Retrieved from https://www.amazon.co.uk/d/cka/Psychological-Contract-Developing-Professional-developing-professional-Organizational/0335216129#reader_0335216129

Morse, G., Salyers, M. P., Rollins, A. L., Monroe-DeVita, M., & Pfahler, C. (2012). Burnout in mental health services: A review of the problem and its remediation. *Administration and Policy In Mental Health, 39*, 341–352. doi:10.1007/s10488-011-0352-1

Reicher, S., & Haslam, A. (2017). Writing for impact. *The Psychologist, 30*, 36–41.

Salter, L. (2015). From victimhood to sisterhood – A practice-based reflexive inquiry into narrative informed group work with women who have experienced sexual abuse. *European Journal of Psychotherapy & Counselling, 17*, 402–417. doi:10.1080/1364253 7.2015.1095215

Stake, R. E., & Trumbull, D. J. (1982). Naturalistic generalizations. *Review Journal of Philosophy and Social Science, 7*(1–2), 1–12.

Stratton, P. (2003a). Causal attributions during therapy I: Responsibility and blame. *Journal of Family Therapy, 25*, 136–160. doi:10.1111/1467-6427.00241

Stratton, P. (2003b). Causal attributions during therapy II: Reconstituted families and parental blaming. *Journal of Family Therapy, 25*, 161–180. doi:10.1111/1467-6427.00242

Tracy, S. J. (2010). Qualitative quality: Eight "abig-tent" criteria for excellent qualitative research. *Qualitative Inquiry, 16*, 837–851. doi:10.1177/1077800410383121

The researcher in the field – some notes on qualitative research in mental health

Jarl Wahlström

ABSTRACT

In this published response to five studies in the present special issue, all representing qualitative research in the field of mental health, this research is approached as cultural and social practice. The five studies are looked upon as informative examples of research activity in mental health, and it is asked how that particular field is conceptualised as a form of human activity, how the authors position themselves in relation to the field, why they ask the questions they seek to answer and how epistemic queries concerning knowing and not-knowing manifest themselves and are addressed in the studies. The paper seeks to contribute to the debate on the uses of qualitative methodology in mental health research by explicating some of the differences and some of the similarities between the pieces of research at hand.

EL INVESTIGADOR EN EL CAMPO: Notas acerca de la investigación cualitativa en salud mental

Esta es una respuesta a los cinco artíulos publicados en el presente número acerca de la investigación cualitativa en el campo de la salud mental, considerando dicha investigación como una práctica social y cultural. Se analizan los cinco estudios como ejemplos informativos de la actividad investigativa en salud metal y se pregunta: cómo ese campo particular se conceptualiza como una forma de actividad humana, cuál es la posición de los autores con relación al campo, por qué hacen las preguntas a las cuales esperan respuestas, cómo se manifiestan las dudas epistémicas concernientes al saber y al no-saber y cómo éstas se presentan en los estudios.

Con este artículo se desea contribuir al debate acerca de los usos de la metodología cualitativa en la investigación en salud mental, al explicar algunas de las diferencias y algunas de la similitudes entre las piezas de investigación disponibles.

Il ricercatore sul campo – Alcune note sulla ricerca qualitativa nell'ambito della Salute Mentale

Questo contributo costituisce una risposta ai cinque studi del presente numero speciale dedicati alla ricerca qualitativa nell'ambito della salute mentale, una ricerca simile ad una pratica culturale e sociale. I cinque studi devono essere considerati come esempi esplicativi dell'attività di ricerca in questo ambito, e ci si chiede in qual modo tale ambito è concettualizzato come una forma di attività umana, quale posizione gli stessi autori assumano rispetto al campo di ricerca, per quali ragioni si pongono le domande a cui cercano di rispondere, e come interrogativi epistemici relativi al sapere e al non-sapere si svelano e sono indirizzati in questi studi. Il documento si propone di contribuire al dibattito sulla metodologia qualitativa nella ricerca nell'ambito della salute mentale per esplicitare differenze e somiglianze tra le ricerche proposte.

Le chercheur sur le terrain – Quelques notes sur la recherche qualitative dans le domaine de la santé mentale

Cet article est une réponse aux cinq études présentées dans ce numéro représentant toutes des travaux de recherche qualitatives dans le champ de la santé mentale, recherche abordée en tant que pratique sociale et culturelle.

Les cinq études sont considérées comme des exemples fournissant des informations quant à l'activité de recherche dans le champ de la santé mentale. L'article pose la question de savoir comment ce champ particulier est conceptualisé en tant que type d'activité humaine, comment les auteurs se positionnent en relation avec ce champ, pourquoi ils posent les questions auxquelles ils souhaitent avoir des réponses et comment les questions épistémiques concernant le savoir (et l'absence de savoir) se manifestent et sont adressées dans ces travaux. Cet article a pour objectif de contribuer au débat sur l'usage de méthodologies qualitatives dans la recherche en santé mentale en expliquant certaines des différences mais également les similitudes entre les travaux proposés.

Ο ερευνητής στο πεδίο- Σημειώσεις για την ποιοτική έρευνα στην ψυχική υγεία

Σε αυτό το απαντητικό σχόλιο προς τις πέντε ποιοτικές έρευνες στο πεδίο της ψυχικής υγείας που φιλοξενούνται στο παρόν ειδικό τεύχος, η έρευνα προσεγγίζεται ως πολιτισμική και κοινωνική πράξη. Οι πέντε έρευνες αντιμετωπίζονται ως ενημερωτικά παραδείγματα της ερευνητικής δραστηριότητας στη ψυχική υγεία και τίθενται ερωτήματα για την τοποθέτηση των ερευνητών στο πεδίο, την επιλογή των ερωτημάτων που θέτουν, και τον τρόπο με τον οποίο οι επιστημονικές ερωτήσεις αναφορικά με τη γνώση και την απουσία της δηλώνονται και κατονομάζονται στις έρευνες. Το άρθρο αποπειράται να συμβάλει στη συζήτηση για τη χρήση της ποιοτικής μεθοδολογίας στην έρευνα της ψυχικής υγείας, επεξηγώντας κάποιες διαφορές και κάποιες ομοιότητες ανάμεσα στα άρθρα.

In their joint editorial to the previous special issue of this journal devoted to developments in qualitative research in mental health, Loewenthal and Avdi (2016) somewhat provocatively asked whether research in psychotherapy and counselling is a waste of time. Having been asked to write a published response to the five studies in the present special issue I would like to subscribe to Loewenthal's and Avdi's notion that research should be looked upon as cultural and social practice. I will not, however, attempt an answer to their question. Rather, I will look upon the five studies as informative examples of research in mental health, with the intention of taking a closer look at what might be going on in that practice. I will, in particular, ask how, in those studies, some concrete instances of human encounters are constructed as occasions of mental health work, worthy of shedding some light on questions pertinent to that field; how the authors appear to position themselves in relation to the field, why they ask the questions they seek to answer and how epistemic queries concerning knowing and not-knowing are addressed – or fail to be addressed.

Encounters in mental health

Let me start this 'investigation' by presenting the 'basic data'. The five papers included in this special issue offer us, as readers, accounts of the following encounters between people:

- In the UK a female counselling psychologist was contacted by a man, presently employed in an enterprise, but with an earlier work history of five years of military service in elite forces (Challenor, 2017). The reasons he gave for making contact were his feelings of anxiety and panic, his thoughts about committing suicide and his fear of breaking down psychologically. They agree to start meeting regularly at the psychologist's independent practice, thus establishing a professional psychotherapeutic relationship. After 12 months of treatment, the relationship is unilaterally ended by the male client, much to the surprise and even shock of the practitioner.
- In Italy a family therapy team, working in a private institute, was approached by a married, academically educated and professionally active couple (Salamino & Gusmini, 2017). The couple requested consultation regarding the trouble they experienced with their 15 years old adoptive son. The therapeutic team meets the parents twice and all the three family members seven times during a period of ten months in therapy sessions of two

hours' duration, and later at two follow-up meetings 18 and 34 months respectively after the end of treatment.

- In Ireland, a male university lecturer and psychoanalytic practitioner went to units – acute inpatient settings, day hospitals and community services – of adult psychiatric services to observe how staff members act and interact with patients in so called critical incidents, and to talk with them, both informally and in more formal interviews, about those incidents and their experience of them (Moore, 2017). He defines critical incidents as sudden and unexpected events outside the range of normal experience which may lead to a sense of threat and loss of control.
- In the UK two female clinical psychologists invited staff members from crisis resolution home treatment teams to talk to each other in so called focus groups (Iliopoulou & Sacks, 2017). The task of the staff is to respond rapidly and appropriately to people experiencing a mental health crisis. In their work staff meet with high risk situations almost daily and the intent of the invitation to the focus groups was to offer them an opportunity to talk about the risks met and managed by the teams. The staff members meet in groups of four or five and have their discussions facilitated by one of the researchers.
- In the UK a female systemic psychotherapist working in a small island community has been involved with establishing and facilitating support groups for women who have been sexually abused (Salter, 2017). She is in many ways participating in the life of the community and of the women attending the support group and has talks with them in different settings. She starts to give her activities the title 'conversational inquiry', and to ponder on the interrelations of her positions as practicing therapist, group facilitator, member of the community and doctoral researcher.

There are some observations we as readers can make on these encounters. Although in many respects different and even unique, they have some shared features. Since they have been reported in a scientific conference we can be confident that they have actually taken place. The persons involved and the events described are not fictions. The social context of all the encounters is professional, and in this sense public. And more precisely, the professional context of each encounter relates somehow to the societal institutional field of 'mental health'. As such they involve two categories of participants – practitioners and clients. The interests and reasons for participating in the encounters are different for the representatives of those two categories. They have dissimilar roles and positions with respect to the institutional task of the encounters.

Yet another common feature of these encounters is that they have been taken as source for data for qualitative inquiry into some aspect of professional activities in 'mental health'. From the myriads of encounters going on in that field, these have been selected to shed some light on what is going on in such encounters, to answer some question concerning mental health work practices. It also appears that beyond asking questions is an intent, at least implicitly, to draw conclusions about some of those practices, to validate and encourage or to criticise and discourage their use.

The lifeworld and the field

The description above of the human encounters which formed the data basis of the five studies reported in this special issue was intended to be as factual as I could make it. Not factual in the sense of being as comprehensive as possible but factual in the sense of not being 'interpretative'. These were the partici-pants and these were the contexts in which they met. Of course even such a presentation involves 'interpretations'. Using words such as 'therapy', 'anxiety', 'adoptive family', 'critical incidents', 'mental health crisis' and 'sexual abuse', the encounters are already cast into a social world, created by human communica-tion and meaning-making, and identified as particular instances of that world.

What was given above is then not merely an introduction to the *life condi-tions* of the people involved in the encounters but one of the *lifeworld* of the participants. While, according to Kraus (2015), the concept of *life conditions* refers to the material and immaterial circumstances of people's life, by the concept *lifeworld* reference is given to peoples' subjective constructions of reality, which they form under the condition of their life circumstances. Action, knowing and consciousness are embedded in and operating in a world of meanings and pre-judgements that are socially, culturally and historically constituted.

Encounters in psychotherapy and other forms of mental health work become, so to speak, sections of the lifeworld of the participants. I will call such sections *action fields*. Constituting, within the lifeworld of the participants, an encounter as a particular instance of the action field of mental health interventions is an achievement involving both subjective (i.e. private) and social (i.e. collective) meaning-making. The uses of words such as 'treatment', 'panic', 'trauma', 'out of control' etc. establish a communicative medium for the gradual co-ordination of meanings (Pearce, 2007) that are given to the experiences and life-events of (mostly) the client-participants. The participants subscribe to the use of dis-courses which are appropriate to the forms and goals of the encounter in its distinctiveness as an instance of mental health work. (In animal-assisted ther-apy, the dog or the dolphin may be experienced by the client as 'therapeutic', and even denoted as a 'therapist', but it is unlikely that these ascriptions in any way would correspond to the animal's experience – it may enjoy the situation, though!).

Now, how do the participants in mental health work, as *players* in that par-ticular subfield of their lifeworld, identify and (co-)create their common activities as instances of the appropriate social forms of that field? What kinds of actions are more successful in achieving outcomes that are perceived to be desira-ble, and what kinds of actions are less successful? Are there forms of activities which could be seen as 'effective' from some point of view but considered as undesirable from even unethical from a wider perspective? To what extent do the 'players' need to have a shared understanding of their joint meaning-making? These are the kind of questions that present themselves as particularly appropriate to be addressed by the methodological means of qualitative inquiry.

Obviously none of the five studies attempt to answer all of these questions. When designing his/her study, each researcher has made choices concerning how the relevant field of study is defined and delimited, what are the pertinent questions to be asked and what methods of inquiry are appropriate for eliciting trustworthy reconstructions of the study participants' lifeworld within the particular action field under investigation. Some of these choices have been conscious and deliberate, and accounted for in the study report. Others may have been less reflected upon by the researcher.

The researcher and the field

The social action field of mental health work and interventions is established, maintained and transformed through social practices by numerous 'players' in a large variety of contexts, go on many 'levels', taking different roles and positions. Things go on, events unfold, deeds are done, words are spoken – 'the whole hurly-burly of human actions' (Wittgenstein, 1981, No. 567). How can this in its overwhelming multitude be appropriated by research?

It cannot. For the purpose of scholarly inquiry, the researcher needs to delineate from the multitude of activities a set of practices, chosen to be the object of interest of the investigation. Doing this, the researcher takes an outsider perspective on the field. Some activities – things done or things said – are considered to be more relevant than others. How and why? Mostly this is done by the researcher or the research team in their capacity as 'players' on another field, i.e. the social field of mental health research.

Still, since the many mental health researchers are also practitioners in the field, an interesting intersectionality is established. And what is more – many do research on their own professional work. Of the five studies this was the case in three pieces of research (Challenor, Salamino & Gusmini, Salter). Apparently also Iliopoulou and Sacks are closely affiliated to the organisation they are investigating. Only Moore, a trained psychoanalytic practitioner, seems to have an outsider position with respect to the practices he is reviewing.

This intersectionality means that the choices of the researcher are profoundly affected by how his/her lifeworld is constituted. The researcher's understanding, allegiances and the discourses he/she subscribes to influence the total research process. The complexity of research into mental health interventions is further accentuated by the fact that these are intersectional in themselves. On the one hand, they have the societal status of professional and hence public activities, whilst on the other hand mental health interventions necessarily dig deep into the private lifeworld of clients, and cannot fail to touch also those of the practitioners.

Obviously, for the researcher, having the double position of a 'player' in the field of practice who takes the step over into the field of research has both advantages and disadvantages. An insider has access to tacit knowledge and understandings of the field which open possibilities of comprehending what is going on that perhaps never are available to an outsider researcher. Such pre-understanding of the many subtleties of, let us say, interaction in psychotherapy may be a prerequisite for any analysis of therapeutic processes. Then again, an un-reflected stance towards one's perceptions of the practices under scrutiny, may make the researcher blind to significant features of the interactions which easily stand out for researchers whose observations are guided by some other tradition of conceptualising human encounters. There is a complex dialectic between *preunderstanding* and *not-knowing* (Bleicher, 1980) in qualitative research on mental health.

Roles and positions in the five studies

Roles define the expectancies participants in institutional encounters have of the actions performed by themselves and others (Suoninen & Wahlström, 2009). The differences between the roles of a practitioner and a client in mental health are relatively clear, as are the differences between a researcher and a study participant in qualitative research. However, when taking up a role and adhering to it, a person can still adopt a large variety of *positions* in regard to whatever is encountered while performing the role.

In two of the five studies (Challenor; Salamino & Gusmini) the writers adopted the double role of being both therapist-participants and researchers. The positions they took with respect to the therapy cases under investigations were, however, quite different. The motivation for Challenor to look in close detail at the present case appears to have been her experience of the treatment as having an unexpected and unsatisfactory outcome. Using concepts from inter-subjective, relational psychoanalysis, she seeks to throw light on the client's choice to leave treatment without the consent of herself as therapist, and much to her disappointment. This study, then, carries two contributions. First, to give the author (and readers) a new and deepened understanding of the events that took place, and second to elaborate on the applicability of some theoretical concepts (here especially the relational understanding of dissociation).

The motivation for the Salamino and Gusmini case study is different. The intent is to present a case with satisfactory outcome and use it as a demonstration of a particular therapeutic approach. The authors use the case study as one instance of confirmation of the plausibility of their approach and even its advantage over another one. The specific argument here is that in adoptive families too much concern about the adopted child's (supposed) inadequate early attachment relationships will lead to attributions and explanations of the child's problematic behaviours that are counterproductive for finding solutions to the present-day difficulties. Focusing on current relationships and patterns of mutual connection in the present is given as a more viable alternative.

The studies by Moore and by Iliopoulou and Sacks have in common that both are concerned with complicated encounters between staff and patients in mental health institutions. In both studies the authors adopt the role of researchers approaching 'the field' from outside. But again the positions taken by the researchers in the two studies are very different. Moore goes into the organisation as a non-participant observer and occasional interviewer, and furnished with a very specific conceptual instrument: a lens informed by specific, mainly Freudian and Lacanian, aspects of psychoanalysis. This lens enables him to see events (critical incidents) and detect meanings in them that are in some respect hidden from the staff members themselves as 'players in the field'.

Iliopoulou and Sacks on the contrary invite the staff to focus groups and ask them to discuss how they manage risks in their work with clients in the home environments of these clients. Apart from defining the theme of the focus groups, the researchers do not bring into the formation of the data any conceptual framings of their own. They state as their intent to help the team to understand how they presently manage risks and to generate ideas to aid them manage risk better in the future. Using Interpretative Phenomenological Analysis when reading the data, the researchers mainly 'give back' the discussions to the participants, but now more conveniently ordered and opened up as categories of themes.

The role and position of Salter in her study is quite complex. She defines her investigation as 'inside research', and it appears that this 'insider' position takes many forms. First, the women with whom she has conducted what she names as 'conversational inquiries' are women she has either co-facilitated groups with or who have attended those groups. In this sense, she is researching her own practice. But then actually not so because her interest is in the activities of these women as members in the community of which she also is a member, and as members with a particular point of view (which she also shares): that of women who have experiences of oppression and abuse, and who have, in spite of that, found their ways of 'going on' in their lives. Third, the paper itself is, at least in my reading, not actually a report on the findings of those 'conversational inquiries' but has perhaps more the character of an essay or even a testimonial on the role and position of the researcher as an insider.

Epistemic asymmetry

The position of a qualitative researcher with respect to the actors of the particular field of study is often compared to that of an anthropologist entering an exotic society. In such an ethnographic approach the researcher is expected to acknowledge his/her unfamiliarity with the social practices of the action field and the actors' understandings of them. This notion of the researcher taking up a not-knowing position with respect to the field of study is problematic in research on psychotherapy and other mental health interventions at least for two reasons. First, as noted above, most researchers are actual practitioners in the field and are necessarily informed in their investigations by quite elaborate preunderstandings, not easily *bracketed* (Fischer, 2009) from the analysis. Second, the phenomena related to mental health exhibit in themselves an intriguing condition of *epistemic asymmetry* (Weiste, Voutilainen, & Peräkylä, 2015).

Mental health problems are usually manifested in a person's sense of psychological distress and difficulty to master some aspects of his/her life. Such a sense of lost agency (Wahlström & Seilonen, 2016) is in psychological theories attributed to some kind (and there are a plenty on offer) of deficiency in the function of the person's 'mind'. In psychological interventions, clients are invited to observe and reflect on the workings of their 'minds', and in that process it is, at least implicitly, accepted that the person in the role of therapist or some other kind of mental health practitioner has somehow some kind of access to the client's 'mind'. Such an epistemic asymmetry, where the professional knows something about the client's way of experiencing and relating to that experiencing that is not known to the client him/herself, is subtly subscribed to by the participants in therapeutic relations.

For practitioner-researchers in the mental health field, there arise then tensions between the somewhat idealistic notion of the researcher as a not-knowing but hermeneutically able 'visitor' to the lifeworld of the actors in the field and as an actor in his/her own right with inside knowledge of the social practices involved, and even such knowledge of some other actors' (clients or other study participants) grounds for their actions that is not fully accessible to themselves. How are these tensions manifested in the present five studies?

For Challenor the challenge in the clinical situation was to help her client to gain access to and reframe violating and abusive experiences from his childhood and to relate them in a meaningful way to his present conduct in adult life – a typical instance of epistemic asymmetry in psychotherapy. When it turned out, in the therapeutic process, that this course of action, meant to be helpful, actually made the therapy turn into a threat to the well-being of the client, Challenor redirected her curiosity. Now, taking the position of a researcher, she started to inquire into her own conception of the psychological phenomenon supposed to be at work, i.e. dissociation. By reading the literature on dissociation, informed by relational psychoanalysis, and applying those conceptualisations, she constructed an account of the therapeutic process that made new sense of what happened. The 'epistemic gain' gathered from this process is what we as readers are given.

Salamino and Gusmini, in their study (and in their practice), criticise the use of attachment theory as a ground for preunderstanding predicaments adoptive families may find themselves in, especially with respect to the conduct of the adoptive child. This could be seen as a confrontation of the notion of epistemic asymmetry in therapeutic relations, in favour of a more egalitarian setting in which therapists and clients together set out for a joint exploration of the field of relational patterns in the families involved (the biological family, the adoptive family, the extended families of the adoptive parents). What we actually find, however, when reading the study, is that the therapists use, with considerable force, very definite tools for interpretations when challenging the family members' understandings and attributions – the most prominent being 'a non-individual, non-innate triadic way of understanding'. In my view, the use of these tools, beneficial as it seems, introduces a structure of epistemic asymmetry in the process.

Moore as researcher, on his part, positions himself as possessing tools for interpretation not accessible to the actors in the field of his study. Here we meet an unapologetic recognition of epistemic asymmetry grounded on the psychoanalytic notion of unconscious motivation. The study in itself does not include any intervention but suggests that supervision, aimed at reassuring staff to use their natural skills of understanding, and applying an interpretative psychoanalytic stance, would have an effect of making the interaction between staff and patients in mental institutions more open, free and human. What one finds oneself asking is: how can interpretations, taken from a position of knowing, be validated? In what sense is e.g. the talk about a vomit stain on a carpet somehow 'really' connected to the unconscious wish of the staff to get rid of a recalcitrant patient? Some proponents of psychoanalytic hermeneutics (e.g. Laplanche, 1992) would hold that the only criterion of validity is whether the communication between analyst and analysand is restored – a criterion Moore could not use in his study. Restoring communication could be equated to a momentary alleviation of the epistemic asymmetry which then reemerges when further analytic work is required.

Iliopoulou and Sacks appear as the two researchers who most clearly adopt a position of not-knowing when approaching the lifeworld of the actors in their field of study. They put an open question concerning risks met and managed by staff in the home service. It is interesting, then, that even when there were many kinds of experiences that could have been discussed in response to the question groups focused on two areas, namely aggression and violence and challenging suicidal behaviour. There seems to have been in the groups some kind of a shared understanding of what is meant by 'risk'. This could be because these situations are the most common ones actually met by staff in their work. But then again, this shared (pre)understanding could cover other possible issues worth of consideration.

Salter is the second author in this selection, beside Moore, who takes an unapologetic stance with respect to her position of knowing as a researcher. Her standpoint is, though, quite different from that of Moore's. Her knowing is the shared knowing of individuals who occupy similar positions in the community, in this case the position of sexually abused women who have experienced the double abuse of not having their experience validated at the level of relationship, community or society. In relation to this group of actors in the field the researcher places herself within perfect epistemic symmetry. The epistemic asymmetry is constructed with regards to the rest of the community, those who either actively disregard the experience of the abused and oppressed members or who do it passively by not paying attention. From the point of view of political action this is, obviously, a justified stance. From the point of view of research, however, one could argue that the total pattern of meaning-making on which the unjust social practices are being maintained is not revealed in its whole complexity.

Some conclusions

The most obvious 'finding' of my small investigation into practices of doing qualitative research in mental health, exemplified by the five studies in this special issue, is that this is a set of procedures with great diversity. This is of course nothing novel or surprising but perhaps my minor exercise can contribute to explicate some of the differences and some of the similarities between pieces of research.

In all of the studies the authors were closely connected to the action field of mental health, actually having as their main occupation some kind of practice in that area. This seems to be the rule, with few exceptions, in this range of research, especially in studies employing qualitative methodology. From this follows that most of those undertaking such investigations, actually are 'lay-researchers'. This was the case in most of the present five studies. The advantage of having practitioners doing research is that they possess valuable insight into the social practices of the field. But this, of course, is a two-edged sword, since it may prevent the researcher perceiving what in those practices might present itself as strange, and even undesirable, when looked upon and experienced from another perspective.

It goes without saying, that the lay position of the researcher also has some bearing on the quality of research as an academic performance. It is not my prerogative to comment on the five studies from this point of view. What I would like to take note of is that the multitude of human activities within the action field of 'mental health' actually are representative of many aspects (i.e. also non-clinical) of the human condition, and can as such be of interest to academics in human sciences at large, even when their main orientation is towards basic research. One would like to see more of fruitful collaboration between practitioner-researches and 'professional' researchers.

When it comes to the motivation and intent to do research one could observe clear differences between the five studies. Some of the studies were oriented towards looking at particular interventional practices, either with the aim of critically examining a certain practice or to propagate the use of some practice in the field. Other authors were concerned with institutional routines or procedures in mental health organisations, or social attitudes towards those affected with mental health problems. What all of the studies had in common, was the intention not only to describe a certain state of affairs, but to have an impact on how practices are performed. Such an emancipatory interest was more clearly articulated in some studies, but was nevertheless observable in all of them. Laudable as such goals are, I did find myself wishing for even more detailed descriptions of what actually 'was going on' in the encounters.

From a philosophical point of view, what seemed to create the greatest difference between the studies was the authors' stance towards the epistemic polarity between knowing and not-knowing. In hermeneutics, the division is thought to be bridged when knowing is conceptualised as pre-knowledge, a necessary precondition for the not-known to be known. I have drawn upon the notion of 'epistemic asymmetry' to deliberate on how this is being actualised in therapeutic encounters. It seems that a difference in knowing between therapist and client is essential for therapeutic progress, even as such differences also may lead to unintended and even abusive practices. The dilemma of pre-knowledge, both in the relationship between practitioners and clients and between researchers and study participants, was present in all the studies but did not, in my judgement, get the mindful attention it would have deserved.

Returning then to my point of departure, I find that it is definitely appropriate to look at the five studies as social practice, i.e. as acts meant to be meaningful and to have an impact on the lived world and the lifeworld of people 'playing' as actors in the social field called 'mental health'. I would like to invite the reader to make a thought experiment: how would a study on e.g. Challenor's data look like if it was conducted by Salter; or a study on Iliopoulou and Sacks data as analysed by Moore? It is obvious that the same concrete human encounters would afford different researchers to do different things with them. So what in the end might be the benefit of doing qualitative research in mental health? Perhaps, as Salter might put it, – to find new ways to 'go on'.

Disclosure statement

No potential conflict of interest was reported by the authors.

References

Bleicher, J. (1980). *Contemporary hermeneutics; Hermeneutics as method, philosophy and critique*. London: Routledge & Kegan Paul.

Challenor, J. (2017). 'Not dead … abandoned' – A clinical case study of childhood and combat-related trauma. *European Journal of Psychotherapy & Counselling, 19*.

Fischer, C. T. (2009). Bracketing in qualitative research: Conceptual and practical matters. *Psychotherapy Research, 19*, 583–590. doi:10.1080/10503300902798375

Iliopoulou, M., & Sacks, M. (2017). The impact of professional role on working with risk in a home treatment team. *European Journal of Psychotherapy & Counselling, 19*.

Kraus, B. (2015). The life we live and the life we experience: Introducing the epistemological difference between "Lifeworld" (Lebenswelt) and "Life Conditions" (Lebenslage). *Social Work and Society. International Online Journal, 13*. Retrieved from http://www.socwork.net/sws/article/view/438

Laplanche, J. (1992). Interpretation between determinism and hermeneutics; A restatement of the problem. *International Journal of Psychoanalysis, 73*, 429–445.

Loewenthal, D., & Avdi, E. (2016). Is research in psychotherapy and counselling a waste of time? *European Journal of Psychotherapy & Counselling, 18*, 311–315. doi: 10.1080/13642537.2016.1261651

Moore, G. (2017). Critical incidents in mental health units may be better understood and managed with a Freudian/Lacanian psychoanalytic framework. *European Journal of Psychotherapy & Counselling, 19*.

Pearce, W. B. (2007). *Making social worlds: A communication perspective*. Oxford: Blackwell.

Salamino, F., & Gusmini, E. (2017). A shift in narratives: From "attachment" to "belonging" in therapeutic work with adoptive families. A single case study. *European Journal of Psychotherapy & Counselling, 19*.

Salter, L. (2017). From victimhood to sisterhood part II – Exploring the possibilities of transformation and solidarity in qualitative research. *European Journal of Psychotherapy & Counselling, 19*.

Suoninen, E., & Wahlström, J. (2009). Interactional positions and the production of identities: Negotiating fatherhood in family therapy talk. *Communication & Medicine, 6*, 199–209.

Wahlström, J., & Seilonen, M.-L. (2016). Displaying agency problems at the outset of psychotherapy. *European Journal of Psychotherapy & Counselling, 18*, 333–348. doi: 10.1080/13642537.2016.1260616

Weiste, E., Voutilainen, L., & Peräkylä, A. (2015). Epistemic asymmetries in psychotherapy interaction: Therapists' practices for displaying access to clients' inner experiences. *Sociology of Health and Illness, 38*, 645–661. doi:10.1111/1467-9566.12384

Wittgenstein, L. (1981). *Zettel* (2nd ed.). (G.E.M. Anscombe & G.H.V. Wright, (Eds.)). Oxford: Blackwell.

Index

abuse 9–10, 34–5, 173, 175, 222, 225, 228, 291–2, 294–5, 298–9, 320
accent 79, 105, 214, 240
acceptance 56, 94, 134, 190–1, 193, 195, 204, 234
accident 9, 64, 181, 183–6, 190–1, 194–5, 204–5, 216, 266, 280
action field 156, 269–70, 289, 294, 298, 317–18, 321, 323
actors 124, 169, 171, 320–4
adolescents 33, 117, 120, 238, 240, 244, 248
adoption 241–3, 250, 254–5, 8, 307
adoptive families 10, 238, 241–43, 254, 307, 317, 319, 322; case study 241–55
adults 9, 17, 135, 231, 293, 299, 305, 316, 321
affections 88, 114, 120, 128
agency: constructions 170, 176; display 171, 175, 177–8; human 9, 209, 215, 219; problems 9, 165, 203
agent 15, 37, 160, 168–9
agentic 165, 168–72, 174, 176, 178, 204, 219
aggression 114, 119, 124, 126–8, 245, 264–5, 277, 281, 285–6, 322
agreements 20, 68–9; collective 65
alcohol 17, 231, 247–8
altruism 251–4
ambivalence 32, 83, 117, 120, 202, 233
American Psychiatric Association 242
analyst 264, 266, 269, 322
anxiety 89, 137, 141, 170, 174–6, 8, 222, 229–31, 233–4, 259, 265–6, 268, 270, 284, 209, 315, 317
apology 282, 285
appraisal 188
art 215; and psychotherapy 217–18
articulation 151, 154, 157–8

ASD (autism spectrum disorder) 193, 195
assessments 31, 65, 68, 70, 94, 172, 230–1
asylums 151, 160, 205
attachment 10, 53, 134, 238, 241–3, 245, 248, 251–2, 255
attributions 173, 175–7, 203, 240, 243–8, 253–5, 308, 320, 322
attunement 71–2, 228, 234
audio 5, 15, 33, 187
autobiographies 27, 29, 33, 39, 140
autonomy 39, 84, 117–18

BACP (British Association for Counselling and Psychotherapy) 42, 47
barriers 6, 52, 101, 127, 303, 311
behavioral adjustments 157
behaviour 7, 30–32, 34, 66–7, 88, 108, 111, 117, 170, 174, 190, 242–5, 247–8, 252, 259, 264, 269–70, 273, 283, 285, 320; suicidal 277, 281, 285, 322
beliefs 15, 63, 80–1, 90, 107–8, 110, 185, 190, 229, 231, 263–5, 271, 273, 283
believer 86–7
belonging 8, 10, 131, 136–7, 142–5, 208, 238, 251
biases 2, 194, 292, 297–98, 300, 310
biographies 32–4, 36, 38
body image 33–5, 37, 39
body language 71, 283
body movements 64, 66–7, 71–2
body positions 66, 71
bonds 53, 119, 269; social 120, 122, 153–4
BPS (British Psychological Society) 47
breakdown 141–2, 222
breaking down 232, 234
British Association for Counselling and Psychotherapy (BACP) 42, 47
British Psychological Society (BPS) 47

Bromberg's theory of multiple self-state trauma and enactments 229–30
bulimia 36

CA (conversation analysis) 6–7, 60, 65–6, 68, 72
capacity 69, 92, 96, 143, 222, 225, 229, 231, 234–5, 318
care 16, 117–18, 126–7, 207, 216, 230, 234, 242, 245, 251, 266–8, 271
caregiver 54, 242, 245, 249
case study 9–10, 12, 15, 152–3, 168, 177–8, 205, 225–6, 235, 254, 306–7; adoptive families 238–40, childhood and combat related trauma 222–4; encounter 315–16
catalyst 51, 96, 143, 194
causal attributions 9, 165, 168, 171, 173, 176–7, 219, 244, 246, 308
CCD (Christ Church Deal) 138
chance and fate 34–5
change processes 16–17, 30, 32–3, 36, 39, 107–8, 168, 262
child 8–9, 34, 117, 124–5, 127, 201, 203, 228–9, 243, 245, 248, 254, 293, 295; adopted 10, 250, 319
childhood 9, 34, 50, 222, 228–9, 297, 321; combat-related trauma (case study) 222–36
children 114, 117–18, 120–1, 126–30, 172, 192, 242–3, 297; therapeutic community and 114–28; 201–2
Christ Church Deal (CCD) 138
Christians 85, 87, 89–90
classes 173–4, 195, 204, 253
client members 136–8, 144
client-participants 170, 178, 317
clients 3–4, 12–25, 44–5, 48–57, 94–6, 136–40, 167–74, 176–8, 203–4, 206–8, 219–22, 224–27, 229–30, 284–6, 319–22
clinical practice 5, 7, 10, 89–90, 107, 114, 117, 126–7, 303, 305–7
clinical supervision 1, 226, 230, 270–1, 273
clinicians 3, 5, 109–10, 230, 235, 268, 305, 307
combination 84–7, 140, 308–9
commentary 7, 106–7, 112, 199, 213, 219, 272, 311
commitment 215, 269, 293
communication 5, 44, 51, 55, 86, 100, 202–3, 243, 264–5, 270, 322

community 101, 121, 124, 138, 140–4, 151, 193–4, 201–3, 205, 207–8, 217–18, 294–7, 299, 316, 323; meetings 125, 136; members 137, 207
Community Psychosocial Centres 151–2, 159, 205
community services 263, 316
competence 231, 295 professional 81
complexity 107–9, 112, 144, 153, 206–7, 209, 217, 225, 241, 243, 289, 292, 294, 318, 323
conceptions 31, 34, 118, 144, 321
conduct 12, 15–17, 24–5, 273, 321–2
conflicts 20, 81, 89
congruent environment 8, 131, 140, 143, 145
consciousness 50–1, 55–6, 141, 154–6, 225, 229–30, 264, 317
consent 227, 256, 319; informed 33, 65, 67, 171
constructionism 168, 178, 298–9
consultations 60, 62, 64–5, 67–9, 71, 186, 202, 245–7, 255–6, 315
contemplation 27, 34, 37–9
contradictions 32, 37, 77, 82, 89, 154, 202
convergence 47–8, 64
conversational inquiries 291, 293, 310, 316, 320
conversations 1, 66–69, 106, 111–12, 137, 152–3, 169–70, 263, 267, 291, 294
coping strategies 185, 189, 204, 217
counselling 1–2, 9, 92–4, 165, 169–70, 171, 176–8, 203, 213, 215, 219–21, 315; psychotherapy 2–3, 83, 94, 96
counsellor 7, 42–4, 46–7, 77–9, 81–9, 95, 101, 192; person-centred approach (PCA) 77–90
couples 3, 34, 70, 159, 170, 203, 207, 250, 298, 315
creation 30, 114, 121, 134, 158, 160–61, 238, 243
credibility 92, 98–9, 168, 216, 306–9
critical incidents 259, 262, 264–6, 269–72, 309, 316–17, 320
critique 2, 10, 31, 79, 83, 93, 109, 308
cruel 123–4, 128
culture 2–3, 5, 122, 155, 161–3, 193–4, 209, 265, 294
curiosity 56, 218, 243, 251, 256, 321

danger 110, 208–9, 231, 233, 235, 251, 298
data: analysis 48, 82, 99, 136, 187, 212, 303, 308; collection 47, 82, 98, 109, 136, 187, 216, 280, 307–9

deadlocks 117, 122, 127, 148, 161, 201
death 70, 87, 89, 155
debriefing 187, 283, 285–7
defence 52, 228–9, 231, 265–6, 268, 272
deinstitutionalization 148, 151, 154, 160–1, 205–6
democracy 4, 135, 311
dependency 39, 46
depression 7, 60, 64–5, 68, 172; diagnosis of 72, 98, 280
deviant behaviors 245–6
disciplines 2, 5, 9, 81, 219
discourse analysis 6–7, 77, 81, 210
disorder 32, 108, 137; acute stress 181, 193
display 66–7, 69–72, 88, 168–9, 215
dissociation 222, 224, 226–33, 235, 319, 321
distress 4–5, 9, 14–16, 18–19, 51, 68, 81, 111, 188, 190–1, 193, 195, 206
diversity 3, 5, 9, 109, 201, 306, 323
divine 85–6
dreams 42, 45, 50, 57, 188, 233
drunk-driving cases 177

eating disorders (ED) 6, 27–30, 33, 37, 39, 95, 106–7, 109. 137
emotions 67, 69, 136, 142, 155–6, 158, 185, 190, 228–9, 232, 234
empathy 63–4, 72–6, 85, 134, 286, 307
engagement 3, 70, 96, 106, 263; social 151, 158, 160
ethics 3, 160, 306
ethnocentrism 86
ethnography 199, 208
everyday life 3, 9, 12, 15–16, 19–22, 24–5, 95, 13 psychotherapy and 215–17
excitement 53, 56
exclusion 8, 127, 144, 148, 205, 250, 261; social 138, 154, 298
expertise 81, 107, 126–7, 143, 208, 268, 306
experts 4, 15, 25, 94, 100, 108, 121, 124, 203, 311
exploration 4, 56, 105–6, 181, 183, 185, 209, 269, 271, 290, 300, 305
expression 8, 48, 60, 64, 66, 67, 69, 72, 81, 98, 131, 133, 137, 142, 144–5, 152–5, 169, 268

facilitator 51, 82, 121, 123, 125–6, 194, 281, 295, 310
failure 37, 109, 117–18, 127, 144, 231, 233, 259, 268, 270, 272–3, 292, 309
families/family 36, 117, 121, 123–8, 140, 191–2, 201, 204, 238, 241–6, 248–50,

252–5, 297–9, 322; members 17, 294, 308, 315, 322
family therapists 203, 241, 243
family therapy 12, 238, 241–4, 249, 254
fantasies 63, 123, 228, 233, 235
fate 34–5, 242
feedback 6, 138, 186, 291
feminists 292, 294
fieldwork 205–6, 208, 227, 263
five aspect model: causal attribution 173, 176; historicity 174–5, 177; intentionality 174, 177; 177; reflexivity 175, 177; relationality 172–3, 176
fluid hierarchie 8, 131, 138, 144–45
focus groups 277, 281–2, 285–7, 308, 316, 320; client perspective 284–5; difficult emotional experience 284; professional role 282–3 responsibility283–4
football metaphor 206
formation 156, 271, 320
formats 47, 99–100, 140, 216
formulations 31, 98, 167–8, 173, 202–3, 226, 230, 306
Foucault, M. 80, 89, 128, 151, 154, 270, 299
fragments 36, 122, 141, 152, 207
freedom 77, 82, 84, 88, 90, 118, 127, 139–40
Freud, S. 5, 10, 118, 143, 241–2, 259–73, 320
frustration 89, 117, 124, 128, 217–18, 294
functional adaptation 27, 34, 36, 38

gaze 66 106, 108
gender 5, 65, 138, 186
general practitioners (GPs) 7, 60–2, 64–5, 67–72, 98, 111, 202, 230, 283–5; with depression patients 60–72
generosity 86, 256
genesis 118, 155
gesticulations 71
God 190–1, 204, 296
grounded theory 8, 131–3, 139, 199–200, 206
groups 51–52, 65, 121, 124, 136–8, 159, 161, 259, 270–4, 280–5, 291, 293–9, 310, 320, 322–3
guilt 77, 85, 117, 127, 174, 259, 265

happiness 233
healing 8, 55, 131, 206, 210, 255
health problems mental 134, 205, 283, 285–6, 321, 324

health professionals 98, 139, 172, 202, mental 117, 194, 204
health services 151, 160, 195, 279
health setting 299, 305
Hegel, G. W. F. 114–16, 118, 201–2
helplessness 124, 172, 177, 201, 204, 233, 235
hermeneutics 6, 218, 227, 281, 324–5
hermetic 148, 161
heuristic value 148, 157, 161
hierarchies 135, 138, 144, 208
historicity 9, 165, 169, 171, 174–5, 177, 219
history 136, 144, 156, 163, 174, 206, 252, 263–4, 268, 281, 294
hospital 15, 19, 36–7, 117, 127, 135, 141, 144, 184, 190, 206, 208, 268, 279–80
HTT (Home Treatment Team) 10, 277–81, 285, 303, 305, 308, 316
human agency 9, 209, 213, 215, 219
human beings 80, 83–5, 88, 155, 256, 262, 292
humour 51–2, 232
hurt 34, 134, 140, 207
hurting 8, 34, 70, 131, 134, 140, 206–7, 210

ICD-10 criteria for depression 65
ICPS (Institute of Counselling and Psychological Studies) 82
identification 66, 87, 120, 122–3, 133, 270, 272
ideology 3, 5, 7, 80–1, 85, 87–9
illness 37, 151, 153, 169, 192, 268, 283
images 50, 89, 118–19, 124–5, 128, 173, 176, 204, 273
imaginary identifications 119, 122–3, 126–8
implementation 72, 85–7, 110, 153
imposition 259, 261, 265, 270, 273
incidents 45, 216, 226, 231, 259–60, 263, 265–8, 270–1, 282–4, 309, 316
inclusion 136–7, 143, 186; social 137
individuality 194
individuals 4, 53, 80, 87, 89, 135–7, 140, 142–3, 148, 156–61, 262, 323
infants 54, 118
initiative 25, 27, 29, 34–6, 38, 65, 72, 173
innovations 135, 199, 206, 209, 307
inquiry 10, 92, 94, 97, 99, 219, 226, 291, 299–300, 318; qualitative 8, 213, 215, 316, 318
insecurity 87, 153, 174

insider research 10, 291–3, 303, 310
insider researcher 10, 292, 296, 299–300, 303, 309, 311
Institute of Counselling and Psychological Studies (ICPS) 82
institutionalization 152–3, 160
institutional network 8, 33, 37, 114, 117, 123–4, 127–8, 201; social 158, 262, 265
integration 83, 156, 180, 228; social 151, 153
intensity 49, 53, 67–9, 71; emotional 46
intentionality 9, 63, 165, 168, 171, 174, 176–8, 219, 248, 262
intentions 6, 31, 85, 88, 171, 174, 176–8, 219, 245, 250, 296, 300, 315, 324
interactions 12, 14, 60, 63–4, 66, 111, 135–7, 203–4, 238, 240, 319, 322
interpretations 88–9, 97, 99, 104, 106–7, 109–12, 122, 175, 202–3, 217–18, 226, 285
inter-subjectivity theories 227–81; Bromberg 229–30; Stolorow 227–8
interviews 15–18, 23, 31, 33, 37, 47–8, 82–3, 136–40, 181, 186–7, 204, 206, 208, 210, 263
intimacy 22, 39, 52
intrusion 51, 120, 195
investigation 93–4, 98, 203, 263, 268, 315, 318–21, 323
IPA (interpretative phenomenological analysis) 42–4, 46–7, 218, 227, 277–8, 280–81, 308, 320
Islam 190–1

job 68–9, 100, 153, 160, 205, 282–7
judgement 54, 114, 134, 324
justice 1, 17, 116, 206, 293; social 292, 294, 298, 300, 310

kindness 89, 142
Klein, M. 5, 272
knowledge 4–6, 37, 80, 85–6, 89–90, 96, 98–9, 121, 126, 128–29, 160–61, 268, 292, 298–9, 321

Lacan, J. 8, 10, 117–19, 121–2, 124, 126–7, 201–2, 262, 264–6, 268–70, 272–3, 320
language 8, 47, 63, 67, 82, 119–20, 122, 127, 296–8, 306
Larkin, M. 43–4, 46, 94, 218, 227, 280, 286
learning 20–1, 23–2, 4, 84, 100–101, 209, 272 see also everyday life

legacy 247, 251, 297, 310
life situation 165, 168–9, 171, 173
literature 7, 9–10, 39, 45–6, 94, 97–8, 127, 194. 263, 267, 273, 280, 286, 309
lived experience 8, 98, 104, 109–12, 217, 227
loneliness 232, 250, 268
love 4, 82, 88–9, 108–9, 126, 268, 270
loyalty 231, 251–3

Malaysian Muslim 9, 181, 204; coping strategies 204–5
marital rape 293
marital status 186
marital sub-system 249
markers 10, 33, 300, 306–8, 311
meditation 191, 204
members 2, 20, 22, 117, 122, 134–8, 143–4, 204, 262–4, 269, 282, 285, 291, 294–5, 320, 323
memories 50, 69, 141–2, 191, 202, 230
mental disorders 151, 154, 158, 193
mental health 4–5, 8–10, 148, 154, 156–8, 161–3, 205–6, 210–12, 315–16, 319, 323–4; encounters 331–2; see also qualitative research
mental health care 8–9, 148, 151, 156–8, 160–1, 262; Brazilian context 151–61; cultural-historical approach 154–61; educational actions 157–61; 205–6; therapeutic environments 206–8
mental health interventions 134, 142, 145, 317–18, 321
mental health services 135, 138–40, 144, 148, 151, 153–4, 157–9, 181, 185, 189, 193, 195, 262, 264, 294–5; relational context 131–45
mental illness 72, 123, 127, 143, 153, 156, 193
mental states 14, 63–4, 70–2
metaphors 50, 55, 95, 206, 256
mirroring 7, 60, 64–9, 72, 107, 226
motor vehicle accident (MVAs) 181–2, 184–5, 189–91, 194–7, 204, 216
MVAs (motor vehicle accident) 181–2, 184–5, 189–91, 194–7, 204, 216

narratives 10, 108, 111, 176, 190–1, 204, 238, 249, 251–5, 300, 307
negative feeling 123, 131, 259, 272
neutrality 251, 297–8, 310

non-agentic 169, 171–2, 174, 176, 178, 219
nurses 98, 121, 137, 139, 192, 265–6, 269, 280, 283

object relations theory 272 see also Klein, M
occasions 2, 20, 33, 100, 235, 245, 315
organisation/organization 66, 110, 230, 262, 264, 291, 309, 318, 320
otherness 118–19, 294

pain 139, 190–1, 225, 231–3, 235, 242, 256, 265, 296
parents 8, 35–8, 109, 114, 116–17, 121–8, 172–4, 192, 201–3, 228, 242–5, 249–50, 252, 254–6; adoptive 10, 243, 245–6, 322
participants 7, 32–3, 46–57, 65, 81–9, 99–100, 105–12, 138–40, 158, 185–95, 204–5, 263, 273, 280–5, 316–17
patients 27, 29–30, 32–3, 36–7, 39–40, 60, 62–72, 74, 111, 142, 259, 261, 265–74, 277–8, 282–7; recalcitrant 267–8, 270, 322
PCA (person-centred approach) 7, 77–9, 81–9; freedom discourse 84–5; libidinal attachments 87–8; militarism 86–7; philosophical discourse 83–4; religion/ spirituality discourse 85–6
perceptions 56, 63, 112, 119, 123, 128, 243, 264, 319
personal agency and initiative 34–7
personality disorder 135, 280
person-centred approach (PCA) 7, 77–9, 81–9; libidinal attachments 878
phenomenology 2, 42, 46, 56, 83–4, 88
philosophy 83, 88
post traumatic stress disorder (PTSD) 181, 185, 193–8, 216, 228
post traumatic stress symptoms 181, 185, 188–9, 193
power dynamics 108
power imbalances 52, 144, 298
practitioners 1, 7, 42, 45–7, 56, 60, 95, 98, 100–1, 300, 315–16, 318–19, 321, 323–4
pre-contemplation 27, 30–1, 34, 37–9
prescriptions 157, 172, 268
pressure 50, 112, 245, 254
problems 12, 17, 27, 30–4, 36–9, 108–10, 117, 153–4, 161–2, 168, 170–4, 176, 210–11, 244–9, 255
professionals 5, 10, 32, 35–6, 65, 72, 114, 121, 124, 126–8, 138–9, 152, 201, 256, 285

psychiatrists 7, 60, 64–5, 67–72, 98, 111, 121, 123, 135, 153; with depression patients 60–72
psychiatry 66, 111, 163, 206, 271
psychoanalysis 87, 122, 178, 226, 262–4, 271, 273–6, 320
psychologists 42, 46–7, 121, 172, 202, 280, 315
psychology 4, 64, 155, 164, 180, 201, 271
psychosis 104, 118–20, 127, 201–4, 280 *see also* Lacan
psychotherapists 1–2, 33, 46–7, 95, 101, 121–2, 158, 218, 245, 291–2, 295, 297, 316; systemic 292, 295, 297, 316
psychotherapy 7, 9, 12, 94–6, 4, 47, 165, 180, 202–3, 210–11, 215–21; agency problems 165–79; 203–4
psychotherapy research 25, 64, 168, 216–18 *see also* research
PTSD (post traumatic stress disorder) 181, 185, 193–8, 216, 228

qualitative analysis 7, 39, 199, 244
qualitative research: description and interpretation 217–18; encounters case studies 315–16; issues of theory and practice 91–101; psychotherapeutic innovation and diversity 199–210; transformation and solidarity 289–90, 307–16
qualitative researchers 94, 98–100, 107, 201, 263, 299, 305, 320
questionnaires 39, 138
questions 2–7, 10, 15, 16, 31–3, 48, 82, 94–7, 99–101, 108, 124, 109, 112, 127, 138, 141, 175, 203, 208, 226–7, 263–4, 273, 281, 291–2, 298–9, 315–16, 318
Quran 187

rationality 88
recognition 55, 118–20, 125, 233, 262, 269
reflexivity 3, 9, 89, 97, 165, 168, 171, 175–8, 219, 250
relationality 9, 169, 171–2, 175–7, 178, 219
relationships 8, 119–20, 125–26, 131, 134–5, 139–40, 142–3, 159–60, 173, 201, 207–9, 245
relief 230–1, 233
religion 85, 89, 191, 193, 204
research 7, 95–8, 100–1, 108, 112, 152, 197, 291–2, 294–5, 297, 305–7, 309–11, 318, 323

researchers 10–11, 97–9, 101–2, 107–8, 110–12, 152, 201–2, 205–6, 210, 263–5, 286, 291–2, 297–300, 305–11, 318–24
research participants 104, 107, 109, 210, 310
research process 97–8, 108, 152, 303, 310–11
research questions 6, 108, 226–7
resistance 51–2, 55, 87, 89, 156, 264, 267, 270, 273
resonance 49, 293, 306–9, 311
responsibility 36, 90, 174, 219, 281–3, 285–7, 308, 311–12

sadness 68, 86, 124, 160, 201, 233
safeness 235
safety 139–40, 142, 228, 268, 271, 283
secular 85–6, 204
self 51, 85, 89–90, 96, 111, 120, 139–40, 168–69, 171, 176–8, 228–31, 235, 273
self-reflection 174, 226, 307
services 3–6, 8, 10, 124, 131, 135, 138–40, 144, 148, 150–4, 157–60, 170–2, 181, 183, 185, 189, 193, 195, 199, 201, 203–5, 207, 210, 225, 230, 259, 261, 262–265, 268, 273, 279–80, 282, 285, 294, 295, 306, 309, 315, 316, 322
service users 4–6, 135, 148, 153, 158, 160, 199, 207, 210, 285, 294
service workers 159
sexual abuse 295–7, 293, 299, 310, 317
shame 85, 123, 139, 142, 229, 230, 235, 295
shock 53, 56, 225, 315
signifiers 122, 124–5, 272, 304
sinking ship 268–9, 270
sisterhood 10, 289, 296–7, 306 *see also* victimhood
slave 114, 118, 121, 124, 127–8
smoking 30–1, 136–7
SOC (stage of change) categories 34, 37
social interactions 135–8
social media 192, 205
social sciences 155, 201, 218
social support 191, 193, 195, 204
social worlds 80, 140, 268, 280, 293–4, 310, 317
society 47, 80, 101, 119, 122, 128, 153, 161, 205–6, 228, 262, 273, 294, 299, 320, 323
solidarity 10, 136–7, 207, 289, 291, 294–6, 298, 300
spirituality 190–1, 193, 204
staff approach, critical incident 265–70

stages of change (SOC) categories 38, 95
stigma 193, 205–6, 283, 294, 297
stress 9, 21–2, 50, 68, 70, 117, 134, 181–3, 185, 188–9, 191, 193–5, 204–5, 216, 228, 286–7
superordinate themes 42, 48, 51
supervision 1, 56, 90, 222–4, 226, 230, 270–1, 273, 307, 322
support group 293–5, 316
surprise 17, 53, 56, 225, 315
survival 87, 139, 207–8, 222, 228, 232–3
syllables 68–70
symbolism 50, 54–55
symptoms 32, 37, 72, 153–4, 173–4, 181, 185, 188–9, 191, 193, 195, 205, 216, 218, 222, 225, 230, 266–7, 269, 271–3, 306
synchronicity experiences 6–7, 42, 45–7, 49–56, 95, 106, 110
synchrony 64, 71

temporality 222, 226, 229
tensions 7, 9, 32, 36, 64, 95, 104, 108, 213–14, 218, 226, 295, 321
thematic analysis 53, 109, 199, 208, 226, 307
therapeutic communities (TC) 8, 117, 125, 134–5, 138, 144, 147, 201, 206–8, 216–18
therapeutic relationship 42, 46, 52, 54–6, 58, 81, 84, 107, 111–12, 134, 143, 222, 228, 230
therapists 3–4, 18–20, 23–5, 31–3, 45–58, 95–6, 110–11, 134, 203–4, 219, 229–30, 241–2
therapy 12, 15–20, 22, 24–5, 42, 94–7, 106–7, 80, 215–17, 225–8, 232–6, 241–2, 244–5; five aspect model 171–9; synchronicity analysis 42–57
therapy session 15, 18, 21–2, 24, 45, 51, 169, 171, 209, 216, 244, 254, 308, 315
threat 117, 205, 234, 262, 264, 316, 321
TMC (Transtheoretical Model of Change) 6, 27, 29–31, 35–7, 39, 108
tobacco pouch 265–6, 270
traditions 1, 66, 91, 101, 118, 208–9, 218–19, 319
training clinic 170
transcribed verbatim 48, 122, 136, 181, 187, 281
transcripts 18, 48, 82, 114, 121–3, 170, 172, 201, 203, 210, 245, 256
transferability 169, 176, 203
transference 10, 58, 227, 229, 235, 259, 263–73, 309

transformation 10, 56–57, 142–3, 151, 289–91, 295
trauma 5, 108, 198, 222, 224–30, 233, 239, 244, 296, 303–6, 317
treatment 12, 14–16, 18, 31, 117, 120, 124, 127, 131, 135, 140, 151–3, 168, 170, 181, 195–7, 204, 207, 228, 265–66, 269, 315–17, 319; residential 117, 127
triadic 238, 243, 249–50, 252–3
troubles 12, 16, 19–25, 29, 173–5, 177–8
trust 19, 21, 49, 83, 97, 99, 124, 139, 142, 208, 231, 270
truth 1, 4, 11, 32, 77, 80, 83–4, 86, 88, 107, 139, 266, 269, 273, 294

UK Council for Psychotherapy (UKCP) 2, 47
UK Mental Health Act 138
UKMMC (University Kebangsaan Malaysia Medical Centre) 185–6; Ethics Committee 186
UK's National Health Service 203
UK universities 2
United Kingdom Council for Psychotherapy (UKCP) 2, 47
United States 185, 193
unity 63, 86, 119, 154, 156–7, 294
University Kebangsaan Malaysia Medical Centre (UKMMC) 185–6
University Research Ethics Committee 47
utility 38, 46, 110, 208, 219

validation 84, 264, 281
validity 2, 31–2, 81, 97–98, 187, 218, 225–6, 291, 322
vehicle 52, 185, 191
Venn diagram 187, 192
victimhood 10, 289, 296, 306, 310 see also sisterhood
videos 3, 65–67, 100, 111, 187, 203
violence 4, 185, 225, 228, 277–8, 280–1, 283, 285–7, 322
vocal expressions 64
vocal intensity 68–71
vocal tone 60, 64
vomit stain 267–68, 270, 322
vowels 67–68
vulnerability 10, 248, 250

weight 34–35, 97
withdrawal 120, 235, 306

women/woman 10, 27, 33, 35, 39, 172, 210, 289, 291, 310, 316, 320, 323
word constraints 310
workers 94, 148, 152, 160; social 123, 125, 245, 254, 280
World Health Organisation (WHO) 184, 264
worldview 39, 52, 292

World War II 135, 144
worries 23, 32, 174
wound 242–3, 255, 249

yes/no responses 31
yippee 70
youth counseling 17

For Product Safety Concerns and Information please contact our EU
representative GPSR@taylorandfrancis.com Taylor & Francis Verlag GmbH,
Kaufingerstraße 24, 80331 München, Germany

Printed and bound by CPI Group (UK) Ltd, Croydon, CR0 4YY
01/05/2025
01858507-0001